Instructor's Manual to Accompany Clinical Decision Making

Case Studies in Pediatrics

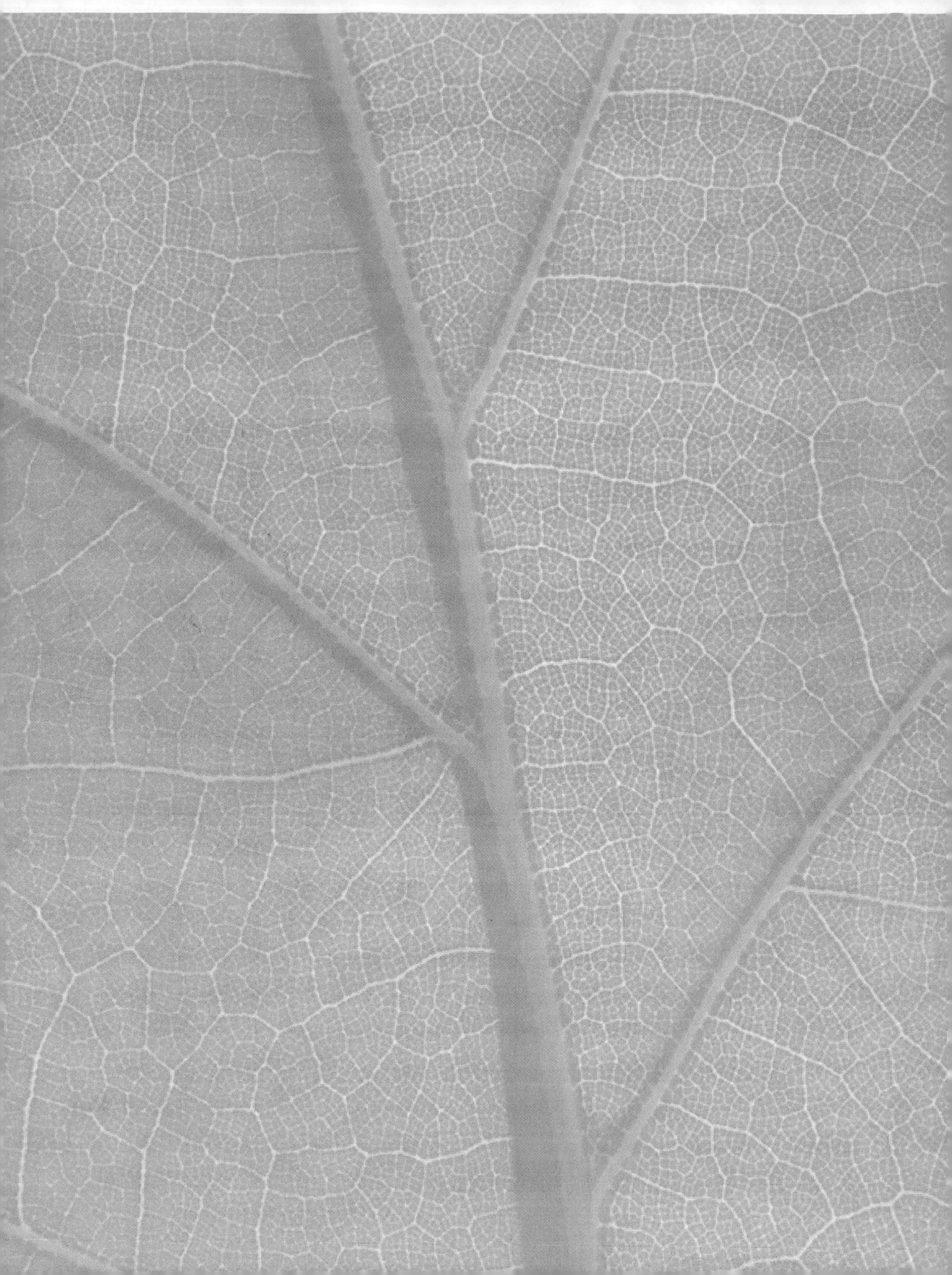

Instructor's Manual to Accompany Clinical Decision Making

Case Studies in Pediatrics

Bonita E. Broyles
RN, BSN, MA, PhD

Instructor
ADN Program, Piedmont Community College,
North Carolina

THOMSON
DELMAR LEARNING™

Australia Canada Mexico Singapore Spain United Kingdom United States

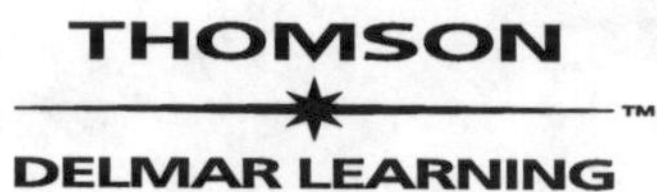

Instructor's Manual to Accompany Clinical Decision Making: Case Studies in Pediatrics

by Bonita E. Broyles

Vice President, Health Care Business Unit:
William Brottmiller

Editorial Director:
Cathy L. Esperti

Executive Editor:
Matthew Kane

Developmental Editor:
Maria D'Angelico

Editorial Assistant:
Michelle Leavitt

Marketing Director:
Jennifer McAvey

Channel Manager:
Tamara Caruso

Marketing Coordinator:
Michele Gleason

Production Director:
Carolyn Miller

Production Editor:
Jack Pendleton

Printed in United States of America

2 3 4 5 6 7 XXX 08 07 06

For more information, contact Thomson Delmar Learning, 5 Maxwell Drive, Clifton Park, NY 12065-2919
Or you can visit our Internet site at http://www.delmarlearning.com

ISBN 1-4018-2632-6

Contents

Reviewers

Jane H. Barnsteiner RN, PhD, FAAN
Professor of Pediatric Nursing
University of Pennsylvania School of Nursing
Philadelphia, Pennsylvania

Diana Jacobson MS, RN, CPNO
Faculty Associate
Arizona State University, College of Nursing
Tempe, Arizona

Nancy Oldenburg RN, MS, CPNP
Clinical Instructor
Northern Illinois University
DeKalb, Illinois

Deborah J. Persell MSN, RN, CPNP
Assistant Professor
Arkansas State University
Jonesboro, Arkansas

JoAnne Solchany RN, ARNP, PhD, CS
Assistant Professor, Family & Child Nursing
University of Washington
Seattle, Washington

Preface

Thomson Delmar Learning's Case Studies Series was created to encourage nurses to bridge the gap between content knowledge and clinical application. The products within the series represent the most innovative and comprehensive approach to nursing case studies ever developed. Each title has been authored by experienced nurse educators and clinicians who understand the complexity of nursing practice as well as the challenges of teaching and learning. All of the cases are based on real-life clinical scenarios and demand thought and "action" from the nurse. Each case brings the user into the clinical setting, and invites him or her to utilize the nursing process while considering all of the variables that influence the client's condition and the care to be provided. Each case also represents a unique set of variables, to offer a breadth of learning experiences and to capture the reality of nursing practice. To gauge the progression of a user's knowledge and critical thinking ability, the cases have been categorized by difficulty level. Every section begins with basic cases and proceeds to more advanced scenarios, thereby presenting opportunities for learning and practice for both students and professionals.

All of the cases have undergone expert review to ensure that as many variables as possible are represented in a truly realistic manner and that each case reflects consistency with realities of modern nursing practice.

How to Use This Book

Every case begins with a table of variables that are encountered in practice, and that must be understood by the nurse in order to provide appropriate care to the client. Categories of variables include age; gender; setting; culture; ethnicity; pre-existing conditions; co-existing conditions; significant history; cultural, communication, disability, socioeconomic, spiritual, pharmacological, psychosocial, legal, ethical, prioritization, and delegation considerations; and alternative therapy. If a case involves a variable that is considered to have a significant impact on care, the specific variable is included in the table. This allows the user an "at a glance" view of the issues that will need to be considered to provide care to the client in the scenario. The table of variables is followed by a presentation of the case, including the history of the client, current condition, clinical setting, and professionals involved. A series of questions follows each case that ask the user to consider how she would handle the issues presented within the scenario. Suggested answers and rationales are provided for remediation and discussion.

Organization

The cases are grouped into parts based on topics. Within each part, cases are organized by difficulty level from easy, to moderate, to difficult. This classification is somewhat subjective, but they are based upon a developed standard. In general, difficulty level has been determined by the number of variables that impact the case and the complexity of the client's condition. Colored tabs are used to allow the user to distinguish the difficulty levels more easily. A comprehensive table of variables is also provided for reference, to allow the user to quickly select cases containing a particular variable of care.

Praise for Thomson Delmar Learning's Case Study Series

I would recommend this book to my undergraduate students. This would be a required book for graduate students in nursing education, women's health, or maternal-child programs.

—Patricia Posey-Goodwin, M.S.N, R.N., Ed.D (c),
Assistant Professor,
University of West Florida

This text does an excellent job of reflecting the complexity of nursing practice.

—Vicki Nees, RNC, MSN, APRN-BC,
Associate Professor,
Ivy Tech State College

. . . the case studies are very comprehensive and allow the undergraduate student an opportunity to apply knowledge gained in the classroom to a potentially real clinical situation.

—Tamella Livengood, APRN, BC, MSN, FNP
Nursing Faculty,
Northwestern Michigan College

I commend the effort to include the impact of illness on the growth and development of the child, on the family's cohesiveness and on the subsequent health problems that will affect the child in years to come. Inclusion of questions that focus on the nurse's perceptions, biases and beliefs are extremely important when training nurses to provide comprehensive care ... Often one system illness will affect another health system and this has been demonstrated numerous times [in this text].

—Diana Jacobson, MS, RN, CPNP
Faculty Associate,
Arizona State University College of Nursing

These cases and how you have approached them definitely stimulate the students to use critical-thinking skills. I thought the questions asked really pushed the students to think deeply and thoroughly.

—JoAnne Solchany, PhD, ARNP, RN, CS
Assistant Professor, Family & Child Nursing,
University of Washington, Seattle.

The use of case studies is pedagogically sound and very appealing to students and instructors. I think that some instructors avoid them because of the challenge of case development. You have provided the material for them.

—Nancy L. Oldenburg, RN, MS, CPNP
Clinical Instructor, Northern Illinois University

[The author] has done an excellent job of assisting students to engage in critical thinking. I am very impressed with the cases, questions and content. I rarely ask that students buy more than one pediatrics book ... but, in this instance, I can't wait until this book is published.

—DEBORAH J. PERSELL, MSN, RN, CPNP
Assistant Professor,
Arkansas State University

This is a groundbreaking book that ... will be appropriate for undergraduate pediatric courses as well as a variety of graduate programs ... One of the most impressive features is the variety of cases that cover situations from primary care through critical care and rehabilitation. The cases are presented to develop and assess critical-thinking skills ... All cases are framed within a comprehensive presentation of physical findings, stimulating critical thinking about pathophysiology, developmental considerations, and family systems. This book should be a required text for all undergraduate and graduate nursing programs and should be well-received by faculty.

—JANE H. BARNSTEINER, PHD, RN, FAAN
Professor of Pediatric Nursing,
University of Pennsylvania School of Nursing

Note from the Author

These case studies were designed to assist nursing students of all levels develop and strengthen their critical thinking skills to provide the best care for this very special client population. I have thoroughly enjoyed writing this work of heart.

About the Author

Dr. Broyles began her nursing career in 1968, working as a student nursing assistant while pursuing her Bachelor of Science degree in nursing from The Ohio State University in Columbus, Ohio. She graduated with her BSN in 1970 and continued for the next 13 years staffing and teaching on obstetrics and gynecology. From 1972 to 1976, she taught in the Associate Degree Nursing Education program at Columbus Technical Institute (which is now Columbus State). During her 5-year position as Patient Teaching and Discharge Planning Coordinator for Obstetrics and Gynecology at Mt. Carmel Medical Center in Columbus (1976–1981), she published her first professional writing. At this juncture, she decided to expand both her mind and nursing skills into the medical-surgical arena of nursing where she has staffed and taught nursing since that time to present. With her husband, Roger, she moved to North Carolina in 1985. She has been an educator in the nursing education department of Piedmont Community College in Roxboro, North Carolina since 1986 and is currently the course coordinator for Maternal-Child Nursing (teaching the pediatric component of the course), Adult Nursing II, and Pharmacology. Dr. Broyles received her Master of Arts in Educational Media from North Carolina Central University in 1988, and her Doctorate of Education in Adult Education from LaSalle University in 1996. Her dissertation research concerned critical thinking in Associate Degree Nursing Students and was the largest study published on this topic. In 2004, Dr. Broyles received her PhD from St. Regis University with further study in adult education. Dr. Broyles has published nursing texts in the areas of pediatrics, medical-surgical nursing, and pharmacology.

Acknowledgments

The author wishes to express her appreciation to all who contributed to the development of these cases. Without the love, support, encouragement, and diligence of my husband Roger this project as with those past would not be the success I believe this will be. I also thank the many friends and colleagues who helped me through their love, support, encouragement, and expertise. Thank-you Mama Lou, Papa Joe, Pat, Alisa, Kelly, and Colman.

The author also wishes to acknowledge the Associate Degree Nursing Education students who serve as continuing inspiration to produce student-friendly textbooks that help them learn this most important content for their safe nursing practice.

For the opportunity to be involved in this project, the author wishes to thank the people at Thomson Delmar Learning for their support, encouragement, and editorial guidance during the writing of the Pediatric Case Studies. Special thanks goes to Matt Kane, who continues to believe in me as a nursing author, and to Michelle Leavitt, whose enthusiasm and flexibility helped make this project so enjoyable.

Finally, the author wishes to thank the reviewers of this work for their time and expertise evident in their constructive comments and suggestions. Having been a book reviewer for 5 years, the author appreciates the time and effort of the reviewers as they share their knowledge and expertise to help make this edition a worthy educational tool.

Bonita E. Broyles

PART ONE

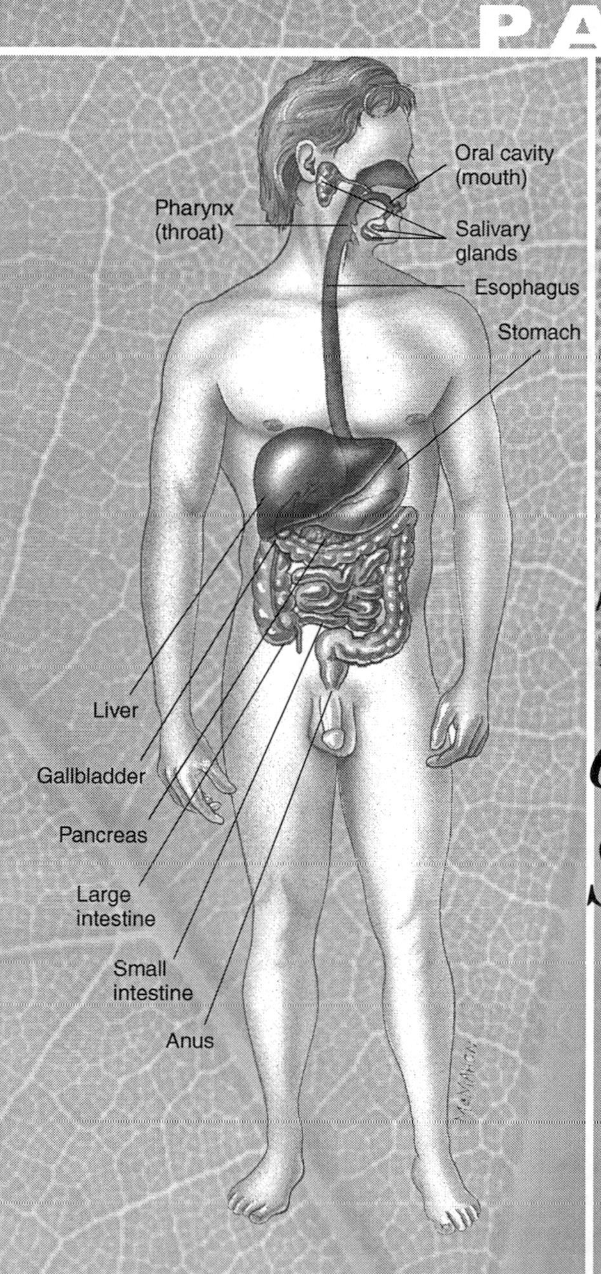

The Digestive and Urinary Systems

CASE STUDY 1

Shelly

EASY

GENDER

F

AGE

4

SETTING

- Home/clinic

ETHNICITY

- White American

CULTURAL CONSIDERATIONS

PREEXISTING CONDITIONS

COEXISTING CONDITIONS

SIGNIFICANT HISTORY

COMMUNICATION

DISABILITY

SOCIOECONOMIC

SPIRITUAL

PHARMACOLOGIC

- Acetaminophen (Tylenol)
- Trimethoprim-sulfamethoxazole (Bactrim)

PSYCHOSOCIAL

- Fear

LEGAL

ETHICAL

ALTERNATIVE THERAPY

PRIORITIZATION

- Yes

DELEGATION

- Client teaching

THE URINARY SYSTEM

Level of difficulty: Easy

Overview: This case requires knowledge of growth and development, as well as an understanding of the client's background, personal situation, and parent–child relationship.

Client Profile

Shelly is a 4-year-old preschooler who lives with her parents and younger brother. She and her brother attend a local daycare center during the week while their parents are at work. In the evenings she and her brother take a bath and then their parents read to them before bedtime at 8:00 P.M. Shelly's daycare class includes many children her age and she enjoys playing outside with them. Although snack times are planned, Shelly would rather play and does not always finish her beverages.

Case Study

Shelly's mother calls the pediatric clinic in town and tells the nurse that Shelly has been "running a fever of (101° F) for the past 2 days" and although her temperature decreases to 37.2° C (99° F) with acetaminophen, it returns to 38.4° C (101° F) within 4 hours of each dose. Further, her mother says that Shelly complains that "it hurts when I pee-pee." Shelly's mother also has noticed that her daughter seems to be in the bathroom "every hour." She makes an appointment to see the pediatrician this afternoon.

Questions and Suggested Answers

1. **Discuss the significance of Shelly's clinical manifestations.** Urinary frequency and pain or burning on urination are classical manifestations of a urinary tract infection. An elevated temperature of 38.3°C (101° F) also indicates the presence of infection.
2. **What other assessment data would be helpful for the nurse to have to prepare Shelly's care plan?**
   a. Urine for culture and sensitivity
   b. Urine specific gravity
   c. Vital signs
   d. Breath sounds to rule out an upper respiratory infection
   e. Shelly's normal fluid intake and usual bladder habits
   f. Whether Shelly knows the proper method of wiping following urination and/or defeation
   g. Has Shelly had a UTI in the past? If so, what were her symptoms and how was the condition treated?
3. **Discuss Shelly's anatomic risk factor(s) for developing a urinary tract infection (UTI).** The urethra of very young girls is only 2 cm (0.8 in.) in length, allowing a short pathway for bacteria to enter the urinary tract. The closure of the urethra after urination can trap bacteria in the urethra. The bacteria then move up the urinary tract, and this can lead to cystitis, ureteritis, and pyelonephritis (see Fig. A-1). In addition, in very young girls the anus is closely approximated with the urethra, resulting in increased risk of urinary tract contamination from bacteria excreted in the stool during defecation.
4. **Discuss the relationship between Shelly's hygiene habits and her risk for developing a UTI.** Bathing in tubs is a high risk factor for the development of UTIs. Even if the bathtub is cleansed between each use, some bacteria remain on the tub's service and become mobile when water is placed in the tub. In addition, when the child sits down, the warm water dilates the urethra, allowing bacteria and water to enter the urinary tract. Furthermore, a common habit is to add bubble bath to the child's bath water, which further increases the risk of UTIs. If Shelly's brother is not toilet trained and urinates in the bath water, the risk increases. Children should be taught as early as possible to shower, because in showering the water is moving at all times and does not remain stagnant (as with tub water), which would provide an ideal medium for bacterial growth.
5. **Discuss how Shelly's level of growth and development places her at risk for developing a UTI.** The peak incidence of UTIs occurs in 2- to 6-year-olds, and is higher in girls than in boys. Preschoolers frequently delay

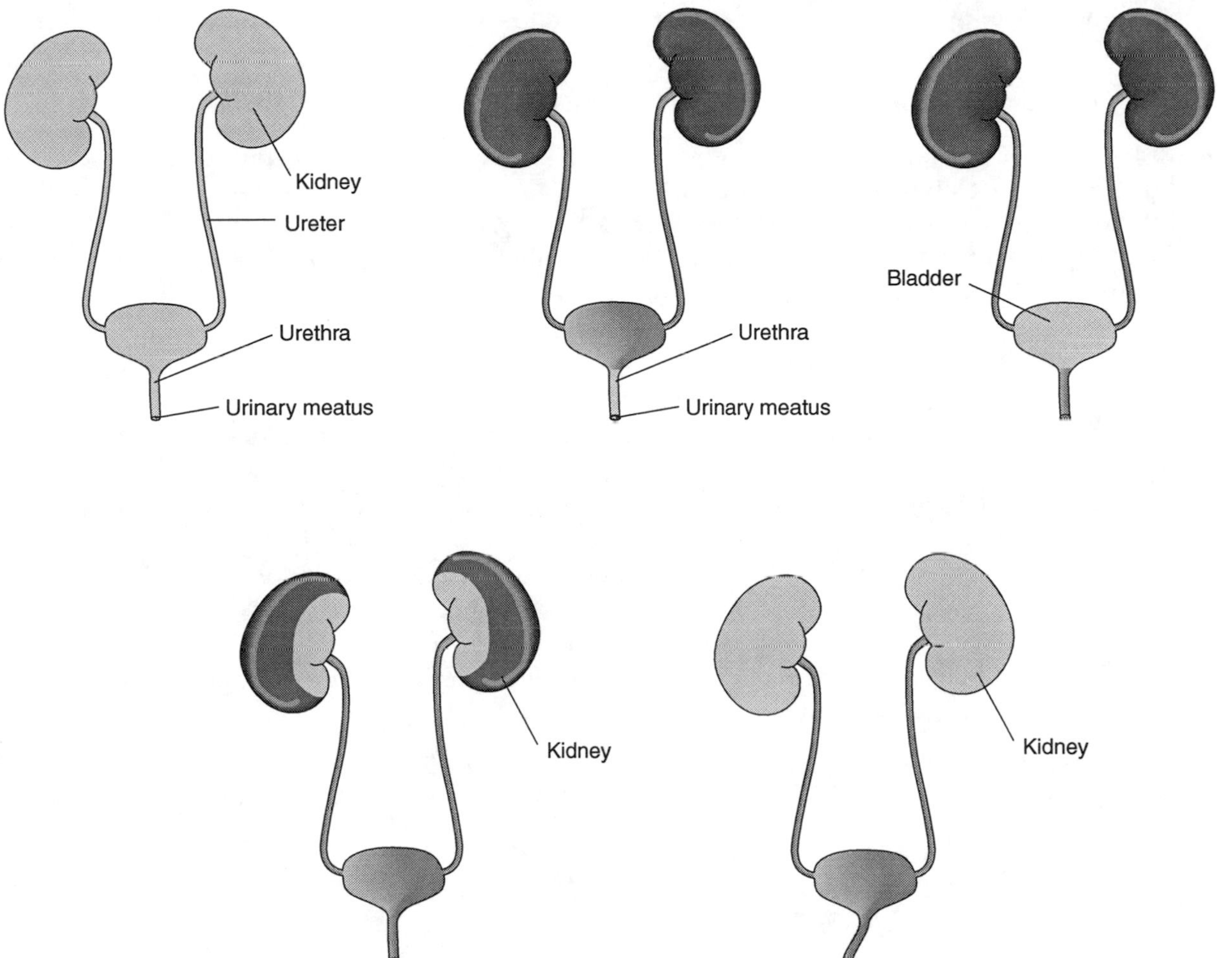

Figure A-1 *Sites of urinary tract infections.*

urinating because of their involvement in play. When they do go to the bathroom, they commonly hurry, leading to incomplete emptying of the bladder and stasis of urine. Further, they may not wipe from front to back or even wipe at all. Because of their focus on socialization and playing with friends, they may not recognize the need to urinate, which leads to both stasis of urine and overdistention of the urinary bladder. For young girls, underwear that is too tight also increases the risk of UTIs.

6. **Shelly's urine culture returns positive for *Escherichia coli.* What is the significance of this finding?** This bacteria is responsible for 80% of all UTIs. It is a common bacteria of the intestines and is excreted in the stool.

7. **What are the priorities for Shelly's care?**

    a. Risk for injury, complications (pyelonephritis) of presence of bacteria in the urinary tract
    b. Risk for deficient fluid volume related to decreased fluid intake
    c. Acute pain related to nerve irritation from the presence of bacteria in the sterile urinary tract
    d. Deficient knowledge related to UTIs and their prevention and treatment

8. **Shelly is prescribed trimethoprim-sulfamethoxazole 60 mg every 12 hours for 10 days. What is this drug and is her prescribed dose safe? Shelly weighs 15 kg (33 lb).** Trimethoprim-sulfamethoxazole (Bactrim, Septra) is a sulfonamide antibacterial agent that acts by blocking essential nucleic acids and protein necessary for bacterial cell synthesis. This causes the death of the bacterial cells. The safe dose of this drug for children is

8 mg/kg per day in two divided doses every 12 hours. At 33 lb, Shelly weighs 15 kg, so her safe dose every 12 hours is 60 mg.

9. What are the teaching priorities for Shelly and her mother prior to her discharge from the clinic?

a. Risk factors for developing UTIs and providing instructions as needed to avoid risk factors including:
   (1) Appropriate technique for perineal care
   (2) Avoidance of tub baths, using shower instead
   (3) Daily fluid intake of >1,250 mL until antibiotics completed, then 1,250 mL/day (100 mL/kg for first 10 kg [22 lb] and 50 mL/kg for next 10 kg); water and cranberry juice
   (4) Need to empty bladder when urge is present; should not hold urine
   (5) Having Shelly urinate every 1–2 hours
   (6) Use of cotton rather than nylon underwear
b. Medication administration including importance of completing the prescribed medication regimen even though signs and symptoms may disappear after 1–2 days of therapy
c. Signs and symptoms of adverse effects of medications (primarily hypersensitivity reactions)
d. Signs and symptoms of worsening of condition
e. Contact phone numbers to report signs and symptoms or if family has questions
f. Importance of regular handwashing and appropriate technique
g. Importance of follow-up with health care provider to reculture urine
h. Allowance of adequate time for Shelly's parent to ask questions, answering them honestly
i. Documentation of teaching and father's response

10. Shelly is scheduled for a return visit to the clinic in 2 weeks. What is the purpose of this appointment? The return visit is for a follow-up urine culture. This is the definitive method of determining that the UTI is no longer present.

References

Centers for Disease Control and Prevention. *http://www.cdc.gov*

Daniels, R. (2002). *Delmar's manual of laboratory and diagnostic tests.* Clifton Park, NY: Thomson Delmar Learning.

North American Nursing Diagnosis Association. (2005). *Nursing diagnoses: Definitions & classifications, 2005–2006.* Philadelphia: NANDA.

Potts, N. and Mandleco, B. (2002). *Pediatric nursing: Caring for children and their families.* Clifton Park, NY: Thomson Delmar Learning, pp. 617–620.

Spratto, G.R. and Woods, A.L. (2005). *2005 Edition: PDR nurses's drug handbook.* Clifton Park, NY: Thomson Delmar Learning.

Wong, D.L., Perry, S.E., and Hockenberry, M.J. (2002). *Maternal child nursing care* (2nd ed.). St. Louis: Mosby, p. 1250.

CASE STUDY 2

Justin

GENDER

M

AGE

Neonate

SETTING

- Hospital

ETHNICITY

- White American

CULTURAL CONSIDERATIONS

PREEXISTING CONDITIONS

COEXISTING CONDITIONS

SIGNIFICANT HISTORY

COMMUNICATION

DISABILITY

SOCIOECONOMIC

SPIRITUAL

PHARMACOLOGIC

PSYCHOSOCIAL

- No prenatal care
- Teenage mother

LEGAL

ETHICAL

ALTERNATIVE THERAPY

PRIORITIZATION

- Yes

DELEGATION

MODERATE

THE DIGESTIVE SYSTEM

Level of difficulty: Moderate

Overview: This case requires knowledge of the impact of TEF, growth and development on mother and son, as well as an understanding of the client's background, personal situation, and mother–child attachment relationship.

Client Profile

Justin is a neonate whose mother, Danielle, is a 16-year-old young woman who lives at home with her mother and 14-year-old sister. Danielle is in her 36th week of pregnancy and has not received any prenatal care because "we can't afford it." She stopped going to school last month because she was self-conscious of her appearance. The father of her unborn child does not live in the area, and from the time she told him of the pregnancy he has shown no interest in her or the unborn child.

Case Study

Danielle is admitted to the hospital in active labor, and 10 hours later Justin is born. His Apgar score is 4 at 1 minute and 6 at 5 minutes. He is cyanotic and coughing, and chokes on his oral secretions. He is admitted to the nursery and examined by the pediatrician on call. He is diagnosed with tracheoesophageal fistula (TEF) and transferred to the pediatric intensive care unit for monitoring. He is scheduled for surgery to repair his TEF.

Questions and Suggested Answers

1. **What is the meaning of Justin's Apgar score?** Apgar scoring is a method of performing a rapid assessment of the neonate immediately after birth to assist in evaluating the neonate's adaptation to extrauterine life. It is based on five categories: (1) heart rate, (2) respiratory rate, (3) muscle tone, (4) reflex irritability, and (5) color. The maximum score for each category is 2, with 10 as the highest possible Apgar score. Apgar scores between 7 and 10 are considered normal and reflect that the neonate is not in distress and should adapt to extrauterine life without complications. Scores of 4–6 mean moderate distress and scores of 0–3 indicate severe distress. Justin's scores reflect moderate distress. His 5-minute Apgar score is congruent with higher infant mortality. Justin's clinical manifestations are consistent with tracheoesophageal fistula (TEF).

2. **Discuss esophageal atresia and TEF.** Esophageal atresia is a congenital anomaly of the esophagus in which the esophagus ends in a blind pouch and thus does not provide a connection with the stomach (see Fig. A-2). TEF is the most common and the most life-threatening of the atresias with the esophagus connected and emptying into the trachea. Congenital TEF is the most common and causes moderate to severe respiratory distress in the neonate. The clinical manifestations of TEF include the three C's (coughing, choking, and cyanosis), excessive oral secretions, regurgitation, and abdominal distention. The fistula between the esophagus and the trachea is usually at the distal end of the trachea. The fact that this location is the closest to the bronchi and then the lungs poses a high risk for aspiration and respiratory distress in the neonate.

3. **How common is TEF and what causes it?** TEF is a common congenital anomaly occurring in one of every 2,000–4,000 live births. The exact cause of TEF is unknown; however, it is associated with chromosomal abnormalities including trisomy 21 (Down syndrome), trisomy 18, and trisomy 13. Approximately 10% to 15% of infants with TEF die.

4. **How is TEF diagnosed?** Initial suspicion of TEF is based on both clinical manifestations and the inability to pass a feeding tube or suction catheter. The presence of polyhydramnios on prenatal ultrasound is an indicator of the possibility of esophageal atresia. Chest radiography is performed following birth that serves as the final confirmation of TEF.

5. **Discuss the problems associated with Justin's mother not receiving prenatal care.** A preliminary diagnosis of esophageal atresia with TEF can be made with prenatal ultrasound. Characteristics usually noted include polyhydramnios, fluid-filled stomach, lower than expected fetal weight, a distended pouch, or the tissue connection of the esophagus and the trachea. Adolescence is a time of establishing identity, achieving a sense of belonging from peers, becoming sexually active, and, as a means of emancipating from the parents,

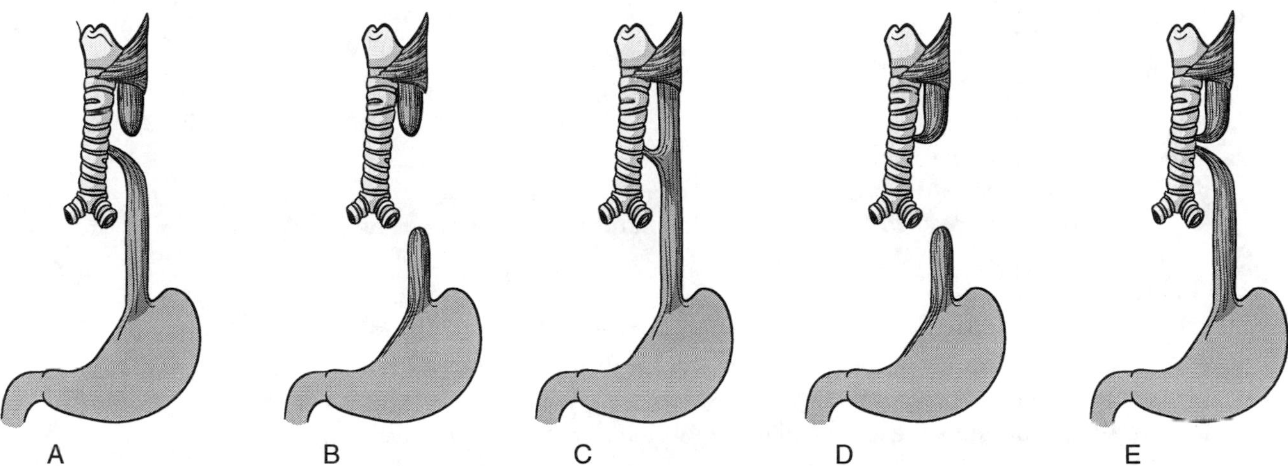

Figure A-2 *Types of esophageal atresia and tracheoesophageal fistula. A. Esophageal atresia with distal tracheoesophageal fistula; B. Isolated or pure esophageal atresia; C. Tracheoesophageal fistula without esophageal atresia; D. Esophageal atresia with proximal tracheoesophageal fistula; and E. Esophageal atresia with proximal and distal tracheoesophageal fistula.*

risk-taking behavior. Because of the growth spurt associated with adolescence, nutrition is a health concern. Without proper instruction, adolescents may make unhealthy choices about what they eat. The stress of pregnancy increases this already stressful time, and adequate nutrition is required for both mother and fetus. One of the focuses of prenatal care is nutritional guidance. Psychosocial support also is offered during prenatal visits that is especially important for a pregnant teenager, who, in trying to establish her identity, naturally focuses on herself and has difficulty focusing on an unborn child. Prenatal care provides regular monitoring of the health of both the mother and fetus and has been correlated with a reduced incidence of maternal and infant mortality.

6. Identify the priority nursing concerns for Justin.

- **a.** Risk for aspiration related to ineffective airway clearance
- **b.** Risk for imbalanced nutrition: less than body requirements related to lack of oral intake
- **c.** Risk for deficient fluid volume related to suctioning of stomach contents and NPO status
- **d.** Deficient knowledge, maternal, related to neonate's condition and treatment

7. Discuss the appropriate priority nursing interventions for Justin.

- **a.** Prevent aspiration and respiratory distress.
  - **(1)** Provide warmth by placing the neonate in a heated isolette.
  - **(2)** Maintain NPO.
  - **(3)** Monitor respiratory status continuously and place on cardiopulmonary monitor.
  - **(4)** Monitor continuous oxygen saturation via pulse oximetry and administer oxygen to maintain prescribed oxygen saturation.
  - **(5)** Suction as indicated by neonate's condition.
  - **(6)** Place in semi-Fowler's position.
- **b.** Maintain adequate infant nutrition
  - **(1)** Neonates require 108 kcal/kg of body weight daily.
  - **(2)** Collaborate with health care provider to establish alternate method of feeding.
  - **(3)** Establish and maintain intravenous access, monitoring hourly.
  - **(4)** Administer intravenous fluids as prescribed.
  - **(5)** Maintain strict intake and output.
  - **(6)** Weigh at least daily.
  - **(7)** Administer enteral feedings as prescribed.
  - **(8)** Provide pacifier to satisfy sucking needs.

c. Maintain fluid balance
   (1) Assess hydration status every 1–2 hours while the neonate is in the PICU.
   (2) Maintain patency of IV access, monitoring hourly.
   (3) Administer intravenous fluids as prescribed.
   (4) Monitor strict intake and output.
   (5) Monitor urine specific gravity.
   (6) Administer enteral feedings or hyperalimentation as prescribed, providing site care according to facility protocol.

d. Maternal client teaching
   (1) Encourage maternal visits, allowing the mother to hold the neonate if condition allows.
   (2) Explain all monitoring equipment, allowing sufficient time for questions.
   (3) Actively listen to the mother's concerns.
   (4) Provide preoperative teaching, allowing sufficient time for questions.

8. **Because of Justin's condition, Danielle has had difficulty bonding with him. Discuss the concept of bonding (attachment) and your impressions of its importance.** In 1967, Reva Rubin first introduced the concept of maternal-infant bonding and its importance to the well-being of both mother and infant (Klaus and Kennell, 1983). Bonding is the process of attachment between mother and infant and often begins during pregnancy. According to Rubin, following birth, bonding occurs in identifiable stages or phases that she referred to by name and characteristic behaviors (Martell, 1996). **Taking in** occurs immediately after birth and is characterized by the en face position (Wong et al., 2002) in which the mother and infant face each other and the mother gazes intently on the infant. This represents identifying the infant as hers. **Taking hold** takes place during the first to third day following delivery and represents the mother caring for her infant and "taking hold" of her concept of being the infant's mother and responsible for his or her care, acknowledging that the infant is a part of the family unit. **Letting go** is the final phase and involves multiple events over the course of a lifetime when the parents must allow the child to progress in autonomy and independence that is very difficult at times for most parents. Bonding solidifies the reality of childbirth. Other researchers (Klaus and Kennell, 1983; Martell, 1996) have continued to study this process. Because of cognitive and developmental challenges, the process of bonding faces increased interference in the adolescent mother. Separation immediately following birth as a result of maternal or infant distress can interrupt the process of attachment. Bonding is established by close proximity and frequent interactions between parents and infant. Therefore, health care facilities that provide maternal–child care should make every effort to foster the maternal–infant attachment, allowing and encouraging mothers to visit their children in the critical care environment, supporting them to practice hands-on care of their children during hospitalization. Given the inherent problems of an adolescent mother and the lack of contact with the infant, it may be difficult for Danielle to identify Justin as her infant and take hold of her mothering responsibilities. This may cause the infant to experience difficulties such as failure to thrive, psychosocial delays in development, attachment issues, and mental health problems.

9. **Justin's TEF is surgically repaired when he is 1 day old and a D-tube is placed. Why would Justin require enteral feedings during his surgical recovery?** Initially the neonate with TEF receives nothing by mouth and is provided with parenteral fluids. Once the repair of the TEF is completed, the suture lines must be allowed to heal; however, nutrition must be provided. A tube placed in the duodenum allows elemental nutrition to be provided while the sutures heal. A nasogastric tube is also placed and attached to low intermittent suction to maintain gastric decompression. The suction removes any stomach contents including gastric secretions (hydrochloric acid) that could erode the surgical wound.

10. **Danielle was discharged when Justin was 2 days old. She visited him once a day with her mother. Justin is 5 days postop with an anticipated discharge in 2 days. How can the nurse assist with maternal–infant bonding and prepare Danielle for Justin's care at home?** The nurse should schedule to spend time with Danielle when Danielle visits Justin, monitoring Danielle's nonverbal as well as verbal questions. Danielle plans to

continue living with her mother indefinitely following Justin's discharge, so the nurse should suggest that both Danielle and her mother visit Justin together so that discharge instructions can be communicated to both. Because of the cognitive immaturity and developmental stressors of adolescence, teaching all those involved in the care of the infant will increase the chances that the instructions will be heard and understood. Assuming Danielle's mother is planning to form an attachment to her grandson and participate in his care, she would be an important asset in helping Danielle bond with her infant son. During the visit, the nurse can serve as a role model for bonding behavior and give gentle guidance and positive reinforcement to Danielle as she interacts with Justin. Encouraging Danielle and her mother, if possible, to room-in with Justin prior to discharge also will help with the mother–infant bonding process. In addition, collaborating with the health care provider for a home health nurse referral would provide continuity of care for this new family following discharge.

References

Daniels, R. (2002). *Delmar's manual of laboratory and diagnostic tests.* Clifton Park, NY: Thomson Delmar Learning.

Esophageal Atresia and TEF. *http://www.eatef.org*

Josephson, D.L. (2004). *Intravenous infusion therapy for nurses: Principles & practice.* (2nd ed.). Clifton Park, NY: Thomson Delmar Learning.

Klaus, M. and Kennell, J. (1983). *Bonding: the beginnings of parent-infant attachment.* St. Louis: Mosby.

Klaus, M. and Kennell, J. (1982). *Parent-infant bonding* (2nd ed.). St. Louis: Mosby.

Martell, L. (1996). Is Rubin's "taking-in" and "taking hold" a useful paradigm? *Health Care Women Int.* 17(1): 1–13.

Maternal-Infant Bonding. *http://www.neonatology.org*

North American Nursing Diagnosis Association. (2005). *Nursing diagnoses: Definitions and classifications, 2005–2006.* Philadelphia: NANDA.

Wong, D.L., Perry, S.E., and Hockenberry, M.J. (2002). *Maternal child nursing care* (2nd ed.). St. Louis: Mosby, pp. 558–559.

CASE STUDY 3

Beth

MODERATE

GENDER

F

AGE

4 months

SETTING

- Clinic

ETHNICITY

- White American

CULTURAL CONSIDERATIONS

PREEXISTING CONDITIONS

- Preterm birth

COEXISTING CONDITIONS

SIGNIFICANT HISTORY

COMMUNICATION

DISABILITY

SOCIOECONOMIC

- Middle class

SPIRITUAL

PHARMACOLOGIC

PSYCHOSOCIAL

- Parental anxiety
- Caregiver stress
- Breastfeeding support

LEGAL

ETHICAL

ALTERNATIVE THERAPY

PRIORITIZATION

- Yes

DELEGATION

- Yes

THE DIGESTIVE SYSTEM

Level of difficulty: Moderate

Overview: This case requires knowledge of infant feeding, association between preterm birth and gastroesophageal reflux, as well as an understanding of the client's background, personal situation, and mother–child attachment relationship.

Client Profile

Beth is a 4-month-old infant who was delivered by Cesarean section at 35 weeks' gestation weighing 2.3 kg (5 lb) and measuring 42.5 cm (17 in.) in length. She is the first child for Robert and Janice Carter. Since birth Beth has been a "fussy" baby who frequently "throws up after almost every feeding and cries all the time." Janice stays home and cares for Beth while Robert works; however, when he comes home from work each day, he helps with Beth's care. Beth is clean and obviously well cared for by her parents, who appear to have bonded well with her and love her very much. During her recent 4-month check-up Beth was diagnosed with gastroesophageal reflux (GER) following a battery of diagnostic tests in response to Beth's history of frequent regurgitation following feedings. Janice's parents live in the same town as Janice and Robert and his parents live a 30-minute driving distance away.

Case Study

Janice and Robert bring Beth in for a 2-week weight check at the pediatrician's office. During the nurse's family assessment, Janice and Robert appear exhausted and anxious. Janice comments, "I feel like it's my fault that Beth is not gaining weight as she should. I get so frustrated because she is still throwing up after at least two breastfeedings a day. I try but I don't think I'm a very good mother. Maybe I should give up breastfeeding and give her a bottle." Robert further states that his family has a history of gastric ulcer disease and asked if he "gave this stomach problem to her." The couple comment that they are not sure they are doing the right things for Beth and question how they are going to manage caring for her. At this visit Beth weighs 3.4 kg (7.5 lb), her posterior fontanel is closed, and her anterior fontanel remains opened and level with suture lines.

Questions and Suggested Answers

1. **Discuss your impressions about the above situation.** The clinical manifestations that Beth has (crying, "throwing up" after feedings) are consistent with a diagnosis of gastroesophageal reflux (GER) (see Fig. A-3). The parents' concern and frustration are very common, especially for the mother who is breastfeeding because following a feeding, the mother's milk supply is not sufficient to simply feed the infant again immediately. Anxiety is common in new parents, especially with their first child. For Beth's parents this is complicated by her GER. Many parents see how their infant eats, gains weight, and responds as reflections of how well they are parenting. Guilt is a common emotion in parents whose infants are not "perfect." The fact that Beth was preterm increases her risks of GER owing to immature development of the lower esophageal sphincter (LES).

2. **What is the incidence and etiology of GER in children?** GER is the most common esophageal disorder in infants, affecting approximately 5 in 1,000 live births. "It affects boys three times more frequently than girls." (Potts and Mandleco, 2002, pp. 668–669). GER also is more common in preterm infants. Although the exact cause of GER in infants is not known, it is considered by researchers to result from immature development of the LES or "impaired local hormonal control mechanisms" (Potts and Mandleco, 2002, p. 669).

3. **How does GER differ from pyloric stenosis?** Although some clinical manifestations are similar between GER and pyloric stenosis including lack of appropriate weight gain, vomiting during or after feedings, and fussiness, the pathophysiology is different in the two conditions. GER occurs as a result of an incompetent LES causing regurgitation or back flow of stomach contents during or after feedings. Pyloric stenosis results when the circular muscle surrounding the pylorus thickens or is not elastic. This prevents stomach contents from moving through the sphincter and entering the duodenum of the small intestines for final digestion. Although both GER and pyloric stenosis pose a risk of aspiration for the infant, GER is characterized by regurgitation, whereas pyloric stenosis is reflected by projectile vomiting. Pyloric stenosis more commonly requires surgical repair as opposed to GER, which the infant usually outgrows.

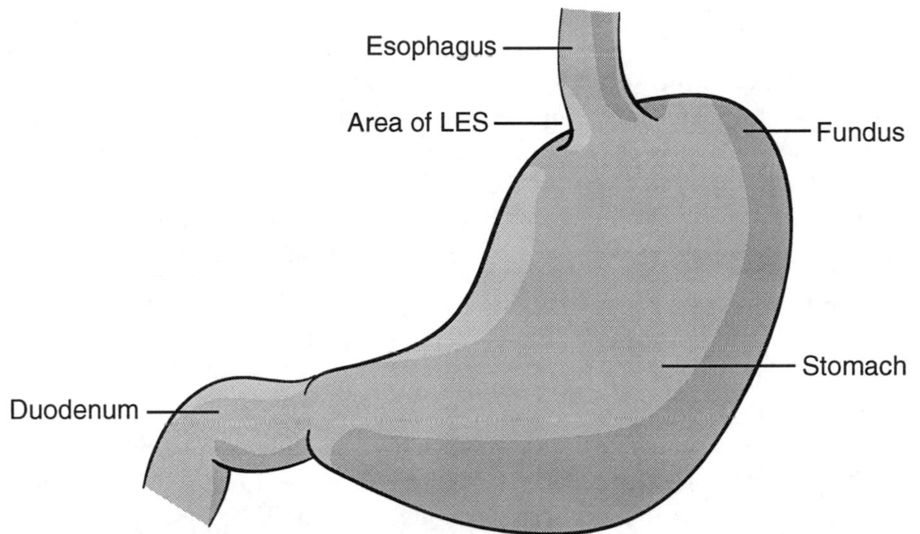

Figure A-3 *Stomach contents are refluxed into the esophagus through the lower esophageal sphincter (LES) in GER.*

4. **Identify the priority nursing concerns for Beth and her parents.**
   a. Risk for aspiration related to reflux of gastric contents into the esophagus and mouth
   b. Imbalanced nutrition: less than body requirements related to decreased nutrient entry and absorption into the duodenum
   c. Risk for deficient fluid volume related to vomiting of gastric contents and electrolytes
   d. Anxiety (parental) related to infant regurgitation, crying, and lack of weight gain
   e. Deficient knowledge related to infant's condition

5. **Discuss the nurse's findings concerning Beth's fontanels.** As a 35-week premie, Beth probably still had an open posterior fontanel at birth as this allows for increased head growth. As she is 5 weeks preterm, it may take as long as 18 months for her to be at the appropriate level of growth and development, meaning that at 4½ months of age, she may display characteristics of infants 5 weeks younger than she is. The posterior fontanel normally closes by 6–12 weeks after birth, so the closure of Beth's posterior fontanel is normal. The anterior fontanel is the primary fontanel for head growth and is usually closed by 12–18 months of age. Beth's being open is normal, as are the characteristics of the fontanel being diamond-shaped, soft, and flat.

6. **Discuss the relationship between Beth being preterm, her birth weight, and her current weight.** During the last 4–6 weeks of the normal 40-week gestation fetal weight gain is approximately 0.24 kg (0.5 lb) per week. The birth weight of a full-term infant is approximately 2.5 kg or 2,500 g (5 lb, 8 oz) to 4 kg or 4,000 g (8 lb, 13 oz), with boys typically weighing 0.24 kg (8 oz) more than girls. The weight is significantly affected by both the age of gestation and parental build, as this is a trait that can be transmitted to the fetus. Beth weighed 2.3 kg or 2,272 g (5 lb) at birth, with a possible projected weight of 1.1 kg (2.5 lb) more had she been delivered at term. Normally infants lose 10% of their birth weight by the third or fourth day of life and then regain this loss by 2 weeks of age. The normal weight gain for an infant is approximately 0.5–1 kg or 1.1–2.2 lb per month, calculated according to the accepted characteristic of doubling the birth weight by 6 months and tripling it by 1 year. Beth should weigh approximately 9.4–13.8 pounds, so her weight gain is lagging, probably because of her GER not being diagnosed until she was 4 months old, resulting in inadequate nutrition for weight gain.

7. **How would you respond to Janice's concern about breastfeeding and Beth's GER?** Research indicates that because of the digestive compatibility between infants and breast milk, breastfed infants have a lower incidence of GER. No national organization recommends stopping breastfeeding as a result of GER.

Head elevated positioning during and following feedings is the most accepted standard of care, as well as frequent bubbling during feedings and immediately following each feeding. Formula-fed infants may be placed on hypoallergenic formula without iron; however, breast milk is naturally hypoallergenic. Reassurance for Janice may not be sufficient, so the nurse can recommend to Janice that she pump her breasts and then add 1 tablespoon of rice cereal to each 2 ounces of expressed breast milk. This is a recommendation of the National Institute of Diabetes & Digestive & Kidney Diseases of the National Institutes of Health for breast-fed infants with GER. The nurse also should reinforce the information that most infants outgrow GER and that the condition has no relationship to the mother's parenting abilities.

8. **During the nurse's assessment of Beth's growth and development, she finds that Beth can put her hand to her mouth, lift her head up from a prone position, turn and look for sounds, focus on the face of the person speaking to her, and that the head lag is present when she is pulled to sitting position. Beth's rooting reflex is not present, nor is the moro reflex and tonic neck. Her sucking reflex is still present as well as her step, Babinski, ciliary, and grasp reflexes. How would you interpret these findings?** As noted in the previous answer, Beth being born at 35 weeks may delay her growth and development by approximately 5 weeks compared to the "normal" until she is 18 months to 24 months old. The nurse also needs to understand that the "normals" are not absolutes but averages. Infants from 1 to 3 months of age can put their hands to their mouths, lift their heads up in a prone position, and exhibit a head lag when being pulled to a sitting position. Turning and looking for sounds is appropriate for the 3- to 6-month-old infant, as is focusing on the face of the person speaking to her. The rooting, moro, and tonic neck reflexes are usually absent by 3–4 months of age. Sucking as a reflex usually diminishes by 4 months of age, as does the step reflex. The Babinski reflex does not disappear until approximately 9 months of age and the ciliary reflex lasts indefinitely. From the assessment, Beth's growth and development appears to be appropriate for her age.

9. **How would you respond to Janice and Robert's concerns about how Beth developed GER and their feelings of blame?** Guilt and self-blame are normal emotions for new parents of an infant with a health alteration. This is especially true of first-time parents. The nurse needs to reassure Janice and Robert that the exact cause of GER is unknown, but that Beth being born at 35 weeks was probably a contributing factor. There is no research evidence to support the presence of gastric ulcer disease in the family history as a contributing factor. Janice and Robert need a great deal of support and education to help allay their feelings of self-blame. The nurse also may discuss the impact of their anxiety on Beth's disposition because increased anxiety in an infant's environment will usually result in sensory overload and crying by the infant.

10. **Discuss the teaching plan for Beth and her parents.**
    - **a.** Assess Beth's parents' level of knowledge about GER. The grief process (shock and denial) was probably in play during their teaching session following her diagnosis. This would dramatically limit (up to 50%) how much of the teaching was heard and retained.
    - **b.** Provide verbal and written information concerning:
        - **(1)** Infant feedings NOTE: The National Institute of Diabetes & Digestive & Kidney Diseases of the National Institutes of Health states that most infants outgrow GER and rarely have serious problems after the ages of 12–18 months. They recommend the following treatment to decrease the episodes of GER in infants:
            - "If the baby is bottle fed, add up to 1 tablespoon of rice cereal to 2 ounces of infant milk (including expressed breast milk). If the mixture is too thick for your infant to take easily, you can change the nipple size or cross cut the nipple.
            - Burp your baby after 1 or 2 ounces of formula are taken. For breastfed infants, burp after feeding on each side.
            - Do not overfeed. Talk to your child's doctor or nurse about the amounts of formula or breast milk that your baby is taking.
            - When possible, hold your infant upright in your arms for 30 minutes after feeding."
        - **(2)** Infant positioning. NOTE: The North American Society of Pediatric Gastroenterology and Nutrition state that the prone position after feedings is beneficial in the treatment of GER; however, except in

rare cases, the risk of sudden infant death syndrome (SIDS) is greater in the prone position and is therefore not recommended. Placing infants in an upright position (in an infant seat or holding the infant) for 30 minutes following each feeding or lying them on their right side following feedings will increase stomach emptying as well as decreasing the pressure against the LES.

(3) Medication administration if prescribed

c. Assess Janice's knowledge about breastfeeding, including how often breast-fed infants eat (every 2–3 hours), importance of both mother and infant being relaxed during feedings, importance of Janice having a beverage to drink during breastfeeding (water, fruit drink), importance of Janice having an adequate fluid intake while breastfeeding (2,500–3,000 mL/day).

d. Discuss Robert's role in Beth's care including feeding Beth using pumped or expressed milk that has been placed in a bottle as well as bubbling, holding, and cuddling Beth.

e. Provide adequate time for parental questions.

f. Provide contact phone numbers and encourage parents to call if they have any questions.

g. Document teaching and parent response.

11. What suggestions could you offer Janice and Robert to provide them with support as they care for Beth at home? The nurse needs to pursue the relationship between Beth's parents and her grandparents. With the close physical proximity of Janice and Robert's parents to their home, involving them in Beth's care may allow for some respite time for Janice and Robert as well as provide the grandparents with quality time with Beth. Janice could pump or express breast milk and store it in the refrigerator or freezer for use when Beth's grandparents visit. Sometimes, grandparents feel anxious about not wanting to interfere with their children when there is a new baby in the house, especially a first baby. By encouraging communication, the nurse will help allay this anxiety and provide the new parents with strong support systems.

References

Centers for Disease Control and Prevention. *http://www.cdc.gov*

Children's Digestive Health and Nutrition Foundation. *http://www.cdhnf.org*

Daniels, R. (2002). *Delmar's manual of laboratory and diagnostic tests.* Clifton Park, NY: Thomson Delmar Learning.

North American Society for Pediatric Gastroenterology, Hepatology, and Nutrition. *http://www.nasphan.org*

National Institute of Diabetes & Digestive & Kidney Diseases. *http://www.niddk.nih.gov*

North American Nursing Diagnosis Association (2005). *Nursing diagnoses: Definitions & classifications, 2005–2006.* Philadelphia: NANDA.

Pediatric/Adolescent Gastroesophageal Reflux Association. *http://www.reflux.org*

Potts, N. and Mandleco, B. (2002). *Pediatric nursing: Caring for children and their families.* Clifton Park, NY: Thomson Delmar Learning.

CASE STUDY 4

Jesus

MODERATE

GENDER

M

AGE

4

SETTING

- Hospital

ETHNICITY

- Mexican American

CULTURAL CONSIDERATIONS

- Hispanic

PREEXISTING CONDITIONS

COEXISTING CONDITIONS

SIGNIFICANT HISTORY

COMMUNICATION

- Spanish-speaking

DISABILITY

SOCIOECONOMIC

- Lower Socioeconomic

SPIRITUAL

PHARMACOLOGIC

- Acetaminophen (Tylenol)
- Morphine sulfate (Duromorph)
- Gentamicin (Garamycin)
- Ampicillin sodium/sulbactam sodium (Unasyn)

PSYCHOSOCIAL

- Client anxiety
- Parental fear

LEGAL

- Informed consent

ETHICAL

ALTERNATIVE THERAPY

PRIORITIZATION

- Emergency room care

DELEGATION

- Yes

THE DIGESTIVE SYSTEM

Level of difficulty: Moderate

Overview: This case requires knowledge of appendicitis, growth and development, stressors of hospitalization on children and parents, and appendicitis treatment.

Client Profile

Jesus is a 5-year-old boy who recently moved to the United States with his mother, 7-year-old sister Carlene, and 14-year-old brother Juan to join his father, who is employed as a worker in a packaging company. Mr. Rodriquez joined the company 1 year ago and has been saving money to send for his family. During his employment, Mr. Rodriquez has learned to speak and understand English by taking an "English as a Second Language" course at the local community college. Except for 14-year-old Juan, who has been studying English so he can enter school in the fall, Mr. Rodriquez's wife and children do not speak or understand English. Mrs. Rodriquez plans to attend the same community college as her husband so she can learn to speak English. Jesus' parents are excited to have the family together in their new home, and Jesus and his sister have met a few of the neighborhood children and enjoy playing with them even though the other children are English speaking.

Case Study

Jesus wakes up at 2:00 A.M. crying, telling his mother his "stomach hurts." He has an elevated temperature of 37.9° C (100.2° F) and begins to vomit. His parents administer 120 mg of acetaminophen orally; however, Jesus has emesis 5 minutes later. They continue to monitor him for an hour and then Mr. Rodriquez decides he and his wife should take Jesus to the local hospital emergency room. Mr. Rodriquez wakes Juan and explains that Jesus has to go to the hospital and that Juan must take care of Carleen until one of his parents returns home. Jesus is admitted through the emergency department. On admission Jesus' vital signs are: axillary temperature, 38° C (100.4° F); pulse, 125 beats/minute; respirations, 35 breaths/minute; blood pressure, 119/79; weight, 18.3 kg (40.3 lb); height, 111 cm (44.4 in.). Jesus guards the lower right quadrant of his abdomen and is crying. An intravenous access is established and morphine sulfate 2.0 mg is administered IV for pain control. An abdominal ultrasound is prescribed to confirm his suspected diagnosis. Jesus' leukocyte count is 17,500 cells/mm^3.

Questions and Suggested Answers

1. **Discuss your impressions about the above situation including pathophysiology and potential complications.** Fever, vomiting, and pain in the right lower quadrant of the abdomen are classic manifestations of appendicitis. This area of pain is referred to as ***McBurney's point*** and is located midway between the umbilicus and the anterior iliac crest in the right lower quadrant. In cases of appendicitis it is normal for the client to guard this area. The child may assume a position with the right leg flexed which decreases the abdominal wall tenderness. Although appendicitis is rare in children younger than 4 years of age, the incidence of appendicitis requiring an appendectomy in children of any age is 4 per 1,000 children. NOTE: Normally the temperature elevation for appendicitis ranges between 37.2° and 38° C (99° and 100.4° F, respectively). Temperature elevations greater than 38° C (100.4° F) may indicate peritonitis. The leukocyte count in the presence of appendicitis is usually 15,000–20,000 cells/mm^3.

   The appendix is a finger-like projection located just below the ileocecal valve, and although it does not seem to have any specific function after infancy, it regularly fills with digestive debris and empties into the cecum. If the appendix does not completely empty, its lumen can become blocked. This stimulates the inflammatory response, which can lead to further blockage by the edema associated with inflammation. Calculi comprised of fecal material, calcium- and phosphate-rich mucus, and salts provide an excellent medium and environment for bacterial invasion. The bacteria multiply and can cause ulceration of the mucosal lining of the appendix. In combination with the pressure within the appendix resulting in thinning of the lining, this can cause rupture of the appendix that can lead to potentially life-threatening peritonitis.

2. Compare Jesus' vital signs, height, and weight to the normal readings for a child his age and discuss the possible reasons for any abnormal values. The normal values for a 5-year-old child are:

Temperature: 37° C

Pulse: 75–120 beats/minute

Respirations: 18–28 breaths/minute

Blood pressure: 107–113/69–73

Height: 110 cm (43.3 in.)

Weight: 18.7 kg (41.1 lb)

Jesus is in the 50th percentile for weight and the 55th percentile for height. His temperature is elevated consistent with appendicitis/peritonitis secondary to bacterial infection. The elevation of his pulse and blood pressure are consistent with the increase in metabolism associated with this type of infection. His respiratory rate is elevated as the body attempts to both compensate for the increased metabolic rate and to reduce the body temperature. The presence and location of pain are consistent with a diagnosis of appendicitis.

3. Calculate the safe dosage ranges for the acetaminophen his parents administer and the morphine sulfate administered in the emergency department to determine whether he received safe doses of these two medications. The safe dosage range for acetaminophen is 10–15 mg/kg. Jesus weighs 18.3 kg (40.3 lb), so his safe dosage range is 183 mg (minimum) to 274.5 mg (maximum). The dose of acetaminophen administered by his parents is less than the minimum dose for his weight.

The safe dosage range for morphine sulfate is 0.05–0.1 mg/kg per hour. The safe range for Jesus is 0.9 mg (minimum) to 1.8 mg (maximum) per dose; however, the maximum dose may be as high as 2.6 mg/kg per hour for severe pain. His administered dose is within the maximum safe range for severe pain.

4. The abdominal ultrasound confirms that Jesus has appendicitis. Discuss the following prescribed treatment by the care provider:

a. Bedrest
b. NPO
c. Intravenous fluids of D_5 and .45% normal saline with 10 mEq of potassium chloride at 70 mL/hour.
d. Gentamicin 45 mg IV on call to operating room
e. Morphine sulfate 2 mg IV q1–2h PRN pain
f. K-pad to abdomen
g. Prepare for OR for laparoscopic appendectomy

The standard of care for appendicitis before rupture is rehydration, antibiotics, and surgical removal of the appendix. Rehydration is based on 100 mL/kg every 24 hours for the first 10 kg and 50 mL/kg every 24 hours for the second 10 kg. For Jesus rehydration should be 58.3 mL/hour; however, because of the vomiting he has experienced and his NPO status, the rate should be increased to compensate for these losses. A dose of gentamicin of 2.0–2.5 mg/kg every 8 hours (Gahart and Nazareno, 2005, p. 593) is the safe range and one of the drugs of choice for gastrointestinal infections (usually caused by enterococci). Jesus' safe range is 36.6–45.75 mg/dose. This dose is continued q8h postoperatively with the addition of ampicillin/sulbactam 100–150 mg/kg every 24 hours (Gahart and Nazareno, 2005, p. 100) for mild to moderate infections and 200–300 mg/kg every 24 hours for severe infections. As noted in answer to question 4, the morphine sulfate dose is safe. Emergency surgery is scheduled before complications (rupture of appendix or peritonitis) occur. The nurse should question the order concerning the application of moist heat to the abdomen. This is contraindicated in the presence of appendicitis because the heat increases vascularity to the area, which increases the risk of appendix rupture.

5. The preoperative instructions are given to Mr. Rodriquez, who in turn translates them for his wife and Jesus. Mr. and Mrs. Rodriquez give informed consent and Jesus assents to the surgery after his father explains the procedure to him. How does informed consent of the parents differ from Jesus' assent? Informed consent is the legal and ethical requirement of explaining the invasive procedure to the child and his or her parents

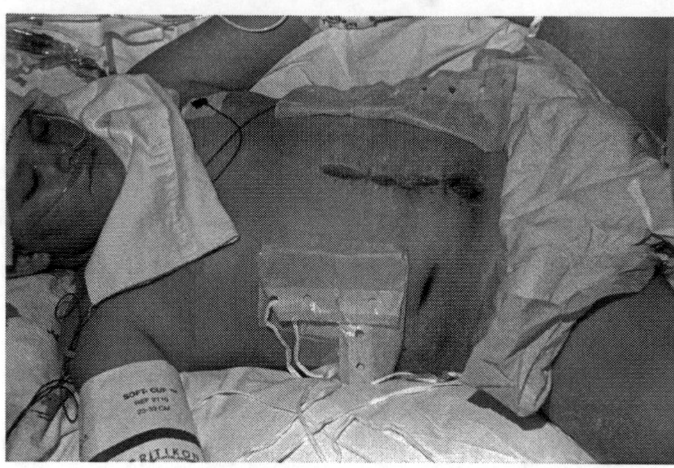

Figure A-4 *Incision healing after appendectomy of a ruptured appendix.*

and having the parents sign a document indicating that they understand the purpose of the procedure and potential risks that could occur during or after the procedure. Assent means the child has been fully informed about the procedure and concurs with the adults signing the informed consent. As informed consent laws vary from state to state, the nurse must become familiar with the laws in the state where he or she practices.

6. **Why is it important to include Jesus in the surgical consent?** Involving Jesus in the surgical consent process is important because if the child understands what he will be experiencing and what to expect, he should be more compliant with care measures, which will assist in his recovery.

7. **Just prior to his transfer to a holding area before surgery, Jesus experiences a sudden relief of pain that is followed by increased pain. What is your impression of this and what is your first action?** Sudden relief of pain is the classic manifestation of appendix rupture or perforation. Children younger than 6 years of age have an incidence of rupture or perforation of 50% to 85%. In younger children, diffuse peritonitis following rupture is more likely because of the underdevelopment of the intestinal omentum. The nurse should notify the health care provider stat and prepare for Jesus' transfer to surgery.

8. **Jesus undergoes an emergency exploratory laparotomy and appendectomy. Discuss the nursing priorities as he recovers from anesthesia.** The nurse's first priority is to address the ABCs—airway, breathing, and circulation. It is imperative to maintain a patent airway and promote effective breathing. This is accomplished through positioning and assessment. Vital signs and oxygen saturation should be monitored continuously. Maintaining patency of the vascular access and intravenous fluids also is crucial (see Fig. A-4). A complete systems assessment should be conducted that includes auscultating breath sounds, heart sound, bowel sounds, and hourly urine output. After a minimum of 1 hour of continuous assessment and assurance that the child is considered stable, he may be transferred to the nursing unit.

9. **Mr. and Mrs. Rodriquez are present in the PACU when Jesus awakens from anesthesia. Discuss the pros and cons of allowing parents in the PACU when children awake from anesthesia.** A child's parents are his or her primary source of security, and in their absence the child's separation anxiety associated with hospitalization is increased. This places increased psychosocial and metabolic stress on the child. Having his parents present when he recovers from anesthesia provides Jesus with a sense of security and lessens the fear and anxiety associated with being in a strange environment with strange sounds and equipment. Most children believe that parents can "fix anything" and having them present assists in their recovery.

10. **After Jesus is transferred to his room on your nursing unit at 5 A.M., Mr. Rodriquez states that he must leave to check on their other children and then must go to work. He says he will return after he finishes work and prepares dinner for Juan and Carlene. How will you communicate with Jesus and his mother in**

Mr. Rodriquez's absence? If the nurse is unable to speak Spanish, he or she should collaborate with other personnel on the nursing unit to see if anyone else can speak the language. If not, the facility's interpreter should be contacted. If an interpreter is not available, discuss the situation with Mr. Rodriquez and enlist his assistance in interpreting words pertinent to adequate care for Jesus and to communicate with his mother. A chart or pictures that depict each word could be posted in Jesus' room. The following are among the required words:

English	*Spanish*	*English*	*Spanish*
Hello	Ola	My name is	Me Ilamo
What is your name?	Como se' Ilama?	Good morning	Buenos diaz
Good afternoon	Buenas tardes	Good evening	Buenas noches
Zero	Zero	One	Uno
Two	Dos	Three	Tres
Four	Cuatro	Five	Cinco
Six	Seis	Seven	Siete
Eight	Ocho	Nine	Nueve
Ten	Diez	One minute	Un minuto
Yes	Si	No	No
Nurse	La enfermera	Doctor	Doctor
Please	Por favor	How are you?	Como esta' usted?
What is wrong?	Que le pasa?	Pain	Dolor
Where?	Donde'	How long?	Por cuinto tiempo?
Fever	Fiebre	Do you have allergies?	Tiene usted alergias?
To what?	A que'?	Stomach	El esto'mago
You will need . . .	Usted necesitara' . . .	Medication	Medicamento
Foley catheter	La sonda vesical o la sonda de la orina		
We will take out the catheter	Quitaremos la sonda		
Incentive spirometry	Espiro'metro		

The nurse should collaborate with the nurse manager to develop a pamphlet or pocket card with key phrases in both English and Spanish that is available to all staff coming in contact with Spanish-speaking clients and their families. More than 8 million people have immigrated to the United States from Spanish-speaking countries and comprise 4.2% of the U.S. population. This translates into the potential for an increased number of hospitalized clients being Spanish-speaking. Nurses must be able to communicate with this group of clients.

11. Discuss how you think you would feel if you were in Mrs. Rodriquez's position with your child in the hospital following surgery and you were unable to speak the language. The answer is a personal one that reflects the student's feelings including those based on similar circumstances. It should, however, address feelings of anxiety, ineffective coping, and powerlessness. Include the importance of assessment of the mother's adaptation and coping mechanisms in this situation.

12. The transfer orders on Jesus include the following:

- **a.** Routine postoperative vital signs
- **b.** Foley catheter to straight drain
- **c.** D_5 and .45% normal saline with 20 mEq of potassium chloride at 75 mL/hour. Medlock when urine output adequate and taking fluids well.
- **d.** Gentamicin sulfate 45 mg IV q8h
- **e.** Ampicillin sodium/Sulbactam sodium 900 mg IV q6h
- **f.** Morphine sulfate 0.5 mg continuous IV and 0.5 mg patient-controlled analgesia
- **g.** Acetaminophen 240 mg q4h per nasogastric tube for temperature >37.5° C (99.5° F)
- **h.** NPO except medications
- **i.** Nasogastric tube (Salem sump) to continuous wall suction
- **j.** Incentive spirometry 10 times each hour while awake
- **k.** Out of bed to chair this afternoon
- **l.** Notify house officer for temperature >38° C (100.4° F)

Discuss the nursing interventions involved in Jesus's care. Routine assessment of vital signs for a child returning to the nursing unit involves hourly monitoring of vital signs for a designated period per facility protocol. Following the hourly vital signs, the standard for routine vital signs is every 4 hours for 24–48 hours. Because Jesus experienced appendix rupture, monitoring his temperature every 4 hours for an extended period may be a nursing consideration. Jesus should be medicated with acetaminophen if his temperature is >37.5° C (99.5° F) and if his temperature exceeds 38° C (100.4°F), the nurse needs to notify the health care provider.

The nurse should monitor Jesus' urine output hourly to ensure his output is >2 mL/kg per hour. The nurse should inspect the catheter for kinks that would impede urine flow and could result in urinary retention and distention. Maintaining the patency of the vascular access is a high-priority nursing responsibility to ensure Jesus receives adequate hydration and antibiotic administration. If the intravenous antibiotics are stored in a refrigerator, they should be removed at least 1 hour prior to administration to warm them to room temperature. The antibiotics should be checked to ensure safe dosage based on Jesus' weight. The nurse should assess Jesus' pain level hourly and proactively encourage Jesus to use the "button" for the patient-controlled analgesia (PCA) dosing to maintain pain control at a level of 0–1/5 on the faces scale.

If acetaminophen is required, the nasogastric (N/G) tube should be flushed with 5–10 mL of normal saline prior to administration, and 5–10 mL after administration; the N/G tube should be clamped for 30 minutes following medication administration. The nurse is responsible for maintaining the nasogastric function. This is accomplished by assessing the tube a minimum of every 2 hours. If it is not suctioning, release the suction and reconnect to relieve suction lock. If this is not successful, 5–10 mL of air should be instilled in the blue air vent to clear the tubing. If this is not successful, Jesus should be repositioned because a common cause of N/G suction malfunction is that the proximal end of the tube is up against the stomach wall. Check for tube placement by inserting 5–10 ml of air into the N/G tube and then the tube may be flushed with 10–15 mL of sterile normal saline and returned to suction. If after these measures the N/G is still not functioning, notify the health care provider.

The nurse will need to reinforce preoperative instructions concerning use of incentive spirometry and encourage Jesus to use this 10 times per hour while awake. The nurse will need to remain with Jesus until he is able to use the spirometer as indicated and should be routinely evaluated to ensure he is compliant.

When preparing to get Jesus out of bed to the chair, the nurse should encourage Jesus to use the PCA "button" to premedicate him with the morphine sulfate to provide adequate pain management through this activity. Coordinating the schedule of his PCA dosing with the activity is prudent. The nurse should follow the principles of body mechanics as they apply to getting a client out of bed as well as facility-specific protocols.

References

Center for Immigration Studies. *http://www.cis.org*

Daniels, R. (2002). *Delmar's manual of laboratory and diagnostic tests.* Clifton Park, NY: Thomson Delmar Learning.

Gahart, B.L. and Nazareno, A.R. (2005). *2005 Intravenous medications* (21st ed.). St. Louis: Mosby.

Intravenous Therapy. *http://www.nursewise.com*

Josephson, D.L. (2004). *Intravenous infusion therapy for nurses: Principles and practice* (2nd ed.). Clifton Park, NY: Thomson Delmar Learning.

North American Nursing Diagnosis Association. (2005). *Nursing diagnoses: Definitions & classifications, 2005–2006.* Philadelphia: NANDA.

Potts, N. and Mandleco, B. (2002). *Pediatric nursing: Caring for children and their families.* Clifton Park, NY: Thomson Delmar Learning.

Rogers, P.T. and Ruiz-Rogers, O. (1997). *Quick medical Spanish* (2nd ed.). Appleton & Lange.

Spratto, G.R. and Woods, A.L. (2005). *2005 Edition PDR for nurses.* Cifton Park, NY: Thomson Delmar Learning

Tucker, J. (2002). Appendicitis. *http://www.emedicine.com/peds/topic127.htm*

CASE STUDY 5

Jamal

GENDER

M

AGE

18 months old

SETTING

- Hospital

ETHNICITY

- Black American

CULTURAL CONSIDERATIONS

PREEXISTING CONDITIONS

- Short bowel syndrome

COEXISTING CONDITIONS

SIGNIFICANT HISTORY

- Single grandmother

COMMUNICATION

DISABILITY

SOCIOECONOMIC

- Middle class
- Single parent

SPIRITUAL

PHARMACOLOGIC

- Yes

PSYCHOSOCIAL

- Parental anxiety
- Grandmother is caregiver

LEGAL

ETHICAL

ALTERNATIVE THERAPY

PRIORITIZATION

- Yes

DELEGATION

MODERATE

THE DIGESTIVE SYSTEM

Level of difficulty: Moderate

Overview: This case requires knowledge of short bowel syndrome and total parenteral nutrition, as well as an understanding of the client's background, personal situation, and family dynamics.

Client Profile

Jamal is an 18-month-old toddler who was born with short bowel syndrome (SBS), weighed 3.2 kg (7 lb), and was 50 cm (19.7 in.) in length at birth. He has lived with his grandmother since his discharge from the hospital 10 months after birth. He has a central venous access device (CVAD) through which he receives home total parenteral nutrition (TPN). His lengthy hospitalization resulted from the severity of his short bowel syndrome; Jamal was born with only 40 cm (15.8 in.) of intestine secondary to jejunal–ileal atresia. He experienced recurrent respiratory infections. Initially his parents visited him every day; however, his father was transferred in his job to a city 3 hours driving distance away when Jamal was 3 months old. Since that time, the parents' visits became infrequent and eventually they gave custody of Jamal to his grandmother because "they just couldn't handle his care." His grandmother has been a very attentive guardian and is very involved in his care. She works for a company that allows her to work from home so she can care for Jamal.

Case Study

Jamal's grandmother brings him to the emergency department of the children's hospital located in the city where they live because of recurrent episodes of fever, irritability, and "temper tantrums." Today the site of his central venous access device (CVAD) was reddened with "some discharge" under the dressing. Jamal is admitted to the pediatric medical nursing unit. His grandmother is very concerned about Jamal's condition and the fact that he required hospitalization. She verbalizes that she feels she is to blame for his current condition. The nurse's assessment reveals the following:

Temperature: 38.6° C (101.5° F)
Pulse: 120 beats/minute
Respirations: 30 breaths/minute
Height: 75 cm (30 in.)
Weight: 10 kg (22 lb)

Questions and Suggested Answers

1. **Discuss your impressions about the above situation.** The fever, irritability, and redness and drainage from Jamal's central venous access device (CVAD) are manifestations of infection at the CVAD site. His growth and development appear to be on track according to the data given. He weighed 3.2 kg (7 lb) at birth and normally an infant's weight triples by 1 year of age. From 1 to 3 years of age the average weight gain per year is approximately 2.4 kg (5 lb). Given his birth weight, Jamal should weigh approximately 10.7 kg (23.5 lb), and he weighs 10 kg (22 lb). He was 50 cm (19.7 in.) long at birth and now is 75 cm (29.5 in.) tall. The normal birth length is 45–52 cm (18–20.8 in.) with average growth of 2.5 cm (1 in.) per month for the first 6 months and 1.3 cm (0.5 in.) per month for 6–12 months of age. Toddlers gain approximately 7.5 cm or 3 in. per year. Jamal is 18 months old, so his height is within normal limits for his age and birth length. The grandmother's concern about Jamal's "temper tantrums" indicates that Jamal is displaying normal toddler behavior in response to the frustration of not being able to verbalize how upset he is. During this time, a child is very egocentric and focused on development of gross motor skills.
2. **What additional data would be helpful for the nurse to have to develop the plan of care for Jamal?**
   - **a.** Complete blood cell count with focus on leukocyte count
   - **b.** Description of the "discharge" at the site of Jamal's CVAD
   - **c.** Serum electrolyte values
   - **d.** Breath sounds, chest x-ray to determine if temperature may be related to his history of recurrent upper respiratory infection (URI)

e. Urinalysis and culture and sensitivity
f. Drainage culture and culture and sensitivity (C & S) from CVAD
g. Information from grandmother concerning how she cares for CVAD at home and her technique for hanging Jamal's TPN at home
h. Other growth and development behaviors to evaluate Jamal's level
i. Jamal's intake and output
j. Did Jamal have surgery to repair his jejunal–ileal atresia?

3. **Discuss the pathophysiology of short bowel syndrome.** Short bowel syndrome (SBS) is the congenital or acquired lack of small (and large) intestines. In children, it is defined as the lack of 30% of the normal length of the bowel. Congenital SBS may be associated with omphalocele or gastroschisis or may be a single anomaly. This leads to malabsorption\malnutrition, dehydration, and diarrhea. This is a complex condition when congenital because the fluid and electrolyte balance in children and especially infants is very fragile. Acquired SBS usually occurs following surgical resection of the bowel in infants and children with necrotizing enterocolitis, Crohn's disease, or volvulus. The small intestine provides final chemical digestion of nutrients and is the primary site of nutrient absorption. Without the small intestine, chyme boluses from the stomach move rapidly through whatever large intestine is available. Although the large intestine attempts to absorb minerals (electrolytes) and water from the fecal matter, limited large bowel surface area and the speed with which the food boluses travel through the intestines limit what the bowel can absorb. The duodenum absorbs iron; the jejunum absorbs carbohydrates, fats, protein, and vitamins; and the ileum absorbs bile salts and vitamin B_{12}. Necrotizing enterocolitis accounts for approximately 41% of SBS cases, jejunal–ileal atresia comprises 14%, and gastroschisis results in 20%.

4. **What is Jamal's prognosis for being weaned from TPN and developing a functional intestine?** According to the University of Michigan's Department of Pediatric Surgery, "Many individuals with 40 cm of small bowel may eventually adapt and transition off TPN." This depends on gastric motility and the condition of the intestines following the trauma of surgical repair of Jamal's jejunal–ileal atresia.

5. **Discuss TPN including indications for use.** TPN is the supplying of all nutrients parenterally (outside the digestive tract). TPN solutions are determined by fluid needs; energy needs; and protein, fat, and micronutrient requirements. TPN is augmented with intralipids to supply fatty acids. Because of the risk of fat embolism, intralipids must be infused concurrently with TPN; however, TPN can be infused without intralipids. Usually TPN is infused over every 24 hours and intralipids are infused over 18 hours every 24 hours.

   Indications for use in infants and children:
   a. Congenital gastrointestinal anomalies (omphalocele, gastroschisis);
   b. SBS
   c. Duodenal atresia
   d. Jejunal–ileal atresia
   e. Necrotizing enterocolitis
   f. Crohn's disease resulting in SBS or malabsorption syndrome

   According to Washington University in St. Louis School of Medicine, guidelines have been established for TPN in children to provide all nutrients for growth and development. The following are the general standards:
   Fluid needs: 125–150 mL/kg per day for infants or using the standard scale of weight <1 kg (2.2 lb) requires 125 mL/kg per day; weight of 1–10 kg requires 100 mL/kg per day; and weight >10 kg (22 lb) requires 2 L/m^2/day (m^2 = square root [weight (kg) × height (cm)/3,600]).
   Energy needs: Because of the growth spurt in infancy, the base solution of TPN is usually 70% dextrose. The standard formula for meeting energy needs is 60 kcal/kg per day for neonates through toddlers.
   Protein needs: Glycine and alanine are the major constituent amino acids in TPN solutions and infant amino acid requirements are 2.0–3.0 g/kg per day; children between infancy and adolescence require 1.5 to 2.0 g of amino acids/kg per day.
   Fat needs: Fatty acids are usually supplied with a 20% lipid solution and the rate is based on 1–2 ml/kg per day.

Electrolyte and mineral requirements: These are based on mEq/kg per day according to the child's age. The following are requirements for children younger than 3 years of age:

Sodium = 3 mEq/kg per day
Chloride = 3 mEq/kg per day
Potassium = 3 mEq/kg per day
Calcium = 1 mEq/kg per day
Acetate = 4 mEq/kg per day
Magnesium = 0.5 mEq/kg per day

Vitamins are usually supplied in a preformulated pediatric solution daily to provide the following for children weighing >3 kg (6.6 lb):

Vitamin C = 80 mg
Riboflavin = 2 mg
Thiamine = 1.2 mg
Pyridoxine = 1 mg
Niacin = 17 mg
Biotin = 20 mcg
Folic acid = 140 mcg
Dexpanthenol = 5 mg
Vitamin B_{12} = 1 mcg
Vitamin A = 0.7 mg
Vitamin D = 10 mcg
Vitamin E = 7 mg
Vitamin K = 200 mcg

Trace elements: Daily requirements for children 3–20 kg (6.6–44 lb):

Zinc = 300 mcg
Manganese = 5 mcg
Copper = 20 mcg
Chromium = 0.17 mcg

The most common cause of mortality in the use of TPN in infants is central line sepsis and hepatic failure secondary to prolonged use of TPN. Other complications include cholestasis, steatosis, and cholelithiasis. Multiple factors may predispose to PN-associated hepatobiliary complications including prematurity, overfeeding, PN dependence, absence of enteral stimulation for gall bladder contraction, short bowel syndrome, and recurrent sepsis. Cholestasis is the most common hepatobiliary complication in children receiving PN (*http:///peds.wustl.edu*).

6. **Why is Jamal at risk for infection?** Infection is the most common complication associated with CVADs because of the catheter entering the central venous system through a puncture insertion site in the skin (intact skin of course is the body's primary protection against infection). The high concentration of dextrose in the base solution of TPN provides an excellent medium for bacterial growth. Catheter-related infections are the primary cause of sepsis in children receiving TPN. A CVAD is required for any dextrose solution >10% in children because of the damage dextrose solutions of higher concentrations cause to peripheral vessels and the small lumen of pediatric peripheral vessels. Hyperglycemia is another complication of TPN associated with the high dextrose concentration of TPN and persistent hyperglycemia has been associated with increased infection rates. The rate of catheter infections is increased in children with SBS because of the prolonged use of TPN. The best types of CVAD for use in administering TPN in children are tunneled

catheters and those made of Silastic material. These have an antimicrobial cuff that helps prevent infection, and the Silastic catheter infections can usually be cleared with intravenous antibiotics.

7. **Jamal's TPN solution has completed; however, the next bag of TPN has not arrived from the pharmacy. What actions should you take at this time?** A temporary solution of 10% dextrose should be administered to prevent a drop in Jamal's blood sugar because his body has adjusted to a high (50%) level of dextrose as his base solution of TPN. The pharmacy should be notified and asked when the TPN will be arriving to the unit. It is important to follow the health care provider's and the facility's protocol.

8. **Identify the priorities of care for Jamal.**
   a. High risk for infection related to altered protection secondary to CVAD, infusion of TPN, child's condition
   b. Risk for imbalanced nutrition: less than body requirements related to inability to tolerate enteral feedings, presence of febrile condition that increases caloric needs
   c. Risk for deficient fluid volume related to febrile state and TPN
   d. Risk for altered growth and development related to child's altered health state
   e. Deficient knowledge related to child's condition, home care needs

9. **Discuss the nursing interventions that are critical in preventing infection when caring for Jamal.** The single most important nursing intervention in preventing infection for Jamal is frequent handwashing using appropriate technique. The alcohol foam canisters designed to be placed on the walls between client rooms have been shown to be more effective in preventing the spread of infection than handwashing alone. The standard of practice is that the hands should be thoroughly washed with soap and water after every tenth use of the alcohol foams. For Jamal, performing CVAD care using strict asepsis is a must. In addition, TPN solution changes should be done under strict aseptic technique including changing the intravenous tubing with each TPN solution change. Jamal's temperature should be monitored at least every 4 hours and antipyretic medication should be administered if his temperature rises above 38° C (100.4° F), as prescribed by the health care provider. Intravenous antimicrobial agents should be administered as prescribed alternating lumens of the CVAD if multiple lumens are present or according to health care provider and facility protocols. Jamal should be placed in a private room and visitors should be screened for communicable diseases prior to visiting Jamal. Age-appropriate toys should be provided for Jamal, but care must be taken to wash toys before and after use.

10. **How do you as the nurse explain Jamal's "temper tantrums" to his grandmother?** The nurse explains that Jamal's "temper tantrums" indicate that Jamal is displaying normal toddler behavior. At this age, toddlers display this behavior in response to the frustration of not being able to verbalize how upset they are. During this time, the child is very egocentric, and focused on self and on development of gross motor skills. This struggle for autonomy and a degree of independence causes the toddler to become easily frustrated when his desires are not consistent with his ability to achieve them or they put him in danger and the adult must set limits. These behaviors result in the typical toddler temper tantrum behavior.

11. **How will you evaluate Jamal's grandmother's ability to care for Jamal at home?**
   a. Assess the grandmother's current level of knowledge concerning Jamal's condition and medical regimen.
   b. Evaluate her ability to perform sterile CVAD dressing changes according to accepted protocol.
   c. Evaluate her ability to administer TPN including infusion changes.
   d. Have the grandmother spend the night in Jamal's room to be sure she understands the intravenous infusion device for Jamal's TPN and how to respond to device alarms.
   e. Provide a nonjudgmental environment for the grandmother to demonstrate her skills.
   f. Gently intervene as needed, providing rationales to increase the grandmother's understanding.
   g. Collaborate with the grandmother and health care provider for home health nurse referral and Social Work referral to provide support systems for Jamal and his grandmother.
   h. Allow adequate time for the grandmother's questions and provide information as needed.
   i. Document your teaching and the grandmother's response.

References

Broyles, B.E. (2005). *Medical-Surgical nursing clinical companion.* Durham, NC: Carolina Academic Press.

Centers for Disease Control and Prevention. *http://www.cdc.gov*

Children's Digestive Health and Nutrition Foundation. *http://www.cdhnf.org*

Daniels, R. (2002). *Delmar's manual of laboratory and diagnostic tests.* Clifton Park, NY: Thomson Delmar Learning.

North American Society for Pediatric Gastroenterology, Hepatology, and Nutrition. *http://www.nasphan.org*

National Institute of Diabetes & Digestive & Kidney Diseases. *http://www.niddk.nih.gov*

Gahart, B.L. and Nazareno, A.R. (2005). 2005 Intravenous medications (21st ed.). Mosby.

IntravenousTherapy. *http://www.nursewise.com*

Josephson, D.L. (2004). *Intravenous infusion therapy for nurses: Principles & practice* (2nd ed.). Clifton Park, NY: Thomson Delmar Learning.

North American Diagnosis Association. (2005). *Nursing diagnoses: Definitions & classifications, 2005–2006.* Philadelphia: NANDA.

Potts, N. and Mandleco, B. (2002). *Pediatric nursing: Caring for children and their families.* Clifton Park, NY: Thomson Delmar Learning, pp. 692–693.

Washington University in St. Louis School of Medicine. *http://www.peds.wustl.edu*

Wong, D.L., Perry, S.E., and Hockenberry, M.J. (2002). *Maternal child nursing care* (2nd ed.). St. Louis: Mosby, pp. 1294–1295.

CASE STUDY 6

Kurt

GENDER

M

AGE

2 days old

SETTING

- Hospital

ETHNICITY

- White American

CULTURAL CONSIDERATIONS

PREEXISTING CONDITIONS

COEXISTING CONDITIONS

SIGNIFICANT HISTORY

COMMUNICATION

DISABILITY

SOCIOECONOMIC

SPIRITUAL

PHARMACOLOGIC

- Acetaminophen (Tylenol)

PSYCHOSOCIAL

- Parental anxiety

LEGAL

ETHICAL

ALTERNATIVE THERAPY

PRIORITIZATION

- Yes

DELEGATION

- Yes

THE DIGESTIVE SYSTEM

Level of difficulty: Moderate

Overview: This case requires knowledge of imperforate anus; anal atresia; colostomy care; growth and development; as well as an understanding of the client's background, personal situation, and parent–child relationship.

Client Profile

Kurt is a neonate who weighed 3.5 kg (7 lb, 11 oz) at birth and was 50 cm (20 in.) long. He is the first child for Karen and Kevin. Karen had an uneventful pregnancy and delivery and breastfed Kurt immediately after birth. Kurt also is the first grandson for both sets of grandparents, who saw him immediately after he was born in the birthing room of the hospital. Kevin has taken paternity leave from his job to stay home with Kurt and Karen for 6 weeks.

Case Study

Within 24 hours of his birth, Kurt is examined by the pediatrician, who determines Kurt has imperforate anus. Following diagnostic testing, the diagnosis is confirmed and Karen and Kevin are informed by the pediatrician that Kurt has a high anal defect that will require surgery and the formation of a colostomy. They are devastated and express concern for their son "going through surgery when he is so young." Kurt's surgery is scheduled for the following day.

Questions and Suggested Answers

1. **How should the nurse respond to Karen and Kevin's concerns?** The nurse should determine what the pediatrician told Karen and Kevin about Kurt's surgery and then proceed with trying to allay their fears. The nurse should present a calm, understanding manner to communicate to them that he understands their concerns, being sure not to say, "I understand exactly how you feel," as this is very inappropriate and nontherapeutic. He should then explain that normally Kurt's surgery is performed on neonates with his condition as soon as possible following diagnosis to prevent complications of bowel impaction. He should reassure them that the staff performing and assisting the surgeon are specialized in caring for children and will monitor Kurt closely before, during, and after the surgery and that they can accompany him to the hold area and following surgery, they can see him in the post-anesthesia care unit (PACU). The nurse also should reinforce that the surgeon will come and talk to them immediately following surgery. Express to them the importance of their role in this process including meeting Kurt's needs to be held and loved.
2. **Discuss imperforate anus, its incidence, and cause.** Imperforate anus, also called anal agenesis or anal atresia, is the incomplete embryonic development of the distal end of intestines (see Fig. A-5). This occurs during the 7th and 8th weeks of gestation with an incidence of 1 in 500–5,000 live births. The incidence is greater in boys than girls and is frequently associated with other anomalies of the gastrointestinal and genitourinary systems. Imperforate anus occurs as either a high anomaly, occurring above the levator ani muscle, or as a low defect occurring below this muscle. These neonates do not have an anal opening so feces cannot be excreted. The etiology of this defect is unknown.
3. **Kurt's parents ask the nurse why Kurt has to have a colostomy. How should the nurse respond?** Whether the surgery involves the actual repair (anoplasty) of the imperforate anus or just the creation of a transverse colostomy, the purpose is to create a mechanism through which feces can be excreted from the body. If the anoplasty is performed at the same time, the colostomy also serves to protect the surgically repaired anus from contamination by feces.
4. **Karen expresses concern about the impact the surgery will have on her ability to breastfeed Kurt. What is the nurse's most appropriate response to Karen's concern?** Neonates who are breastfeeding and need to have this surgery can continue to breastfeed up until approximately 4 hours prior to surgery, and then can resume breastfeeding following surgery as soon as the baby's bowel sounds return and he or she has tolerated at least one feeding of sterile water. If the child must remain NPO for a longer period, the mother can

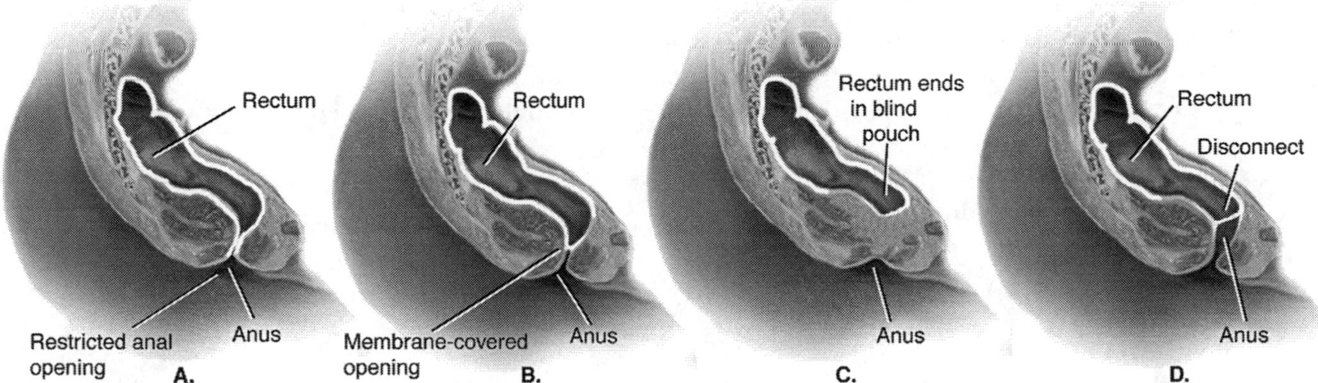

Figure A-5 *Imperforate anus. A. Anal opening is present but constricted; B. Anus and rectum are normal but the anal opening is covered by a thin membrane; C. Rectum ends in a blind pouch; D. Rectum and anal canal are present but not connected.*

be taught to pump her breasts to help establish a milk supply. Usually breast milk does not come in until the third to fourth day postpartum. At Kurt's age, Karen's milk supply has not been established. This should be explained to her to forestall potential fears that Kurt will not "starve" during the time he cannot breastfeed as a result of his surgery. The mother should be given information concerning the storage and freezing of breast milk that is pumped.

5. **Kurt undergoes an anoplasty and a transverse colostomy. What are the priorities for his care following surgery and his return to the pediatric nursing unit?**
   - **a.** Impaired skin integrity related to the colostomy and fecal discharge and anal repair
   - **b.** Acute pain related to tissue trauma secondary to surgery
   - **c.** Risk for deficient fluid volume related to NPO status before and after surgery
   - **d.** Anxiety (parental) related to deficient knowledge of neonate's post operative condition and home care

6. **What precautions should be taken when caring for Kurt following surgery?** Following anoplasty, no rectal temperatures should be performed and no rectal medications given. Because of the natural fragility of the neonates skin, care must be taken to provide adequate means to keep the fecal material excreted from the colostomy away from the child's skin. This may best be accomplished by consultation with the facility's enterostomal therapist who specializes in colostomy care. If an enterostomal therapist is not available, the nursing staff must provide the care. Placing a nonadhering dressing over the colostomy and holding it in place by the infant's diaper is a suggestion.

7. **Kurt's surgeon prescribes acetaminophen for Kurt's postoperative pain. Discuss your impressions of this and the appropriate actions the nurse should take.** Neonates have an acute sense of pain. Their peripheral nerves are not only very sensitive, but they are also very tactile. A common myth among care providers is that neonates do not feel pain, and if they do, they won't remember it. Studies have shown for many years that not only do neonates feel pain, but that it is remembered. Pain increases the stress on the body, causing vital signs to increase and then fluctuate until the pain is controlled. Neonates cry in response to pain which utilizes energy best used for both healing and eating. The nurse should collaborate with the health care provider to obtain a prescription for morphine sulfate intravenously for acute postoperative pain. It should be prescribed in a dosage of 0.1–0.2 mg/kg of body weight (Gahart and Nazareno, 2005, p. 216) to be administered every 1–2 hours. The nurse may need to do some colleague teaching to remove another myth and that respiratory depression secondary to morphine sulfate is uncommon even in neonates. For safety purposes, however, the neonate should be placed on continuous cardiopulmonary monitoring and pulse oximetry during the time opioids are used. The neonate should be medicated proactively for the first 24 hours and then as needed. Opioids are usually only necessary for the first 48 hours postoperatively, but the nurse needs to medicate the child according to his or her assessments.

8. **Kurt's recovery allows him to be discharged to his parents. Discuss the parental teaching necessary for Karen and Kevin prior to Kurt's discharge.**
   a. Assess what Karen and Kevin understand at the time of discharge.
   b. Karen and Kevin should have had colostomy care demonstrated and provided time for a return demonstration prior to the discharge teaching.
   c. Provide verbal and written information and supplies as needed for:
      (1) Colostomy and skin care
      (2) Medication administration to neonates
      (3) Praising parents appropriately regarding care they provide
      (4) Breastfeeding
      (5) Infant care, as needed
      (6) Monitoring of intake and output, stressing that Kurt should have six to eight wet diapers a day
      (7) Signs and symptoms to report to health care provider and contact numbers
      (8) Importance of follow-up care for Kurt
      (9) If available, information regarding Kurt's colostomy take-down surgery
   d. Allow sufficient time for Karen and Kevin to ask questions, answering them honestly and referring questions appropriately as needed.
   e. Document teaching and parents' response.

9. **Kurt is now 2 months old and returns to have a colostomy takedown. He has been breastfeeding well and the skin around his colostomy is clean and dry without any evidence of excoriation. What are your impressions of Kurt's present condition?** Because skin breakdown is the greatest concern with a colostomy, the fact that his skin is dry and intact with no evidence of excoriation indicates that his parents have been adequately caring for Kurt since discharge following his first surgery. It is important for the nurse to commend them and determine what actions they took to keep his skin in such good condition. Skin breakdown can delay his colostomy takedown and may cause him to withstand prolonged hospitalization.

10. **What assessment should the nurse include in her care of Kurt following surgery?** Kurt's vital signs must be monitored every 4 hours for 24–48 hours postoperatively. If possible, place Kurt on continuous cardiopulmonary monitoring and pulse oximetry. His intravenous access and fluid intake must be monitored hourly as well as his urinary output. His bowel sounds should be monitored and his rectal passage of feces appropriately assessed and documented. The abdominal site of the colostomy takedown must be monitored for redness, swelling, and drainage. The nurse needs to encourage Karen and Kevin to be actively involved in Kurt's care and assess the interactions.

References

Gahart, B.L. and Nazareno, A.R. (2005). *2005 Intravenous medications* (21st ed.). St. Louis: Mosby.

North American Nursing Diagnosis Association. (2005). *Nursing diagnoses and classifications, 2005–2006.* Philadelphia: NANDA.

Potts, N. and Mandleco, B. (2002). *Pediatric nursing: Caring for children and their families.* Clifton Park, NY: Thomson Delmar Learning, pp. 519–520, 667–668.

Wong, D.L., Perry, S.E., and Hockenberry, M.J. (2002). *Maternal child nursing care* (2nd ed.). St. Louis: Mosby, p. 664.

CASE STUDY 7

Nathan

GENDER

M

AGE

6

SETTING

- Hospital

ETHNICITY

- Black American

CULTURAL CONSIDERATIONS

PREEXISTING CONDITIONS

- Diarrhea

COEXISTING CONDITIONS

SIGNIFICANT HISTORY

COMMUNICATION

DISABILITY

SOCIOECONOMIC

SPIRITUAL

PHARMACOLOGIC

- Nitazoxanide (Alinia)

PSYCHOSOCIAL

- Fear/anxiety

LEGAL

ETHICAL

ALTERNATIVE THERAPY

PRIORITIZATION

- Yes

DELEGATION

- Client teaching

MODERATE

THE DIGESTIVE SYSTEM

Level of difficulty: Moderate

Overview: This case requires knowledge of diarrhea, acid–base imbalances, fluid and electrolyte balance, client teaching, as well as an understanding of the client's background, personal situation, and mother–child attachment relationship, and of growth and development of the school-age child.

Client Profile

Nathan Woodruff is a 6-year-old first grader who lives with his mother and older brother, 8-year-old Micah. Nathan has been a healthy child with only occasional upper respiratory infections. His mother diligently kept up with his immunizations and all of his pediatric check-ups. He started first grade 2 weeks ago and is always eager to go to school. His level of growth and development is appropriate for his age and he quickly developed friendships with his classmates.

Case Study

Yesterday afternoon when he came home from school, Nathan began having episodes of abdominal pain and diarrhea. His stools have been intermittent, foul smelling, watery, and according to Nathan's mother "float in the toilet." He refused to eat or drink anything since that time so Nathan's mother calls the pediatrician. At the pediatrician's office Nathan is listless, his skin is warm and dry, and he complains that his "tummy hurts." His urine specific gravity is 1.040, his heart rate is 120 beats/minute, his respirations are 30 breaths/minute, and his blood pressure is 78/46. His stool is negative for blood and his complete blood count results are as follows:

Hematocrit: 50%

Hemoglobin: 16.5 g/dL

Platelets: 455,000 cells/mm^3

Red blood cell count: 5.2 million cells/mm^3

White blood cell count: 11,300 cells/mm^3

Because he continues to refuse to eat or drink, the pediatrician recommends that he be hospitalized for further diagnostic testing.

Questions and Suggested Answers

1. **Discuss your impressions about the above situation.** Nathan's clinical manifestations may indicate that he is experiencing a parasitic gastrointestinal infection. His symptoms are consistent with giardiasis, caused by the protozoan *Giardia intestinalis,* the most common intestinal parasitic pathogen in the United States. The infection affects three times more children than adults and is transmitted by the fecal–oral route, but can be transmitted by airborne droplets. Children, especially those in daycare centers or classrooms, are more prone to transmit this infection from one to another primarily because they are still learning handwashing techniques that need to be followed after defecating and they play games involving hand-to-hand and then hand-to-mouth activities.

2. **Because of Nathan's symptoms, the pediatrician prescribes arterial blood gases be drawn. What is the purpose of this prescription and what nursing implications are appropriate prior to drawing Nathan's arterial blood gases (ABGs)?** ABGs are drawn to measure the client's arterial blood pH to determine if he is experiencing an acid–base imbalance. If possible, EMLA (eutectic mixture of local anesthetics) should be applied to the site of puncture 1–2 hours earlier (in the pediatrician's office) in preparation for obtaining the ABGs. Drawing ABGs is painful to the client because of the nerve innervation surrounding the arterial sites.

3. **Nathan's ABG results are: pH, 7.30; Pco_2, 30 mm Hg; Po_2, 90 mm Hg; oxygen saturation, 94%; and bicarbonate (HCO_3), 22 mEq/L. Compare his values to the normal values for a child of Nathan's age.** Nathan's pH reflects acidosis, as the normal range is 7.35–7.45. Values <7.35 indicate acidosis and those >7.45 indicate alkalosis. His Pco_2 level is decreased from the normal 35–45 mm Hg. This may represent the lungs immediate

Related to Respiratory Function   Related to Metabolism of the Body

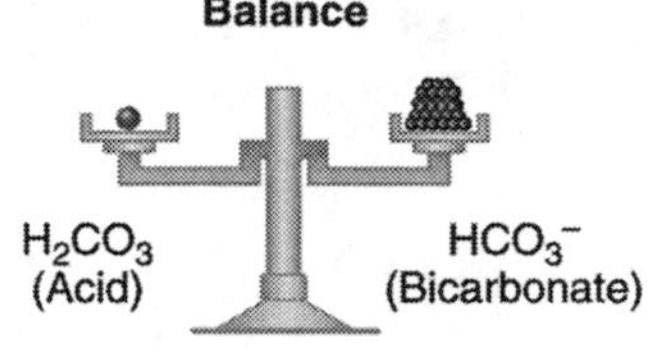

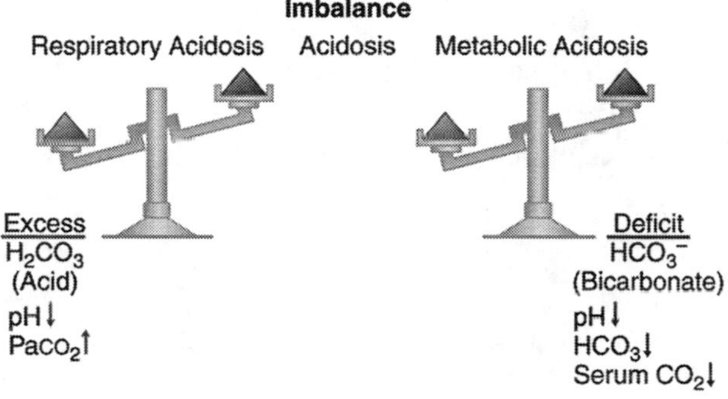

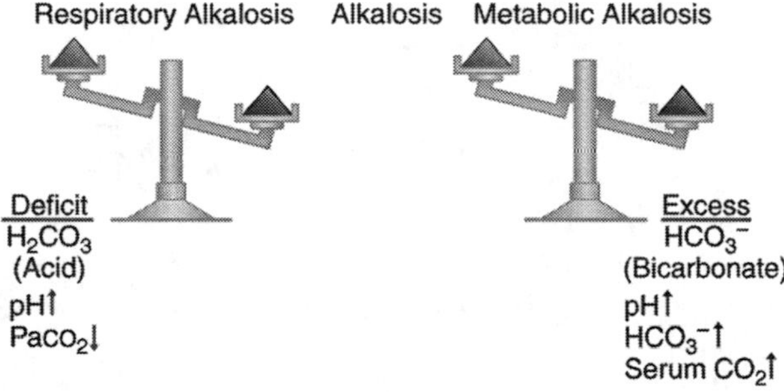

Figure A-6 *Acid-base balance and imbalance*

buffer compensation that takes place to correct acidosis. His partial oxygen is within normal limits of 80–100 mm Hg and his oxygen saturation is slightly below the normal of 95% to 100%.

4. **Discuss Nathan's blood gas values considering his present condition and clinical manifestations.** With his history of diarrhea, his blood gas results indicate he is experiencing metabolic acidosis (see Fig. A-6). His pulse rate and respiratory rates are elevated for a child his age, with normal values being 75–120 beats/minute pulse rate and respiratory rate of 25–28 breaths/minute. Tachycardia, dry warm skin, and tachypnea are consistent manifestations of metabolic acidosis as well as the presence of the underlying condition of diarrhea (a cause of metabolic acidosis).

5. **What is the significance of Nathan's hematological test results and his urine specific gravity?** His hemoglobin and hematocrit are elevated, which when combined with his urine specific gravity of 1.040 indicate he is dehydrated. His loss of fluid in diarrheic stools and his poor oral intake further support this conclusion. Normal hemoglobin and hematocrit levels are 11–16 g/dL and 31% to 41%, respectively. As fluid within the vascular compartment decreases, the concentration of blood products increases as reflected in their elevated levels. This is further supported by his elevated red blood cell count from the normal of 4.5–4.8 million/mm^3. His white blood cell count is slightly elevated above the normal value of 4,100–10,800 cells/mm^3. This also may indicate the presence of an infection. The normal urine specific gravity, which is the weight of urine compared to water, is 1.015–1.030. In dehydrated states, the urine concentrates with solutes, and as fluid volume decreases so does the excretion of water in the urine.

6. **What additional data would be helpful in confirming Nathan's diagnosis?** The following additional data would be helpful in confirming Nathan's diagnosis:
   a. The most helpful information would be obtained from stool samples tested for the microscopic presence of *Giardia.* A *Giardia* enzyme immunoassay (EIS) shows the presence of *Giardia* antigens.
   b. Bowel sounds
   c. Further description of Nathan's abdominal pain
   d. Physical examination

7. **Nathan is diagnosed with giardiasis and is prescribed nitazoxanide. What is this agent and would you question it being prescribed for Nathan?** Nitazoxanide is the only agent approved by the Food and Drug Administration (on December 2, 2002) for the treatment of giardiasis. It is administered in an oral suspension with a recognized dosage of 200 mg every 12 hours for six doses. In clinical trials 85% of clients who received a course of treatment of Alinia (nitazoxanide) responded compared to 80% who received a course of treatment with metronidazole (*fda.gov*). The nurse would not question this prescription given the information here.

8. **What are the nursing priorities for Nathan's care?**
   a. Diarrhea
   b. Deficient fluid volume related to loss of body fluids secondary to diarrhea
   c. Risk for decreased cardiac output related to cardiac rhythm changes secondary to metabolic acidosis
   d. Fear/anxiety related to hospitalization of a child
   e. Deficient knowledge related to condition, treatment, and prevention of reinfection

9. **Nathan begins to respond to therapy and is beginning to eat and drink. What play activities would be appropriate for Nathan while he is hospitalized?** School-age children are involved in both associative and cooperative play. According to Erikson, their focus is to establish a sense of industry versus the development of inferiority. School-age children are aware of rules and need to follow them to achieve a sense of accomplishment. Their fine motor skills are well developed. Given Nathan's condition, computer games could be brought to his bedside and his brother should be encouraged to play with him. If this isn't feasible, the nurse could play with him. Having him throw paper towel balls into the wastebasket would provide a sense of accomplishment as well as range-of-motion exercises for his upper extremities.

10. **What are the teaching priorities you should discuss with Nathan's mother prior to his discharge?**
   a. Assess Nathan's mother's current level of knowledge about Nathan's condition
   b. Provide verbal and written information regarding:
      (1) Proper handwashing as the single most important action to prevent reinfection
      (2) The need to stress to her children the importance of washing their hands after every trip to the bathroom, not only at home but also at school
      (3) Handwashing after children return to the classroom from recess
      (4) Medication administration, if needed, including the importance of completing the entire prescription
      (5) Signs and symptoms to monitor and contact numbers to notify health care provider if Nathan's condition worsens
      (6) Importance of increasing Nathan's fluid intake until all of his symptoms have resolved
      (7) Diet adjustment as prescribed to avoid lactose intolerance post-diarrhea
      (8) Importance of follow-up with the health care provider
   c. Provide sufficient time for Nathan and his mother to ask questions
   d. Document teaching and client and mother's response.

References

Broyles, B.E. (2005). *Medical-surgical nursing clinical companion.* Durham, NC: Carolina Academic Press.
Centers for Disease Control and Prevention. *http://www.cdc.gov*
Daniels, R. (2002). *Delmar's manual of laboratory and diagnostic tests.* Clifton Park, NY: Thomson Delmar Learning.

Food and Drug Administration Website. *http://www.fda.gov*

Gahart, B. L. and Nazareno, A.R. (2005). *2005 Intravenous medications* (21st ed.). St. Louis: Mosby.

KidsHealth. *http://www.kidshealth.org*

National Institute of Allergy and Infectious Diseases of the National Institutes of Health. *http://www.niaid.nih.gov*

North American Nursing Diagnosis Association. (2005). *Nursing diagnoses: Definitions & classifications, 2005–2006.* Philadelphia: NANDA.

Potts, N. and Mandleco, B. (2002). *Pediatric nursing: Caring for children and their families.* Clifton Park, NY: Thomson Delmar Learning.

Wong, D.L., Perry, S.E., and Hockenberry, M.J. (2002). *Maternal child nursing care* (2nd ed.). St. Louis: Mosby, pp. 1264–1267.

CASE STUDY 8

Marissa

GENDER

F

AGE

Neonate

SETTING

- Hospital

ETHNICITY

- Spanish American

CULTURAL CONSIDERATIONS

PREEXISTING CONDITIONS

COEXISTING CONDITIONS

SIGNIFICANT HISTORY

COMMUNICATION

DISABILITY

SOCIOECONOMIC

SPIRITUAL

PHARMACOLOGIC

PSYCHOSOCIAL

- Potential impaired parent–infant attachment

LEGAL

ETHICAL

ALTERNATIVE THERAPY

PRIORITIZATION

- Yes

DELEGATION

- Yes

MODERATE

THE DIGESTIVE SYSTEM

Level of difficulty: Moderate

Overview: This case requires knowledge of cleft lip/cleft palate (CL/CP) surgical repair, growth and development, and parent–child attachment relationship.

Client Profile

Marissa is a newborn weighing 14.2 kg (6 lb, 7 oz) who was born with a cleft lip and palate. She is the third child of Juan and Maria.

Case Study

When Marissa is first brought from the nursery to Maria's room, Maria and Juan are visually alarmed at Marissa's appearance. The nurse notes that Maria holds her daughter in her lap, looking at her while Juan moves from the bedside to a chair next to the bed. Maria begins to cry, "My poor baby. What will happen to her? Everyone will make fun of her. What have we done to her?"

Questions and Suggested Answers

1. **Discuss your impressions of this situation.** Maria and Juan are shocked at the site of their new daughter's cleft lip and palate, especially at the lip. This is a normal reaction toward any baby born with a birth defect, but this defect is especially troubling because it is obvious and changes the appearance of the newborn. Most congenital defects are less visible, which allows the parents more time to accept the baby's flaw. The parents' reaction is a grieving response at the loss of a "perfect" baby. Maria's remarks indicate that she is feeling guilt about Marissa's appearance and also fear that her daughter will experience unkind remarks from others when they see her. Juan is demonstrating denial, another part of the first stage of the grieving process. The student also should address possible cultural factors.
2. **What is the incidence and etiology of cleft lip and cleft palate?** In most cases, cleft lip and cleft palate occur together. Cleft lip can occur with or without cleft palate, and its incidence is approximately 1.5 in 1,000 live births. The incidence of cleft palate occurring without cleft lip is 1 in 2,000 live births. Boys have a higher incidence of cleft lip with or without a cleft palate; however, a cleft palate occurs more often in girls. It is found more often in Asians and in certain Native Americans more than in Caucasians, with the lowest incidence in African Americans. Although the exact cause of cleft lip and cleft palate is unknown, family history, genetics, and environmental factors are implicated. Cleft lip results from failure of the nasal and maxillary process to fuse during the 5th to 8th weeks of gestation. Cleft palate occurs when the palatine plates do not fuse during the 7th to 12th weeks of gestation.
3. **Is the response seen in Marissa's parents unusual?** This is a normal reaction in response to the new parents' loss of the "perfect" baby that is the dream of all expectant parents. This particular defect, referred to as a facial malformation, is especially disturbing to new parents because the cleft lip is so obvious and changes the baby's appearance.
4. **How can the nurse therapeutically respond to Maria and Juan?** The nurse's response must be empathetic and nonjudgmental. The nurse should explain the defect and how it is treated. The best approach, if possible, is to show the parents pictures, available in nursing textbooks and on the Internet, of other children born with cleft lip and/or cleft palate before and after surgical repair. As they are looking at their child during the nurses's explanation, it may be very difficult for the new parents to imagine how the surgical repair will affect Marissa's appearance.
5. **Discuss the standard of care for the surgical repair of Marissa's cleft lip and cleft palate.** The closure of the cleft lip usually occurs between 6 weeks and 3 months of age or when the infant weighs at least 5.4 kg (12 lb). The facial reconstruction is the least complicated of the two surgeries the infant will undergo, but is the most relieving to the parents because the cleft palate is not as externally obvious as the cleft lip. The cleft palate

repair is performed when the infant is approximately 1 year of age and involves a team of surgeons including a neurosurgeon, otolaryngologist, and orthodontist.

6. What are the current priorities of care for Marissa?

- **a.** Risk for aspiration related to structural defect between the nasal septum and the mouth
- **b.** Imbalanced nutrition: less than body requirements related to defect in roof of the mouth interfering with sucking
- **c.** Risk for impaired parent/infant attachment related to visual appearance of infant's congenital defect
- **d.** Deficient knowledge related to infant's condition, treatment, and how to meet Marissa's needs

7. Discuss the impact of Marissa's defect on her growth and development. The greatest impact of the defect on Marissa may be nutritional. Because a newborn normally sucks for a newborn by pressing the tongue against the palate, Marissa will not be able to suck effectively. This can lead to feeding difficulties that can impact or possibly interrupt the mother–child bonding process as feeding time is an important part of the bonding process. In addition, Marissa's primary task during infancy is developing a sense of trust. As long as her needs are met consistently, trust will develop. If bonding/attachment does not occur in a meaningful way for her trust needs to be met, the infant develops mistrust.

8. Discuss the teaching priorities for Marissa's parents prior to her discharge at 5 days of age. Provide parents with information, technique, and time for a return demonstration of ESSR. This is a technique developed by Richard (1991) that involves *E*nlarging the nipple, *S*timulating the suck reflex, *S*wallow fluid appropriately, and *R*est as indicated by the infant. Nipple devices also used for these infants include the lamb's nipple, flanged nipple, and syringe with a rubber tube. The parents need to be taught to feed Marissa in an upright position, assessing for formula escaping through her nose. She also needs to be bubbled frequently because of the tendency to swallow increased amounts of air during the feeding.

- **a.** The parents need to be taught infant CPR in the event of aspiration and allowed sufficient time to demonstrate on the CPR infant manikin.
- **b.** Referrals to home health agency may be necessary, and the parents need information about this service.
- **c.** Contact numbers for parents' questions and to report signs and symptoms of aspiration must be provided for the parents, with encouragement to take advantage of this.
- **d.** The nurse must stress the importance of follow-up visits for Marissa.

9. Marissa returns to the hospital at 8 weeks of age for the surgical repair of her cleft lip. What are the priorities of care for Marissa following her surgery?

- **a.** Risk for ineffective airway clearance related to surgical trauma to the site
- **b.** Impaired skin integrity related to surgical incision
- **c.** Risk for infection related to surgical site
- **d.** Acute pain related to surgical trauma
- **e.** Deficient knowledge related to protecting the surgical site, pain management

10. Discuss the nursing interventions to meet Marissa's care needs.

- **a.** Airway
  - **(1)** Assess airway patency at least hourly.
  - **(2)** Place on continuous cardiopulmonary monitor and pulse oximetry.
  - **(3)** Monitor vital signs every 4 hours following postoperative protocol schedule.
  - **(4)** Administer oxygen as prescribed to maintain oxygen saturation >94%.
  - **(5)** Place in lateral position with head elevated 15–30° as prescribed.
  - **(6)** Maintain NPO status as prescribed.
- **b.** Skin integrity
  - **(1)** Assess incision every 4 hours for redness, swelling, drainage, and approximation.
  - **(2)** Place elbow restraints to prevent the infant from touching the incision line.

(3) Instruct parents that they can remove elbow restraints when holding Marissa as long as they ensure she doesn't put her fingers to her mouth; restraints must be reapplied when Marissa is not being held.
(4) Provide skin care as prescribed.

c. Infection
(1) Refer to skin integrity.
(2) Monitor temperature every 4 hours.
(3) Maintain patency of intravenous access, monitoring hourly.
(4) Administer antibiotics as prescribed.

d. Acute pain
(1) Assess pain level hourly using an infant-appropriate pain assessment tool.
(2) Proactively medicate to maintain pain control.
(3) Monitor for effectiveness of analgesic therapy.

e. Deficient knowledge
(1) Assess parental level of knowledge regarding how to care for Marissa postoperatively.
(2) Provide verbal and written instructions regarding:
(a) Incision care
(b) Medication administration as prescribed
(c) Signs and symptoms of infection including how to monitor Marissa's temperature
(d) Contact numbers to report signs and symptoms or in the event they have questions
(e) Importance of follow-up visits
(3) Provide sufficient time for questions, answering them honestly and providing referrals as needed.
(4) Document teaching and parental response.

11. **Even following Marissa's cleft palate repair, her parents note that she still does not "talk much" and when she does, it is "difficult to understand her." Our other children were very talkative by this age. What should we do?" What actions should the nurse take?** It is common for infants with cleft lip and palate to require speech therapy as they relearn to talk following palate repair. The nurse should assess the infant's ability to verbalize and compare it to the normal standards for her level of growth and development. The findings should be reported to the health care provider and if needed, the nurse should collaborate with the health care provider to obtain a referral to speech therapy.

References

Centers for Disease Control and Prevention. *http://www.cdc.gov*

Cleft Palate Foundation. *http://www.cleftline.org*

Medline Plus. Cleft lip and Palate. *http://www.nlm.nih.gov*

North American Nursing Diagnosis Association (2005). *Nursing diagnoses: Definitions & classifications, 2005–2006.* Philadelphia: NANDA.

Potts, N. and Mandleco, B. (2002). *Pediatric nursing: Caring for children and their families.* Clifton Park, NY: Thomson Delmar Learning, pp. 657–661.

Richard, M. (1991). Feeding the newborn with cleft lip and/or cleft palate: The enlargement, stimulate, swallow, rest (ESSR) method. *Pediatric Nursing* 6(5): 317–321.

Smile Welcome. *http://www.cleft.org*

Wong, D.L., Perry, S.E., and Hockenberry, M.J. (2002). *Maternal child nursing care* (2nd ed.). St. Louis: Mosby, pp. 1279–1283.

CASE STUDY 9

Sandra

GENDER

F

AGE

14

SETTING

- Home/clinic/hospital

ETHNICITY

- White American

CULTURAL CONSIDERATIONS

PREEXISTING CONDITIONS

- Motor vehicle accident
- Acute renal failure

COEXISTING CONDITIONS

SIGNIFICANT HISTORY

COMMUNICATION

DISABILITY

SOCIOECONOMIC

SPIRITUAL

PHARMACOLOGIC

- Prednisone (Deltasone)
- Cyclosporine (Restasis)
- Azathioprine (Azasan)

PSYCHOSOCIAL

- Fear/anxiety

LEGAL

ETHICAL

ALTERNATIVE THERAPY

PRIORITIZATION

- Yes

DELEGATION

MODERATE

THE URINARY SYSTEM

Level of difficulty: Moderate

Overview: This case requires knowledge of acute renal failure and associated complications; growth and development; as well as an understanding of the client's background, personal situation, and family–child relationship.

Client Profile

Sandra is a 14-year-old adolescent who lives at home with her mother, stepfather, and two younger siblings. When Sandra was 9 years old, she was involved in a motor vehicle accident and severely injured. As a result, she developed acute renal failure that eventually progressed to chronic renal failure. She has been receiving peritoneal dialysis for the past 4 years. She is registered with the organ procurement agency in the city 30 miles from her home because her parents have been ruled out as potential donors.

Case Study

Sandra is doing satisfactorily at home, receiving her peritoneal dialysis at night. This allows her to attend school and interact with her friends. She is anxious to receive a kidney transplant so she will not have to continue her dialysis. Sandra's parents receive a phone call from the hospital at 2 o'clock A.M. telling them that the hospital has procured a kidney for Sandra as a result of a motor vehicle crash that killed a 10-year-old boy. Her mother calls Sandra's grandmother to babysit for the younger siblings, and then Sandra's parents take her to the hospital where they are met by the transplant team.

Questions and Suggested Answers

p1076

1. **What is chronic renal failure and end-stage renal disease (ESRD)?** Chronic renal failure is the progressive and "irreversible loss of 30% to 50% of functional nephrons in the kidneys" (Broyles, 2005, p. 712). Chronic renal failure progresses to ESRD causing multiple life-threatening complications. ESRD requires dialysis and can be cured only with a renal transplant.
2. **Discuss the possible connection between Sandra's motor vehicle accident and her development of ESRD.** Motor vehicle accidents frequently result in serious injuries leading to hypovolemia and shock. Shock is hypoperfusion that results in decreased tissue perfusion of oxygen and nutrients to the organs of the body. As a compensatory response to shock, blood is diverted to the brain, heart, and lungs to sustain life. Blood is dramatically decreased to the kidneys in an effort to reduce fluid loss through these primary organs of fluid excretion. As hypoperfusion progresses, the functional cells of the kidneys are gradually lost resulting in acute renal failure (ARF). If the cause of the hypoperfusion is not corrected before sufficient loss of renal function, chronic renal failure results. Sandra probably experienced hypovolemia with resultant hypoperfusion which ultimately led to her chronic renal failure and ESRD.
3. **Discuss the incidence and etiology of chronic renal failure in children.** Statistically, chronic renal failure affects between 1.5 and 3 per 1 million children in the United States. Causes include congenital renal and urinary tract malformation causing obstruction, vesicoureteral reflux that results in recurrent urinary tract infections, chronic pyelonephritis, hemolytic uremic syndrome, and systemic diseases, such as lupus erythematosus. Chronic renal failure also can result from the conditions that cause acute renal failure if they result in ineffective tissue perfusion to the kidneys that leads to nephron destruction. These include hypovolemia, renal trauma, hemorrhage, burns, dehydration, and complications from surgery.
4. **Discuss the complications associated with Sandra's diagnosis.** Unless chronic renal failure is effectively treated with diet and dialysis, a variety of life-threatening complications result, all of which are directly related to the loss of the kidney's multiple functions. Azotemia is the accumulation of nitrogen waste products in the blood stream because they are not excreted. Hyperkalemia that can cause cardiac dysrhythmias results from an accumulation of potassium that is normally kept in check by renal excretion. Hypernatremia resulting in fluid overload is caused by the accumulation of sodium because of the inability of the failing kidneys to excrete it. This can lead to congestive heart failure and hypertension. Hypertension also results from

the loss of the renal system's check on regulation of blood pressure by the renin–angiotensin complex. In renal failure this complex is activated leading to increases in aldosterone secretion causing the blood pressure to rise. Hyperphosphatemia and reciprocal hypocalcemia result from the kidneys' inability to filter and excrete phosphorus. Anemia results from the loss of the production of erythropoietin by the kidneys that is necessary for red blood cell production. Metabolic acidosis occurs because of the loss of the renal buffer for acid–base balance either by decreasing the release or increasing the retention of sodium bicarbonate.

5. **What are the priorities of care for Sandra's ESRD?**
   - **a.** Excess fluid volume related to sodium and fluid retention and inability of the kidneys to excrete
   - **b.** Deficient fluid volume related to third-spacing of fluid (edema), decreased fluid intake, diuretic therapy, and dialysis
   - **c.** Risk for injury, cardiac dysrhythmias related to hyperkalemia and uremic toxins
   - **d.** Risk for infection related to peritoneal dialysis access and uremic toxins
   - **e.** Risk for impaired skin integrity related to edema
   - **f.** Imbalanced nutrition: less than body requirements related to dietary restriction and altered metabolism
   - **g.** Risk for ineffective tissue perfusion related to anemia
   - **h.** Fear/anxiety related to condition, treatment, wait for a transplant
   - **i.** Deficient knowledge related to condition, complications, treatment, and home care

6. **Why is Sandra receiving peritoneal dialysis?** Peritoneal dialysis is the preferred method of dialysis in children because it can be done at home and during sleeping hours, with less disruption of the child's normal schedule (see Fig. A-7). Hemodialysis is usually performed three or four times per week and requires the parents to take the child to a dialysis center that is probably open only during daytime hours, thus interrupting the child's school schedule. Dialysis, also called renal replacement therapy, removes excess fluids and waste products from the body and restores electrolyte and acid–base balance. This is accomplished by moving body fluids through a dialysate fluid composed of glucose, water, sodium chloride, potassium, magnesium, calcium, and sodium bicarbonate. The dialysate fluid draws the toxins and excess fluid out of the body. In peritoneal dialysis, a silicone rubber catheter is surgically placed into the abdominal cavity through which dialysate is infused, drawing the toxins and excess fluid from the body. It functions by diffusion and osmosis across the semipermeable peritoneal membrane, which is rich in capillaries to provide ample access to the vascular system.

7. **Compare the advantages and disadvantages of peritoneal dialysis and hemodialysis in children.** The advantage of peritoneal dialysis is convenience because it can be done at home and parents can easily be taught to do the process. It can be done in the evening so that it does not interfere or disrupt the child's daytime schedule. The primary disadvantages are the high risk of infection related to use of the peritoneal catheter and the longer time required to perform the procedure compared with hemodialysis. Hemodialysis is a faster process, requiring only 3–4 hours per session (three or four times/week) but the client needs to be transported to a dialysis center for each session. The disadvantages of hemodialysis are the high risk of hypotension during dialysis and the inconvenience for many families.

8. **Discuss the impact Sandra's diagnosis may have on her growth and development.** Because she is receiving peritoneal dialysis at home, Sandra should be able to maintain her interactions with her peers at school and attend after school activities. Although the peritoneal catheter is covered by a dressing and not visible to others, it may negatively impact her body image because it makes her "different" from her peers. As she strives for identity and independence, the fact that she requires dialysis can interfere with her need for control. An activity especially common among teen-age girls is going to each others' houses to spend the night. Peritoneal dialysis would interfere with her ability to participate in this. Because Sandra has been undergoing dialysis for 4 years, hopefully she has adjusted to her disease and the demands of her treatment. Dietary changes and medications may negatively impact on Sandra, making her feel different from her friends.

9. **What other assessment data would be helpful for the nurse to have to prepare Sandra's care plan?**
   - **a.** Physical assessment including weight, breath sounds, heart sounds, skin, presence of edema
   - **b.** Complete blood count

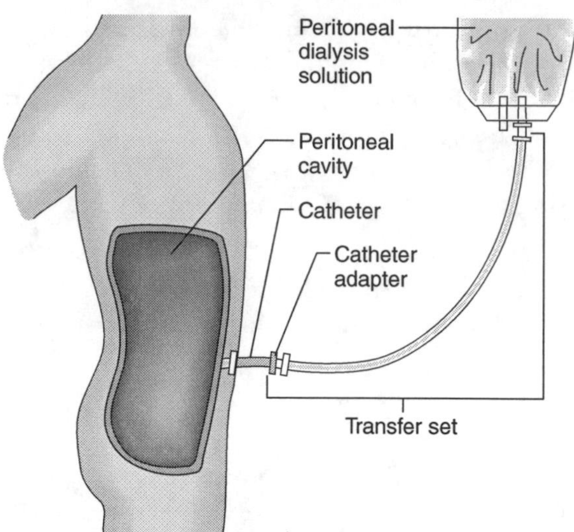

Figure A-7 *Continuous ambulatory peritoneal dialysis.*

c. Blood chemistry (electrolyte levels)
d. Blood urea nitrogen (BUN) and creatinine
e. Which medications she takes
f. How often she undergoes dialysis
g. Assessment of her peritoneal catheter site for indications of infection
h. Who performs her dialysis and catheter care

10. **Discuss the impact of the phone call Sandra's parents received informing them of a kidney donor for Sandra.** Sandra's parents are probably experiencing a combination of feelings ranging from excitement that Sandra will finally receive her kidney transplant, to fear and anxiety about whether the transplant will be effective and what they will need to do to care for her following her transplant, to sadness that Sandra was able to receive a transplant only because the 10-year-old donor died. This is a very emotionally charged time for the entire family.

11. **What is the incidence of renal transplants in a child of Sandra's age?** According to the Organ Procurement and Transplantation Network, "There were 769 pediatric kidney transplant recipients in 2002." Living donor transplants account for more than half of the kidney transplants in children.

12. **Two days following her surgery, Sandra is admitted to the pediatric transplant unit where she received her kidney transplant. What are the priority nursing interventions for Sandra?**
    a. Assess her vital signs every 4 hours.
    b. Assess for signs of rejection:
        (1) Oliguria
        (2) Edema
        (3) Fever
        (4) Increasing blood pressure
        (5) Weight gain
        (6) Swelling and tenderness over transplanted kidney
        (7) Increasing BUN and creatinine levels
    c. Monitor BUN and creatinine levels.
    d. Monitor hourly urine outputs.
    e. Monitor serum electrolyte levels.
    f. Report abnormal findings indicating potential rejection immediately to the health care provider.

g. Maintain patency of intravenous access, monitoring hourly.
h. Administer intravenous fluids as prescribed.
i. Administer immunosuppressants as prescribed.
j. Maintain patency of peritoneal access.
k. Maintain strict universal (standard) precautions.
l. Assess for signs of infection—fever.
m. Monitor vital signs every 4 hours.
n. Report temperature elevations immediately.
o. Monitor complete blood count.
p. Administer antipyretics as prescribed, monitoring temperature after 45 minutes to assess effectiveness.
q. Administer antibiotics as prescribed.
r. Monitor for signs of opportunistic infections (*Candida albicans, cytomegalovirus, Pneumocystis carinii, pneumococcus*).
s. Monitor for signs of septicemia:
   (1) Shaking chills
   (2) Fever
   (3) Tachycardia
   (4) Tachypnea
   (5) Leukocytosis or leukopenia
t. Auscultate over renal artery every 4 hours.
u. Monitor abdomen over transplant site for swelling and tenderness.
v. Assess wound for redness, swelling, tenderness, drainage, and incision approximation.
w. Perform wound care as prescribed.
x. Perform client and parent teaching.

13. **Sandra weighs 49.9 kg (110 lb) and is prescribed prednisone 30 mg by mouth q.i.d., cyclosporine 100 mg by mouth q.i.d., and azathioprine 50 mg by mouth q.i.d. Discuss these medications and if they are safe for Sandra in the doses prescribed.** All three agents are immunosuppressants used following transplantation to prevent rejection. The safe dosage ranges of the medications for Sandra are based on adult doses or body weight. The safe and effective dose for prednisone is 5–60 mg/day (Spratto and Woods, 2005, p. 1010) in divided doses but up to 200 mg/day may be required to prevent organ rejection following transplantation. Cyclosporine can cause nephrotoxicity and is therefore closely monitored following renal transplantation; however, it is still a common agent in the post-transplant immunosuppressant medication regimen. The dosage range by weight is 0.1–2 mg/kg per day (Spratto and Woods, 2005, p. 303). The safe dose for cyclosporine when used to prevent renal transplant rejection is 10–14 mg/kg per day and for azathioprine the safe dose is 3–5 mg/kg per day (Spratt and Woods, 2005, p. 106). These are safe doses.

14. **One month following Sandra's discharge from the hospital, she develops a fever, has decreased urine output, and gained 3.2 kg (7 lb). Her mother calls Sandra's transplant physician and is advised to bring Sandra to the hospital clinic. On arrival her vital signs are: temperature, 38° C (100.4° F); pulse, 90 beats/minute; respirations, 30 breaths/minute; and blood pressure, 140/86. Her blood urea nitrogen (BUN) is 24 mg/dL and her creatinine is 4 mg/dL. Discuss your impressions of Sandra's condition.** Sandra's clinical manifestations, vital signs, and laboratory values indicate renal transplant rejection. When occurring within the first 6 months following the transplant, it is referred to as acute rejection.

15. **Sandra is admitted to the hospital and prescribed prednisone 40 mg by mouth q.i.d, cyclosporine 125 mg by mouth q.i.d., and azathioprine 62.5 mg by mouth q.i.d. Discuss the relationship between Sandra's condition and the increase in her medications.** The first line of treatment for acute rejection is through immunosuppressive therapy. The doses Sandra was receiving to prevent rejection were not the maximum doses she could receive. The current prescriptions represent her maximum doses and would be appropriate for the treatment of her acute rejection.

16. Sandra's acute rejection is successfully treated and she returns home. Three years later Sandra is doing well and her transplanted kidney is functioning well. Does Sandra need to continue her immunosuppressant therapy? If so, for how long? Immunosuppressant therapy following a renal transplant is life-long therapy. Maintenance doses are prescribed as low as possible to decrease the adverse effects while providing adequate immunosuppressant therapy to prevent rejection. The student may address here that the physical changes associated with high-dose steroid therapy to prevent rejection may cause adverse psychosocial effects including disturbed body image.

References

American Society of Transplantation. *http://www.a-s-t.org*

Broyles, B.E. (2005). *Medical-Surgical clinical companion.* Durham, NC: Carolina Academic Press.

Daniels, R. (2002). *Delmar's manual of laboratory and diagnostic tests.* Clifton Park, NY: Thomson Delmar Learning.

National Kidney Foundation. *http://www.kidney.org*

North American Nursing Diagnosis Association. (2005). *Nursing diagnoses: Definitions & classifications, 2005–2006.* Philadelphia: NANDA.

Organ Procurement and Transplantation Network. *http://www.optn.org*

Potts, N. and Mandleco, B. (2002). *Pediatric nursing: Caring for children and their families.* Clifton Park, NY: Thomson Delmar Learning, pp. 643–646.

Scientific Registry of Transplant Recipients. *http://www.ustransplant.org*

Spratto, G.R. and Woods, A.L. (2005). *2005 Edition PDR: Nurse's drug handbook.* Clifton Park, NY: Thomson Delmar Learning.

United Network for Organ Sharing. *http://www.transplantliving.org*

Wong, D.L., Perry, S.E., and Hockenberry, M.J. (2002). *Maternal child nursing care* (2nd ed.). St. Louis: Mosby, pp. 1414–1420.

CASE STUDY 10

Cammie

GENDER

F

AGE

14

SETTING

- Hospital

ETHNICITY

- White American

CULTURAL CONSIDERATIONS

PREEXISTING CONDITIONS

COEXISTING CONDITIONS

SIGNIFICANT HISTORY

COMMUNICATION

DISABILITY

SOCIOECONOMIC

- Upper class

SPIRITUAL

PHARMACOLOGIC

PSYCHOSOCIAL

LEGAL

ETHICAL

- Potential nurse bias

ALTERNATIVE THERAPY

PRIORITIZATION

- Yes

DELEGATION

THE DIGESTIVE SYSTEM

Level of difficulty: Difficult

Overview: This case requires knowledge of eating disorders, growth and development, as well as an understanding of the client's background, personal situation, and parent–child relationship.

Client Profile

Cammie is a 14-year-old adolescent who lives with her mother. Her mother and father were divorced 3 years ago, and she sees her father every other week. Cammie has lost 15.9 kg (35 lb) since her physical exam last year. Despite the weight loss, Cammie has continued to go to school, making the A honor roll. She jogs 2 miles a day regardless of the weather. Her mother works and frequently is not home at dinner time, leaving Cammie to prepare her own dinner. Cammie packs her own lunch for school and often only drinks orange juice for breakfast before leaving for school. She seldom goes out with her friends; however, she talks to her 15-year-old boyfriend on the phone every evening. She weighs herself every morning at the same time, making sure she is unclothed when she gets on the scale. She experienced menarche at the age of 11, but has not had menses for the past 6 months.

Case Study

Cammie's mother accompanies her to her annual physical. Her pediatrician notes that Cammie is small for her age and looks younger than her years. She brings with her a bottle of water and drinks frequently during the visit. During the examination, she denies dizziness or fainting spells and states she feels "fine." When asked about her diet, Cammie becomes indignant saying, "I eat when I'm hungry, but I watch what I eat because I'm fat." Her vital signs are within normal limits for her age and she denies using either drugs or alcohol. Due to the pediatrician's concern, he recommends that Cammie be admitted to the adolescent psychiatric unit at the city hospital. Her mother and father accompany her during her admission.

Questions and Suggested Answers

1. **Discuss your impressions of the above situation.** From the information given, Cammie is experiencing low self-esteem; isolation from peers; and an eating disorder, probably anorexia nervosa.

2. **Discuss the significance of Cammie's clinical manifestations.** Cammie perceives herself as "fat," which is a classic manifestation of anorexia. In addition, she has lost 16 kg (35 lb), does not appear to eat, and is regimented in her daily activity. She does not spend time outside of school with her friends, an example of the isolationism typical of anorexia. She does not have much interaction with either her mother or her father, which can foster her behavior. Her parents are divorced, and as an adolescent girl she may wonder if, had she been a better child, they wouldn't have divorced. Her excelling in school may represent her obsession for perfection to please her parents, whose lack of time with Cammie may be perceived by her that she is not good enough to spend time with.

3. **What other assessment data would be helpful for the nurse to have to prepare Cammie's care plan?**
   - **a.** Cammie's weight and height
   - **b.** Heart and lung sounds
   - **c.** Gastrointestinal assessment
   - **d.** Renal assessment including urinalysis
   - **e.** Characteristics of her menstrual cycle before it stopped
   - **f.** Pregnancy test results
   - **g.** Urine and serum drug screen
   - **h.** Endocrine function
   - **i.** Complete blood count
   - **j.** Exactly what Cammie eats and drinks daily
   - **k.** Cammie's body image

4. **Discuss the difference between anorexia and bulimia.** According to the National Institute of Mental Health of the National Institutes of Health, "An estimated 0.5 to 3.7 percent of females suffer from anorexia nervosa . . . (whereas) 1.1 percent to 4.2 percent of females have bulimia nervosa." In both anorexia and bulimia the clients have an intense fear of gaining weight and perceive themselves as overweight even though they are underweight for their height. Both usually have some obsessive or ritualized behavior that provides them with a sense of control. Among those behaviors is weighing themselves at the same time each day and without any clothing on. However, in the case of anorexia, clients first avoid eating certain foods and then avoid most foods. They do take in fluids, especially water, and exercise to excess. Some with anorexia purge themselves through vomiting. Bulimia is characterized by recurrent episodes of binge eating, followed by purging to prevent weight gain. The purging is manifested as self-induced vomiting and regular abuse of laxatives, enemas, or diuretics. Excessive exercise may be used as a means of purging.

5. **During the interview with Cammie, the nurse notes that Cammie is distant and terse in her answers concerning her perception of herself; however, the teen does confirm that she thinks she is "fat." What is the relationship between body image, need for control, and eating disorders?** The rapid body changes during adolescence can result in a feeling of loss of control over appearance and the feeling of being awkward and unattractive. This also impacts on body image. Some adolescents cannot adjust to these changes in a healthy way and see that all of their friends are going through the same changes. Because by adolescence, eating is basically an independent responsibility, for teenagers, controlling what they eat becomes a control issue and an obsession. Eating disorders including anorexia, bulimia, and obesity can become problems for members of this age group.

6. **What are the priorities of care for Cammie on admission?**
   a. Imbalanced nutrition: less than body requirements related to inadequate food intake
   b. Risk for deficient fluid volume related to insufficient food intake, the main source of fluids
   c. Disturbed body image related to self-evaluation
   d. Risk for delayed development related to inadequate nutritional intake
   e. Deficient knowledge related to condition, self-concept, family relationships

7. **During the interview with Cammie's parents, the nurse notes that both are well dressed and very successful in their respective careers. They state that they have given Cammie "everything." Neither is aware of what Cammie eats or her daily schedule outside of school because they believe that "girls her age need privacy and we try to honor that." Her mother was neither aware nor concerned about Cammie's lack of menses. Both parents exercise regularly and believe that "daily exercise and eating right" is the "key to good health and success." They both state that they are very proud of Cammie and do not understand the pediatrician's concern. Further, they deny that Cammie has ever had any psychiatric problems. Discuss your impressions of this interview and the possible relationship with Cammie's eating disorder.** Cammie's parents seem to be very career oriented, and although they feel they have given Cammie everything, material possessions are not the only thing that a child needs. They do not interact with Cammie sufficiently to be aware of her life. Cammie's obsession with exercise and eating seems to have come from her parents. Further, they don't understand why the pediatrician is concerned about their daughter, possibly because they don't believe being underweight is a problem. Although teenagers do require a degree of privacy as they strive for identity, they also need to feel that they are an important part of a family unit and shown that they are loved and worthwhile as people. Cammie's parents seem to have a misguided impression of what their daughter needs. This is a personal as well as professional evaluation of the interview as it is stated. The student should be encouraged to acquire more information before forming definitive impressions.

8. **Discuss your impression of the communication within this family.** This family does not appear to communicate about topics that Cammie finds important. Her parents have not sufficiently addressed their divorce and its impact on Cammie's self-esteem and her sense of belonging in the family. As noted earlier, the obsession with eating and exercising has definitely had an impact on Cammie and she probably feels that she does not measure up to her parent's expectations. Her mother's lack of awareness of Cammie's menstrual cycle is

evidence that she does not interact with her daughter concerning the normal body changes occurring during adolescence, perhaps leaving Cammie to deal with the issue alone. For some girls, menstruation can be a traumatic adolescent experience that makes them feel like they are not clean or that they have an odor during the monthly cycle. Cammie's father sees her only every other week, which may foster Cammie's feelings of not being worthy. In addition, her mother appears to work long hours in her career, leaving little time for Cammie.

9. **Discuss your biases about adolescents and eating disorders.** Readers should show an understanding of growth and development or lack of knowledge of the needs of this age group. They may feel that eating disorders are a "cop out" from meeting one's responsibilities. Some readers may believe that Cammie is acting out to gain attention. In addition, Cammie and her parents may view Cammie's behavior as a normal phase of development that she will outgrow rather than as a serious disorder. This question requires individual responses, with no answer considered incorrect.

10. **Given your biases, if any, how can you intervene to address the nursing priorities for Cammie?**
    a. Nutrition
        (1) Obtain height and weight and if the client is hospitalized, assess daily weight.
        (2) Maintain intake and output.
        (3) Maintain calorie counts as prescribed.
        (4) Monitor serum electrolytes.
        (5) Assess behavior during meals.
        (6) Collaborate with the health care provider to obtain appropriate consults.
        (7) Collaborate with the nutritional support and psychiatric health care provider to determine behavioral modifications that require nursing assessment and intervention to maintain consistency.
    b. Risk for deficient fluid volume
        (1) Monitor strict intake and output.
        (2) Obtain urine specimens as prescribed.
        (3) Assess to determine Cammie's favorite beverages and obtain these for her.
        (4) Monitor urine specific gravity.
        (5) Weigh daily.
        (6) Assess mucous membranes and skin for indications of dehydration.
        (7) Initiate and maintain patency of intravenous access, if prescribed, monitoring hourly.
        (8) Administer intravenous fluids as prescribed.
        (9) Monitor serum electrolytes.
    c. Body image
        (1) Acknowledge Cammie's assets and positive characteristics.
        (2) Encourage Cammie to verbalize her feelings.
        (3) Encourage her parents to verbalize their feelings.
        (4) Encourage interactions between Cammie and her parents according to health care team guidelines.
        (5) Collaborate with the psychiatric health care provider and family counselor.
        (6) Assess for nonverbal cues indicating ineffective coping strategies.
    d. Development
        (1) Assess Cammie's current level of growth and development.
        (2) Spend time with Cammie, discussing things that are of interest to her.
        (3) Encourage Cammie to have her friends visit her.
        (4) Collaborate with the health care provider for referral to child-life specialist or recreation therapy.
        (5) Provide for activities that are developmentally appropriate.
    e. Deficient knowledge
        (1) Assess the family's current level of knowledge about Cammie's condition and growth and development.
        (2) Collaborate with the health care team concerning specific guidelines for teaching.
        (3) Serve as a role model to Cammie and her parents regarding therapeutic communication.

(4) Stress the importance of nutritional guidelines and the necessity of following them.
(5) Provide information concerning scheduled family counseling.
(6) Provide information concerning support groups including the National Association of Anorexia Nervosa and Associated Disorders (ANAD).
(7) Stress the importance of follow-up evaluations.
(8) Allow sufficient time for client and family questions, answering them honestly.
(9) Document teaching and client and family response and collaborate with the health care team.

References

Centers for Disease Control and Prevention. *http://www.cdc.gov*

Daniels, R. (2002). *Delmar's manual of laboratory and diagnostic tests.* Clifton Park, NY: Thomson Delmar Learning.

National Association of Anorexia Nervosa and Associated Disorders. *http://www.anad.org*

National Eating Disorders Association. *http://www.edap.org*

National Institute of Mental Health. *http://www.nimh.nih.gov*

North American Nursing Diagnosis Association. (2005). *Nursing diagnoses: Definitions & classifications, 2005–2006.* Philadelphia: NANDA.

Potts, N. and Mandleco, B. (2002). *Pediatric nursing: Caring for children and their families.* Clifton Park, NY: Thomson Delmar Learning, pp. 1192–1193.

Wong, D.L., Perry, S.E., and Hockenberry, M.J. (2002). *Maternal child nursing care* (2nd ed.). St. Louis: Mosby, pp. 991–993.

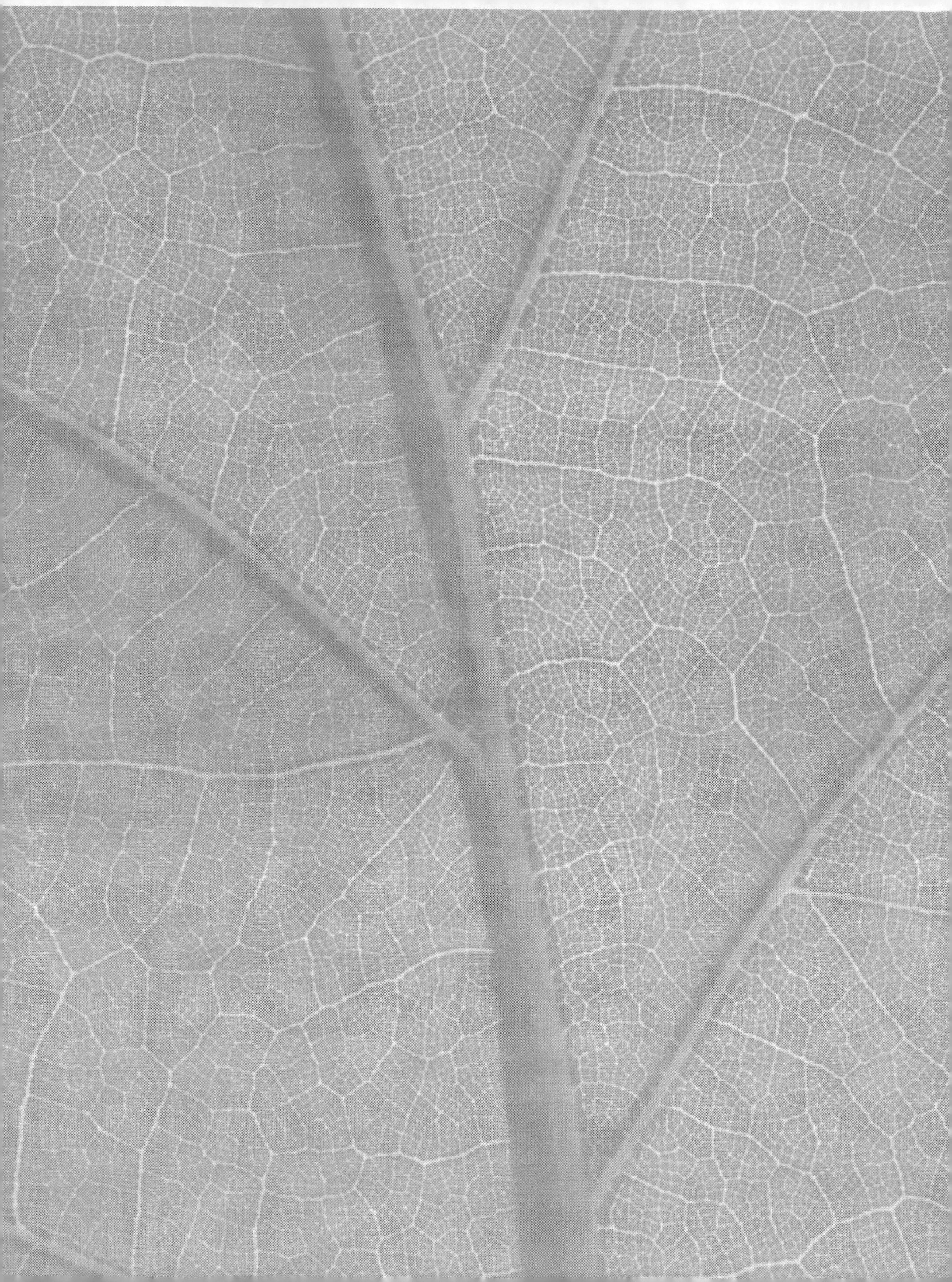

PART TWO

The Respiratory System

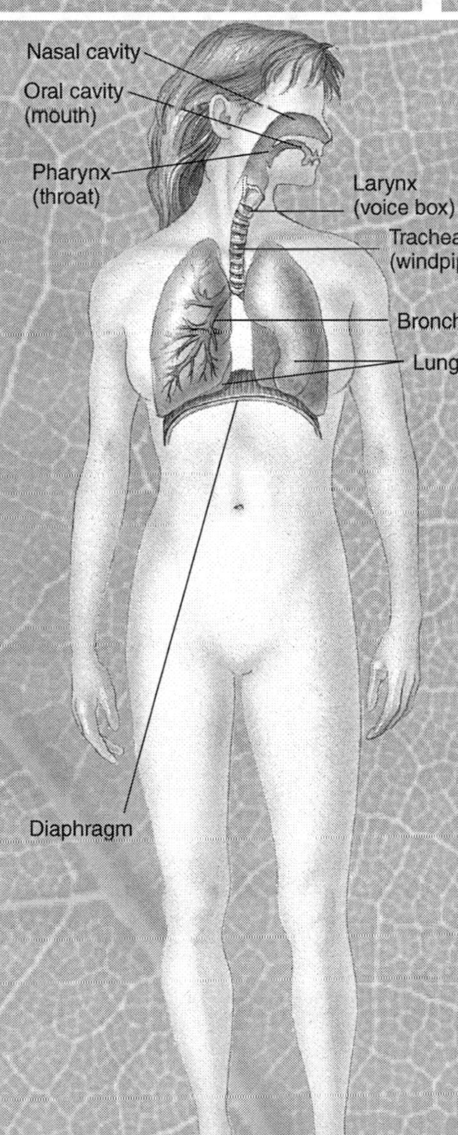

Respiratory system Lungs, nasal cavity, pharynx, larynx, trachea, bronchi, and bronchioles.

CASE STUDY 1

Sara and Mary

GENDER

F

AGE

2 months old

SETTING

- Hospital

ETHNICITY

- White American

CULTURAL CONSIDERATIONS

PREEXISTING CONDITIONS

- Preterm birth

COEXISTING CONDITIONS

SIGNIFICANT HISTORY

COMMUNICATION

DISABILITY

SOCIOECONOMIC

SPIRITUAL

PHARMACOLOGIC

- Acetaminophen (Tylenol)
- Erythromycin lactobionate (Erythrocin IV)

PSYCHOSOCIAL

- Maternal anxiety
- Husband is out of town

LEGAL

ETHICAL

ALTERNATIVE THERAPY

PRIORITIZATION

- Yes

DELEGATION

- Yes

THE RESPIRATORY SYSTEM

Level of difficulty: Easy

Overview: This case requires knowledge of communicable disease, increased risk of infection secondary to preterm birth, intravenous therapy, as well as mother–child attachment relationship.

Client Profile

Sara and Mary are 2-month-old twins born at 35 weeks' gestation and weighing 2,272 g (81.1 oz) and 2,300 g (82.1 oz), respectively. They remained hospitalized for 4 weeks to gain weight and were discharged to home weighing 2,600 g (92.8 oz). They are scheduled to see the health care provider to begin their immunizations at 10 weeks of age. The twins' mother has taken an extended maternity leave to remain home with the twins until they are 4 months old.

Case Study

The twins' mother, Fran, noted that both infants, 9 weeks of age, had "runny noses" when she picked them up from daycare. The twins' father left at 5:00 A.M. for a 5-day business trip and at 6:00 A.M., Fran heard them both coughing. Their coughs sounded dry; however, when she checked them, they both had runny noses and felt warm to the touch. She took their temperatures; Sara's was 37.8° C (100° F) and Mary's was 38° C (100.4° F). She administered 15 mg/kg of acetaminophen. This lowered their temperatures to 37.5° C (99.5° F) and 37.5° C (99.5° F), respectively; however, they continued to cough. Three hours later, both girls began exhibiting a high-pitched, whooping sound when inhaling during their coughing attacks. When Fran noted the girls experienced brief apneic periods during their coughing spells and appeared "bluish" in color, she phoned her pediatrician and was told to go to the nearest emergency department. The girls were admitted to the pediatric nursing unit with a diagnosis of "rule out pertussis." Sara's leukocyte count is 31,000 cells/mm^3 and Mary's count is 32,300 cells/mm^3 on admission. Nasal and throat cultures and serology tests are pending. Intravenous access devices are placed and intravenous fluids of D_5W with 0.225% sodium chloride is initiated at 20 mL/hour. Their oxygen saturations are continuously monitored using pulse oximetry and each is started on 0.5 L of oxygen per nasal cannula in response to oxygen saturation readings of 94% for Sara and 92% for Mary. Arterial blood gases are drawn from each infant with the following results: For Sara: pH, 7.35; P_{CO_2}; 35 mm Hg; P_{O_2}, 90 MM HG; oxygen saturation, 95%; and HCO_3, 22 mEq/L. For Mary: pH, 7.37; P_{CO_2}; 37 mm Hg; P_{O_2}, 85 mm Hg; oxygen saturation, 92%; and HCO_3, 23 mEq/L. On admission Sara weighs 2.9 kg (6 lb, 8 oz) and Mary weighs 3.2 kg (7 lb).

Questions and Suggested Answers

1. **Which child should be seen by the nurse first and why?** Given all the data, the nurse should assess Mary first because her oxygen saturation is below the normal range for neonates. Regardless of the potential diagnosis of pertussis, preterm infants have a higher risk of RSV infections. In addition, their central nervous systems are developing and require oxygen levels adequate to meet these developing needs. Preterm infants have immature nervous as well as respiratory systems and are at higher risk of developing serious and permanent complications.

2. **Discuss pertussis and how it can be prevented.** Pertussis is a bacterial infection caused by the microorganism *Bordetella pertussis*, a gram-negative rod, that affects the upper respiratory tract and is characterized by severe coughing spasms, vomiting (resulting from the coughing spasms), and an inspiratory whooping sound. It is transmitted through droplets from a cough or sneeze of an infected individual through contact with the respiratory secretions of that individual. It occurs in three stages—catarrhal, paroxysmal, and convalescent stages and can last as long as 4–5 months. The catarrhal stage is characterized by symptoms of the common cold and lasts up to 2 weeks; the paroxysmal stage is characterized by coughing spasms stimulated by the need to expel the tenacious tracheobronchial secretions and creating fluid deficit (from vomiting), exhaustion, and possibly decreased tissue perfusion resulting in cyanosis. This stage lasts for up to 6–10 weeks and is followed by the convalescent stage, which is characterized by a gradual recovery from the infection. Erythromycin remains the first-line agent for the treatment of pertussis.

Among the immunizations recommended by the Centers for Disease Control and Prevention and the American Academy of Pediatrics are five immunizations against pertussis beginning at 2 months of age, then one at 4 months, 6 months, 12–18 months, and 4–6 years. The original vaccine against pertussis was developed in the mid-1940s and by 1976 had an estimated effectiveness of 99%. Although the vaccine is believed to have eradicated this communicable disease, 9,700 cases, and affecting both children and adults, were reported in 2002, the highest annual incidence since 1964.

Currently there are three DTaP (diphtheria–tetanus–acellular pertussis) vaccines available in the United States and they are Infanrix, Tripedia, and Daptacel.

3. **What conclusions can you draw about the clients' clinical manifestations and leukocyte counts of the twins?** These two infants have not received their initial immunizations of DTaP so they have no active acquired immunity to a number of communicable diseases including pertussis. The immune cells develop early in gestation; however, they do not become activated for several months after birth. The normal newborn receives passive immunity from the mother that lasts about 3 months. Because of their prematurity, the twins' immune systems are more compromised than those of normal newborns. Classic manifestations of pertussis include runny nose, severe dry (or productive) cough with a high-pitched or whooping sound on inspiration (thus the original name of "whooping cough"), color changes during coughing attacks, fever that is usually below 38.9° C (102° F), diarrhea, vomiting, and choking or severe coughing attacks. Leukocyte counts are usually elevated.

4. **Discuss the leukocyte results for the twins compared to normal values for these infants.** Normal leukocyte count for newborns is 9,000–30,000 cells/mm^3 (Potts and Mandleco, 2002), which is much higher than the 6,200–17,000 cells/mm^3 for children 2 years old and younger and the 4,400–10,800 cells/mm^3 norm for children less than 2 years old compared to Sara's leukocyte count of 31,000 cells/mm^3 and Mary's count of 32,300 cells/mm^3 on admission that are elevated compared to normal values, consistent with a diagnosis of pertussis.

5. **What is the significance of Sara and Mary's arterial blood gas results?** Although Sara and Mary are 9 weeks of age, because they were 5 weeks premature, their growth and development level is that of a neonate. Normal ABGs for neonates and infants are: pH 7.35–7.45; Pco_2 35–44 mm Hg; Po_2, 80–100 mm Hg; oxygen saturation, >94%; HCO_3, 22–28 mEq/L. Consequently, Sara's ABGs are within normal limits, however, Mary's oxygen saturation needs must be addressed and in many health care facilities protocols exist addressing the nurse's responsibility to "administer oxygen to maintain oxygen saturation >94%." These protocols allow nurses to use their knowledge of oxygen therapy and client oxygen needs.

6. **Explain the rationale for prescribing the intravenous fluids prescribed for Sara and Mary.** For young infants, the hardest work they do is eating. When energy is compromised as in the presence of the energy expenditure present with Sara and Mary's coughing spells, infant food intake is usually affected. In addition, the swallowing of respiratory secretions can elicit vomiting that not only poses a threat of aspiration, but also results in fluid loss. The fluid and electrolyte balance of children, especially infants, is very fragile. Imbalances can lead to hypovolemia, acid–base imbalances, and shock. The intravenous solution prescribed is 5% dextrose in water with 0.225% sodium chloride in solution. This is an isotonic solution with an osmolality of 240–340 mOsm, thus providing the same concentration of solutes as blood plasma. This in turn allows for the normal shift of fluid and solutes in and out of vascular and interstitial fluid volume. Isotonic solutions are used to provide for maintenance of daily fluid intake. Infant fluid needs are based on body weight, with a requirement of 100 mL/kg every 24 hours for those with a body weight of 10 kg (22 lb) or less. Sara needs 300 mL/day based on her admission weight and Mary should have an intake of 318 mL/day. This solution will provide 102 kcal of the 650 kcal required by infants daily. To supply the further nutrition, the infants will be provided with either oral or nasogastric feedings.

7. **Should the twins be placed on respiratory isolation to protect the nursing staff? Explain your answer.** Sara and Mary may be placed on respiratory isolation to protect the other clients on the pediatric unit; however, as long as nurses practice universal (standard) precautions, staff is not at risk. Pertussis occurs primarily in children under the age of 4 years who have not been immunized and can result in high morbidity and

mortality in infants. The twins may share a room with each other, but no other infants or children on the unit should be assigned to their room to avoid transmission by droplet of this highly contagious disease.

8. **Identify complications associated with pertussis that Sara and Mary are at risk for developing.** Complications of pertussis include pneumonia, apnea, otitis media, seizures, neurological damage related to hypoxia and/or cerebral hemorrhage, developmental delay secondary to neurological damage, and epistaxis.

9. **Identify the priority nursing diagnosis for Sara and Mary and appropriate nursing interventions.** Because of the high morbidity and mortality in infants with pertussis, impaired gas exchange related to hypoxia secondary to coughing, choking, and apnea occurs. The nursing interventions include but are not limited to:
   a. Place on continuous cardiorespiratory monitoring.
   b. Elevate head of bed (HOB) of crib mattress 15°.
   c. Monitor vital signs at intervals appropriate for clients' conditions.
   d. Monitor oxygen saturation via pulse oximetry continuously.
   e. Administer oxygen, titrating to maintain oxygen saturation within prescribed parameters.
   f. Collaborate with the health care provider for placement of infants in high humidity environment to help liquefy secretions and reduce inflammation of airway secondary to dry, paroxysmal coughing.
   g. Maintain patency of intravenous access for infusion of prescribed fluids.
   h. Maintain strict intake and output, assessing for vomiting and diarrhea (also manifestations of pertussis) and insensible fluid loss through the respiratory system in the presence of tachypnea.
   i. Provide for infants' needs promptly to avoid unnecessary oxygen demand secondary to crying.
   j. If conditions worsen, prepare for transfer to pediatric critical care unit.

10. **The twins' mother is very quiet and appears on the verge of crying. She states, "It's all my fault and now I'm being punished. I shouldn't have worked during my pregnancy, but we couldn't afford for me to quit, and then after the twins came home, I had to go back to work and leave them in daycare because my maternity leave had run out." How can you intervene to assist Fran?** Fran is expressing feelings of guilt, and although this is normal for mothers whose children are ill, she needs clarification about her role in the twins' current condition. The nurse should present a calm, supportive affect. Unless specifically contraindicated, pregnant women can work through the 40th week of pregnancy without endangering the fetus. The nurse should commend Fran for scheduling the twins' immunizations. The nurse should help Fran identify her current support systems and how these systems may be activated. The nurse should also assess for possible financial need, and if it exists, discuss with the health care provider the need for a consult with the social worker.

11. **The twins are prescribed erythromycin lactobionate 13 mg IV every 6 hours. Discuss why this agent is prescribed and if the prescribed dose is safe for Sara and Mary.** Erythromycin is the standard of care for pertussis when diagnosed in the early stages. Erythromycin is effective against the bacteria *Bordetella pertussis,* the causative organism for pertussis. Erythromycin can be administered intravenously and is the appropriate route for these infants. The pediatric dose for intravenous erythromycin is 15–20 mg/kg every 24 hours. Both infants' doses are within the safe range for their weight. Sara weighs 6.5 pounds. Dividing by 2.2 gives Sara's weight in kilograms, or 2.95 kg. The safe range for Sara is 44.25–59 mg every 24 hours (which must be divided by 4 to establish the individual dose range of 11–14.75 mg every 6 hours). Mary's safe range is 47.7–63.6 mg/24 hours or 11.9–15.9 mg/dose. IV erythromycin is very irritating to peripheral veins and should be infused slowly to prevent phlebitis. Once the acute phase of the infants' illness is resolved, oral or nasogastric erythromycin may be prescribed.

12. **The twins respond favorably to treatment, and following a week of hospitalization their health care provider discharges them to home. Fran and her husband Jack are preparing for discharge. Discuss appropriate discharge instructions for this family.** There is deficient knowledge related to homegoing instructions. The nurse should address the following:
    a. Assess Fran and Jack's current level of knowledge about infant care.

b. Provide written and verbal instructions regarding:
   (1) Recommended schedule for immunizations
   (2) Signs and symptoms to report to health care provider:
      (a) Severe cough
      (b) Vomiting
      (c) Diarrhea
      (d) Temperature elevation >38° C (100.4° F)
      (e) Less than six to eight wet diapers per day
      (f) Intake of <650 kcal/day
      (g) Seizure activity
   (3) Formula prescribed by health care provider
   (4) Information related to any referrals made

c. Provide telephone numbers for any questions they may have and for reporting signs and symptoms.

d. Provide sufficient time for questions, providing more information as needed.

e. Document teaching and parents' response

References

Centers for Disease Control and Prevention. (2004). *Epidemiology and prevention of vaccine–preventable disease* *http://www.cdc.gov*

Daniels, R. (2002). *Delmar's manual of laboratory and diagnostic tests.* Clifton Park, NY: Thomson Delmar Learning.

Gahart, B.L. and Nazareno, A.R. (2005). *2005 Intravenous medications* (20th ed.). St. Louis: Mosby.

Intravenous Therapy. *http://www.nursewise.com*

Josephson, D.L. (2004). *Intravenous infusion therapy for nurses: Principles & practice* (2nd ed.). Clifton Park, NY: Thomson Delmar Learning.

North American Nursing Diagnosis Association. (2005). *Nursing diagnoses: Definitions & classifications, 2005–2006.* Philadelphia: NANDA.

Potts, N. and Mandleco, B. (2002). *Pediatric nursing: Caring for children and their families.* Clifton Park, NY: Thomson Delmar Learning.

Schweon, S. (2005). Whooping cough makes its return. RN. 68(2): 32–36.

Wong, D.L., Perry, S.E., and Hockenberry, M.J. (2002). *Maternal child nursing care* (2nd ed.). St. Louis: Mosby.

CASE STUDY 2

Caleb

GENDER

M

AGE

6

SETTING

- Hospital

ETHNICITY

- Black American

CULTURAL CONSIDERATIONS

PREEXISTING CONDITIONS

COEXISTING CONDITIONS

SIGNIFICANT HISTORY

COMMUNICATION

DISABILITY

SOCIOECONOMIC

SPIRITUAL

PHARMACOLOGIC

- Atropine sulfate

PSYCHOSOCIAL

- Anxiety

LEGAL

ETHICAL

ALTERNATIVE THERAPY

PRIORITIZATION

- Yes

DELEGATION

- Yes

MODERATE

THE RESPIRATORY SYSTEM

Level of difficulty: Moderate

Overview: This case requires knowledge of growth and development and its impact on accidental injuries, normal respiratory function, cardiopulmonary resuscitation, mechanical ventilation, intravenous fluid therapy, as well as empathy for parental feelings/expressions of guilt.

Client Profile

Caleb is a 6-year-old boy in first grade. He lives with his mother and father and two siblings, a brother Tyler (8 years old) and a 10-year-old sister, Cherice. Caleb and his family are visiting his grandparents on their 40-acre farm in Minnesota for Thanksgiving. Caleb is an adventurous child who loves being active outdoors and enjoys swimming, fishing, soccer, and school activities.

Case Study

Mrs. Jones was inside the house helping her mother prepare the Thanksgiving dinner, and family were to arrive in 2 hours for the celebration. Mr. Jones was in the garage working on his mother-in-law's vehicle when Tyler came running to the house screaming that Caleb had fallen into the pond while they were fishing. Tyler said he had pulled him out but Caleb wasn't breathing. His father told Tyler to run into the house, call 911, and tell his mother what had happened. Mr. Jones ran to the pond and found Caleb lying face down on the pond bank. He turned Caleb over and confirmed that he was barely breathing. He covered Caleb with his coat, began calling for help, and remained with Caleb. After approximately 10 minutes, paramedics arrived and assessed Caleb. He had stopped breathing "about 5 minutes ago" according to his father. Caleb had a weak, but present pulse of 40 beats/minute. The paramedics performed abdominal thrusts and Caleb began coughing weakly, but remained unconscious. Oxygen was started at 100% per face mask and an intravenous access established. Lactated Ringer's intravenous solution was initiated while Caleb was transported to the local trauma center, where he was treated in the emergency department for immersion syndrome.

In the emergency department, arterial blood gases were drawn and a pulse oximetry sensor was attached. The nurse performed a client history by talking to his parents. According to Mrs. Jones Caleb weighed 24.9 kg (55 lb) and was 1.3 m (4 ft, 2 in.) tall at his routine appointment with his pediatrician last week. His weight is confirmed, he is placed on a cardiorespiratory monitor and atropine sulfate 0.5 mg intravenous is administered. His oxygen saturation was 80% and he is covered with warmed blankets. His vital signs on admission are pulse, 45 beats/minute; respiratory rate, apneic; blood pressure, 50/30; and body temperature, 32.6° C (90.7° F). His arterial blood gas values are pH, 7.29; $Paco_3$, 50 mm Hg; Pao_2, 70 mm Hg; oxygen saturation, 75%; HCO_3, 24 mEq/L. Caleb is intubated and transferred to the pediatric intensive care unit, where mechanical ventilation is established.

Questions and Suggested Answers

1. **What interpretations can you make based on Caleb's ABG results?** The ABGs indicate respiratory acidosis, which is consistent with near drowning. Normal arterial pH is 7.35–7.45 and Caleb's pH of 7.29 represents acidosis. The normal $Paco_2$ is 35–45 mm Hg, representing the respiratory acid–base buffer system. Caleb's $Paco_2$ is 50 mm Hg, which indicates retention of carbon dioxide, consistent with respiratory failure.

2. **Discuss the factors that placed Caleb at risk for near drowning.** According to the Centers for Disease Control and Prevention, 81% of drowning victims are male, and it is the second leading cause of accidental death in children ages 1–14 years. African Americans are 1.6 times more likely to experience near drowning than Caucasians. Drownings and near drownings among children most commonly occur as a result of inadequate parental supervision. All children should receive swimming lessons if they live near water or a swimming pool.

3. **What other diagnostic test would you anticipate the health care provider prescribe for Caleb?** A chest x-ray will show the presence of fluid in the lungs (pulmonary edema) resulting from inhaling water during the near drowning event. Serum electrolytes including sodium, potassium, carbon dioxide, chloride, blood urea nitrogen, creatinine, and blood glucose are used to measure the levels of these, which may indicate tissue

dysfunction. Computed tomography of the head and electroencephalography will determine the extent, if any, of damage to cerebral tissue.

4. **Explain the dive reflex and discuss whether this may have occurred in Caleb's case.** The dive reflex activates if immersion has occurred in very cold water. This reflex slows the heart rate and constricts peripheral vessels, resulting in shunting of blood to the heart and brain. Further, this reflex dramatically lowers body metabolism and the utilization of oxygen in the body. This likely occurred with Caleb because of the geographic locale and the time of year. Minnesota's weather in November usually is characterized by temperatures between –3.8° and 4.9° C (25 and 41° F) with an average daily temperature of 0.55° C (33° F). This suggests the water temperature was probably below 20.9° C (70° F), which is normal in Minnesota. His body temperature was 32.6° C (90.7° F), indicating hypothermia.

5. **Discuss the intravenous fluids prescribed for Caleb including the rationale for their use in his case.** Lactated Ringer's solution is an isotonic colloid fluid used as a volume expander. In Caleb's case it is used to reverse hypovolemia. Although decreased volume may not necessarily be present, hypoperfusion of oxygenated blood to the tissues will elicit the shock response because of lack of oxygen for cellular metabolism. Isotonic solutions have the same osmolality or same solute concentration as human plasma. They don't change the normal flow of fluid in and out of capillaries. By acting like human plasma, the addition of this fluid will expand vascular volume.

6. **Caleb is placed on time-cycled positive pressure continuous mandatory ventilation. Discuss why time-cycled positive pressure ventilation was chosen by comparing it to the other types of positive pressure ventilation.** Positive pressure ventilators are the most frequently used and apply positive pressure to the airway during inspiration. The positive intrathoracic pressure expands the lungs and chest wall. The cessation of gas flow allows the chest and lungs to recoil naturally and the airway pressure to return to normal. Five types of positive pressure ventilators are available for use: time-cycled, volume-cycled, pressure-cycled, high-frequency ventilation, and volumetric diffusion. *Time-cycled positive pressure ventilators* deliver inspiratory flow over a specific preset time. Airway pressures and tidal volumes vary. This type is frequently used in neonates and children. *Volume-cycled positive pressure ventilators* deliver inspiratory flow until a preset volume is achieved. Airway pressures vary depending on airway resistance and lung compliance, and barotrauma is a potential complication. *Pressure-cycled positive pressure ventilators* deliver inspiratory flow until a preset pressure is achieved. Depending on airway resistance and lung compliance, tidal volumes vary and the disadvantages include underventilation or overventilation. Jet ventilation or *high frequency ventilation* delivers small tidal volumes (50–200 mL) at high respiratory rates (60–200 breaths/minute) at lower pressure that decreases problems associated with venous return. *Volumetric diffusion ventilators* deliver inspiratory flow with an oscillating action and are determined by set inspiratory and expiratory times (Broyles, 2005).

7. **Discuss the difference between continuous mandatory ventilation and other types of mechanical ventilation modes.** Continuous mandatory ventilation (control mode) involves a preset tidal volume and rate regardless of Caleb's respiratory effort. Because he is apneic, having no respiratory effort, this mode is used. He cannot initiate a breath or change the ventilatory pattern and usually requires sedation with fentanyl to prevent him from "fighting the ventilator" when his respiratory drive returns. It is used to treat chest trauma, chemical overdose, and near drowning, and is commonly employed during anesthesia.

   The assist/controlled ventilation mode (ACV) allows a client to trigger breathing, but the tidal volume and rate are preset by the ventilator. This mode senses the negative inspiratory force from the client and delivers the present tidal volumes. It decreases the work of breathing and respiratory muscle fatigue since the client needs only to initiate the breath. It is used to treat flail chest and other conditions in which the client has a normal respiratory drive but weak musculature. ACV does have the potential for hyperventilation, and sedation may be required to reduce spontaneous breaths.

   Intermittent mandatory ventilation (IMV) mode is set for 6+ respirations. The client receives 6 (or so) breaths from the ventilator and breathes normally the other times each minute. This allows the client to breathe spontaneously between ventilator breaths; however, the ventilator delivers a predetermined number of breaths per minute regardless of the client's inspiratory effort. This mode is used with clients who have impaired ventilatory drive, such as those with apneic spells.

Synchronized intermittent mandatory ventilation (SIMV) is a version of IMV that synchronizes the ventilator breath with the client's spontaneous breath. The client is able to breathe at his or her own rate and tidal volume. The SIMV senses when the client does not initiate a breath and delivers one. This mode uses the client's own respiratory pattern but is preset so that the breaths are timed to push air into the client's lungs when he or she inhales.

Positive pressure ventilation (PPV) provides positive pressure in response to the client's spontaneous inspiratory breath, augmenting the client's tidal volume and reducing the effort of breathing. This mode is indicated for clients with adequate respiratory drive, but who fatigue easily with the work of breathing.

Finally, continuous positive airway pressure (CPAP) maintains positive airway pressure throughout the entire respiratory cycle, not just during expiration (like positive end expiratory pressure [PEEP]). It is the mode used for weaning clients from other ventilatory modes and for clients with obstructive sleep apnea.

Complications associated with positive pressure ventilation include pulmonary, cardiac, gastrointestinal, infection, immobility, and emotional problems. Pulmonary difficulties include atelectasis, pneumonia, hypercapnia (due to inadequate ventilation), hypocapnia (due to overventilation), oxygen toxicity (resulting in impaired surfactant activity, capillary congestion and edema), tracheal damage related to endotracheal tube, and inability to wean from the ventilator. Decreased cardiac output can occur as a result of increased thoracic pressure which decreases venous return. Muscle wasting, deep vein thrombosis, pulmonary emboli, and decubitus ulcers are complications of imposed immobility associated with mechanical ventilation. Nosocomial respiratory infections, including methcillin-resistant *Staphylococcus aureus* (MRSA), oxacillin-resistant *Staphylococcus aureus* (ORSA), and sinus infections associated with nasal intubations. Stress ulcers and gastrointestinal bleeding result from immobility, and abdominal distention decreases movement of the diaphragm. The inability to communicate verbally combined with the stress of being in the critical care unit causes fear, anxiety, and emotional stress for the client (Broyles, 2005).

8. **Identify three priority nursing diagnoses for Caleb and how endotracheal intubation and mechanical ventilation can assist with treating these problems.** Caleb's priority nursing diagnoses are:
   a. Ineffective airway clearance related to aspiration of fluid
   b. Impaired gas exchange related to presence of fluid in alveoli and washing away of surfactant
   c. Impaired cerebral tissue perfusion related to decreased oxygen to neurologic tissue

   The main purpose of endotracheal intubation is to establish and maintain a patent airway. Mechanical ventilation is initiated to treat impaired gas exchange by supplying oxygen and removing carbon dioxide. Increased oxygenation in the lungs increases oxygenation to the heart to improve cardiac output and increase cerebral tissue perfusion.
   (1) Place on continuous cardiorespiratory monitoring.
   (2) Monitor vital signs at intervals appropriate for client's condition.
   (3) Monitor oxygen saturation via pulse oximetry continuously.
   (4) Administer oxygen, titrating to maintain oxygen saturation within prescribed parameters.
   (5) Maintain patency of intravenous access for infusion of prescribed fluids.
   (6) Monitor intake and output including insensible fluid loss through the respiratory system in the presence of bradypnea.
   (7) Provide for child's needs promptly to avoid unnecessary oxygen demand secondary to anxiety, and pain.

9. **Caleb's father expresses to you that he feels "so guilty about Caleb and I shouldn't have let them go fishing alone." How do you respond to Mr. Jones?** Mr. Jones is expressing feelings of guilt, which may be appropriate because lack of parental supervision is the leading cause of drowning and near drowning in children Caleb's age. However, at this highly stressful time for him and his family, the nurse should present a calm, supportive affect. Although this accident may have been prevented, Mr. Jones' actions following the accident

were appropriate and probably prevented Caleb from sustaining any further injury. He immediately instructed Tyler to call 911 and to explain the incident to his mother. He rushed to the site, turned Caleb over to check his responsiveness, and covered him to prevent any further loss of body heat. The nurse should focus on the positive response Caleb has had to treatment without giving false hope.

10. After 14 days of hospitalization, Caleb recovers completely and is preparing for discharge. What should you include/stress in your discharge teaching? Discharge planning should begin on admission; however, the following should be reinforced prior to discharge:

a. Avoid risk factors for drowning accidents by

(1) Encouraging CPR training for parents if they live near water

(2) Complying with water safety rules

(3) Never swimming alone

(4) Closely supervising children while they are swimming by watching them constantly

(5) Wearing life jackets or vests at all times when boating

(6) Children should wear life jackets or vests when around ponds, rivers, or lakes

(7) Learning to swim and having children learn to swim

(8) Swimming only in designated swimming areas

(9) Learning cardiopulmonary resuscitation

(10) Waiting at least 30 minutes after eating before swimming

(11) Never chewing gum or eating while swimming, diving, or playing in water

b. Provide instructions on any medications Caleb may be prescribed.

c. Emphasize the importance of follow-up with health care provider.

d. The nurse should allow sufficient time for parents' questions and provide clarification as needed.

e. Discharge teaching should be documented including parents' and Caleb's response to teaching.

References

Broyles, B.E. (2005). *Medical-surgical nursing clinical companion.* Durham, NC: Carolina Academic Press, p. 538.

Centers for Disease Control and Prevention. *http://www.cdc.gov*

Daniels, R. (2002). *Delmar's manual of laboratory and diagnostic tests.* Clifton Park, NY: Thomson Delmar Learning.

Gahart, B.L. and Nazareno, A.R. (2005). *2005 Intravenous medications* (21st ed.). St. Louis: Mosby.

Intravenous Therapy. *http://www.nursewise.com*

Josephson, D.L. (2004). *Intravenous infusion therapy for nurses: Principles & practice* (2nd ed.). Clifton Park, NY: Thomson Delmar Learning.

Minnesota Water Temperatures. *http://www.seagrant.umn.edu*

North American Nursing Diagnosis Association. (2005). *Nursing diagnoses: Definitions & classifications, 2005–2006.* Philadelphia: NANDA.

Potts, N. and Mandleco, B. (2002). *Pediatric nursing: Caring for children and their families.* Clifton Park, NY: Thomson Delmar Learning.

CASE STUDY 3

Cara

GENDER

F

AGE

9 months old

SETTING

- Hospital

ETHNICITY

- White American

CULTURAL CONSIDERATIONS

PREEXISTING CONDITIONS

- Preterm birth

COEXISTING CONDITIONS

SIGNIFICANT HISTORY

COMMUNICATION

DISABILITY

SOCIOECONOMIC

- Middle class

SPIRITUAL

PHARMACOLOGIC

- Metoclopramide (Maxolon)
- Albuterol (Proventil)
- Ipratropium (Atrovent)
- Cefazolin sodium (Ancef)

PSYCHOSOCIAL

LEGAL

ETHICAL

ALTERNATIVE THERAPY

PRIORITIZATION

DELEGATION

- Health care team

MODERATE

THE RESPIRATORY SYSTEM

Level of difficulty: Moderate

Overview: This case requires knowledge of bronchopulmonary dysplasia, tracheostomy care and suctioning, growth and development, as well as an understanding of the client's background and personal situation.

Client Profile

Cara is a 9-month-old infant who was delivered by Cesarean section at 25 weeks' gestation secondary to premature rupture of the amniotic membranes. She weighed 1.1 kg (2.5 lb) at birth and required intubation and mechanical ventilation after birth. During her first month of life she required reintubation with each of three attempts to wean her from the ventilator. At 5 months of age, Cara was weaned from the ventilator, but still requires 38% oxygen by tracheostomy collar to maintain her oxygen saturation >92%. Currently, she weighs 4.9 kg (10.8 lb) and receives gastrostomy feedings of 80 mL of Neocate, 24-calorie formula, every 4 hours as a result of severe GER. Prior to her daytime feedings, Cara receives metoclopramide 0.5 mg per gastric tube. The feedings are infused over 2 hours each using a volumetric pump to prevent regurgitation. She requires tracheostomy suctioning every 2 hours for thick yellow-white mucous. She is receiving respiratory therapy with albuterol inhaler every 4 hours and Atrovent (ipratropium), one puff every 8 hours. She also receives an iron supplement. During her hospital stay, Cara experienced two streptococcal pneumonia respiratory infections and required antibiotic therapy to resolve them. At 7 months of age Cara was discharged from the hospital with a diagnosis of bronchopulmonary dysplasia (BPD) into the care of her parents, Carolyn and Josh. Also at home is her 4-year-old brother Alex, who attends preschool three mornings a week.

Case Study

Cara was brought to the hospital yesterday after being seen by her pulmonary specialist at his office following her mother's call that Cara began experiencing respiratory distress at home. Her mother remains with her at the hospital and her father and brother visit every evening. The nurse from the day shift reported that Carolyn is very involved in her daughter's care, insisting on performing her morning care as well at her gastrostomy tube feedings and tracheostomy care and suctioning. The nurse observed Carolyn's care and found it followed appropriate procedures and protocols, but Carolyn is appearing very tired. She leaves only long enough to get a cup of coffee and a snack twice a day. She asks appropriate questions about her daughter's condition and spends all day holding and caring for her.

Questions and Suggested Answers

1. **Discuss your impressions about the above situation.** The data presented indicate that Cara probably has a respiratory infection. Her respiratory distress, in addition to the description of the mucus retrieved with suctioning, are positive indicators of the presence of bacterial growth. As bacteria grow, they shed toxins and dead cells as well as increase the tenacity of the mucus. This interferes with the alveoli's ability to exchange oxygen and carbon dioxide. The decreased oxygen creates hypoxia, and the inability of the alveoli to release carbon dioxide that is trapped in the alveolar spaces can lead to hypercapnia. Her mother is Cara's primary caregiver and does quite well, although the stress of her daughter being hospitalized is taking its toll and causing her to be fatigued.

2. **What is the purpose of Cara being prescribed metoclopramide, and is her current dose safe?** Metoclopramide is a gastrointestinal stimulant that facilitates stomach emptying. This agent is commonly used in both children and adults with gastroesophageal reflux (GER) disease. By more rapidly emptying the stomach, the risk of regurgitation or reflux is decreased. The safe dose for Cara is 0.1 mg/kg per dose. Cara weighs 11 lb, which converts to 5 kg, making her safe dose 0.5 mg, the dose she is prescribed.

3. **What additional data would provide a better understanding of Cara's current condition?**
   a. Sputum culture
   b. Complete blood count with focus on leukocyte count
   c. Vital signs

d. Length at birth compared to present height
e. Assessment of lung sounds
f. Inspection of current tracheostomy secretions
g. History of when she received the last dose of her respiratory agent
h. Are her immunizations up to date?

4. **Discuss the pathophysiology of bronchopulmonary dysplasia (BPD).** Four major risk factors predispose infants to BPD: (1) prematurity, (2) exposure to prolonged and high levels of oxygen, (3) use of mechanical ventilation, especially if prolonged, and (4) the presence of respiratory distress syndrome (RDS). Premature infants usually experience immature lung growth because lung maturity occurs primarily during the third trimester (28–40 weeks of gestation). This immaturity, including the lack of surfactant at birth, places these infants at high risk for respiratory distress or failure. Full-term infants who have experienced meconium aspiration also are at risk for RDS. For these neonates, provisions must be made for adequate gas exchange. This involves supplemental oxygen frequently administered at high concentrations to maintain oxygen saturations within prescribed parameters. The normal oxygen saturation for neonates ranges from 60% to 70% (Daniels, 2002, p. 109). Mechanical ventilation is prescribed to maintain a patent airway, provide supplemental oxygen, and to facilitate gas exchange. However, it increases the pressure in the bronchi and lungs and this damages the epithelial and alveolar surfaces. The damage decreases the structural resistance to microorganism invasion, leading to airway inflammation and edema. The cycle progresses with increased airway resistance and reactivity and increased mucus production. Damage to the alveoli leads to thickening and fibrosis and can decrease the functional alveoli by up to 50%. Atelectasis and fibrotic areas develop in the lungs. This decreases lung compliance and increases the work of breathing that exhausts the neonate. Further, the fibrosis reduces the number of functional cilia available for moving increased mucus secretions. The stasis of secretions combined with the compromised respiratory status can lead to pneumonia. The degree of damage determines how long it will take for the child to fully recover lung function. For some, problems have continued into adulthood.

5. **Is there a relationship between Cara's BPD and her GER?** Both conditions are common in preterm infants because of lack of development of both the lungs and the gastrointestinal tract, especially the lower esophageal sphincter (LES). The GER further places the infant at risk for aspiration and intensifies the respiratory compromise.

6. **Discuss why Cara requires gastrostomy feedings and the formula she is receiving.** The hardest work for a neonate and infant is eating, which requires energy. Cara's respiratory compromise increases her workload on the body and diminishes her energy supply. She would not be able to consume adequate nutrition by mouth for metabolic functions and the increased stress of her condition. By providing enteral feedings through a gastrostomy tube, the increased nutritional needs can be better met. Neocate is a special elemental formula designed for infants with increased metabolic needs and provides free amino acids for cellular growth and maintenance. Cara's Neocate is 24 kcal per ounce, providing increased caloric intake for her metabolic needs. It is comprised of 12% protein, 47% carbohydrates, and 41% fats as well as all vitamins and minerals necessary to meet the increased demands of her condition. It is well tolerated by infants and frequently is used for infants with allergies to other formulas including multiple protein allergies. She is receiving 240 mL or 192 kcal every 4 hours. Normal infants require between 108 kcal/kg of body weight per day; however, Cara requires more owing to her health alterations. The amount she receives is based on metabolic needs and evaluated by weight. Her weight has almost tripled in her first 9 months; however, her estimated weight had she completed full gestation would be >3.6 kg (8 lb), reflecting her lag in weight gain for an infant 9 months old.

7. **What risk factors does Cara have for developing a respiratory infection?** Cara has a tracheostomy that requires suctioning every 2 hours. The tracheostomy itself increases the amount of mucus in the airway, and suctioning increases it even more by stimulation of the secretory cells in the airway wall. This increased mucus provides an excellent medium for bacterial growth, and although tracheostomy care and suctioning is a

sterile procedure, in the presence of a tracheostomy the airway is open to the air through the opening in the skin. This increases the risk of bacterial entry and growth. Because streptococcal bacteria are normal flora in the respiratory tract and the integrity of the skin over the airway is broken, Cara is a susceptible host. Conditions are present for the normal flora to become pathogenic because of an increase in the numbers of bacteria. In addition, respiratory infections normally comprise 80% of all infections in children and Cara has increased risk factors for developing a respiratory infection. Also, her brother attends preschool three mornings a week, which exposes him and eventually Cara to the bacteria carried by other children. Finally, her BPD increases her risk of developing an infection due to her respiratory compromise and the presence of GER increases her risk for aspiration and resultant aspiration pneumonia.

8. **Considering the client's compromised respiratory status, what precautions should be taken when suctioning her tracheostomy?** Tracheostomy suctioning is considered a sterile procedure to prevent the introduction of bacteria into the trachea during suctioning. Rinsing the suction catheter in sterile normal saline before introducing the catheter into the airway for suctioning will help prevent reintroduction of bacteria into the airway. NOTE: The student should provide a discussion of tracheostomy suctioning according to the procedures and protocols of the clinical facility.

9. **Your assessment of Cara's growth and development reveals that she responds to her mother's voice by turning toward the sound and tracking as her mother speaks; she rolls from her back to her side with no evidence of head lag; she is unable to sit without support and does not verbalize; her palmar grasp has disappeared; and she is able to demonstrate a pincer grasp. She is unable to crawl, but moves herself in the crib on her stomach. How does Cara compare to other infants her age?** By 2–3 months of age, palmar grasp is normally replaced by active grasping; head lag normally disappears by 4–5 months of age; infants can normally turn from back to abdomen and can sit leaning forward with both hands by 6–7 months; pincer grasp usually appears between 8 and 9 months; by 6 months the infant recognizes familiar faces and follows voices by tracking; and most infants begin cooing at 1–2 months and are verbalizing two-syllable sounds (mama, dada) by 7–9 months. Cara was born approximately 3 months early and research has shown that these infants usually lag behind other children their age until 2 years, at which time they have caught up with their counterparts. Except for her language, Cara's development is normal for a 6-month-old. Her verbalizations are complicated by the presence of the tracheostomy, so her actual communication skills will be difficult to evaluate until she is decannulated. The student should question whether Cara uses a pacifier to stimulate her orally and maintain her sucking ability.

10. **Following a chest x-ray and culture, Cara was diagnosed with a streptococcal pneumonia and prescribed cefazolin sodium 200 mg IV every 8 hours. Why is Cara prescribed this agent?** Cefazolin sodium is a broad-spectrum first-generation cephalosporin used to treat serious infections caused by staphylococci and streptococci and other gram-positive organisms in the respiratory tract, biliary tract, heart, and gastrointestinal system. It also is used to treat pneumococcal pneumonia. The agent works by inhibiting cell wall synthesis of the organism causing cell death.

11. **Would you question the dosage of cefazolin sodium prescribed? Why or why not?** The safe pediatric dosage range of cefazolin sodium is 6.25–25 mg/kg of body weight every 6 hours or 8.3–33.3 mg/kg every 8 hours (Gahart and Nazareno, 2005, p. 234). Cara weighs 11 pounds, which when converted to kilograms is 5 kg. She can receive 41.5–166.5 mg every 8 hours. Her prescribed dose exceeds this range, so the nurse should question the prescription prior to administering the medication.

12. **How would you respond to Carolyn's fatigue?** The nurse needs to be very empathetic to Carolyn's need to provide care for her daughter and is probably reluctant to trust that anyone can care for her as well as she can. By using therapeutic communication, the nurse should develop a trusting relationship by spending time with Carolyn in Cara's room and be sensitive to nonverbal communication for Carolyn when offering to feed Cara if her mother is resting. Caring for the infant in front of the mother will increase the mother's trust in the nurse's ability. Offering to stay with Cara (stating you need to do your shift assessment) while Carolyn

goes to get a meal encourages her to take her time. Talking to Carolyn about the importance of her receiving sufficient nutrition and rest in order to care for Cara when she is discharged provides Carolyn with an understanding that the caregiver must care for self in order to care for others. Once Carolyn accepts the nurse's offer to spend some time away from Cara and sees that the nurse has cared for her daughter and is at the bedside when she returns, her trust in the nurse may lessen Carolyn's stress. Consulting with the health care provider and Carolyn concerning a referral for a "lap mother" (a hospital volunteer who sits, holds, and rocks infants during hospitalization to provide comfort for the infant in the absence of the parent) may free Carolyn to go home for short periods to rest.

13. **Would a multidisciplinary health care team conference be appropriate for Cara and her family?** A multidisciplinary health care team conference may be beneficial for Cara and her family. The team can discuss the family's support systems and help them best utilize these support people. The scenario does not address the financial status of the family; however, as Carolyn must stay at home with Cara and transport Alex to and from preschool so one could assume she is a stay-at-home mother. Because of Cara's extended hospitalization after birth, Home Health should already be involved in her case. Involving a child-life specialist or pediatric recreational therapist could provide information and techniques concerning appropriate stimulation for Cara that her family could use to assist in Cara's growth and development. A dietician should also be involved in the multidisciplinary team to ensure that Cara's special nutrition needs are being met. Respiratory therapy should be an integral part of the team owing to Cara's risk status for respiratory compromise. Be sure to elicit input from Cara's family in this process so they don't feel they are losing control of the situation into the hands of "strangers." The nurse needs to be both the client and family advocate, but also the liaison between the family and other members of the multidisciplinary health care team.

References

Centers for Disease Control and Prevention. *http://www.cdc.gov*

Daniels, R. (2002). *Delmar's manual of laboratory and diagnostic tests.* Clifton Park, NY: Thomson Delmar Learning.

Gahart, B.L. and Nazareno, A.R. (2005). *2005 Intravenous medications* (21st ed.). St. Louis: Mosby.

Potts, N. and Mandleco, B. (2002). *Pediatric nursing: Caring for children and their families.* Clifton Park, NY: Thomson Delmar Learning.

SHS North American Products. *http://www.shsna.com*

CASE STUDY 4

Erin

GENDER

F

AGE

8

SETTING

- Hospital

ETHNICITY

- White American

CULTURAL CONSIDERATIONS

PREEXISTING CONDITIONS

- Cystic fibrosis

COEXISTING CONDITIONS

SIGNIFICANT HISTORY

COMMUNICATION

DISABILITY

- Chronic disease

SOCIOECONOMIC

SPIRITUAL

PHARMACOLOGIC

- Ceftazidime (Tazicef)
- Gentamicin (Garamycin)
- Vancomycin (Vancocin)

PSYCHOSOCIAL

- Anxiety

LEGAL

ETHICAL

ALTERNATIVE THERAPY

PRIORITIZATION

- Yes

DELEGATION

- Yes

THE RESPIRATORY SYSTEM

Level of difficulty: Difficult

Overview: This case requires knowledge of cystic fibrosis, growth and development, as well as an understanding of the client's background, personal situation, and parent–child relationship.

Client Profile

Erin is an 8-year-old girl who lives with her parents and two younger sisters, Rachel, who is 5 years old, and Samantha, who is 2 years old. They live in a Midwestern community where Erin's father is a bank manager and her mother is a part-time investment broker who works from home, which allows her to stay at home with the children. Both of Erin's parents are very attentive to the children and are very knowledgeable about Erin's cystic fibrosis, which was diagnosed when Erin was 3 months old. Neither of her sisters has the disease. Erin takes pancreatic enzymes with each meal and snack (six doses per day) and she performs breathing exercises twice a day. Her mother performs postural drainage 1 hour prior to breakfast, again when Erin returns from school in the afternoon, and finally each evening prior to Erin's going to bed.

Case Study

During late spring Erin's breathing has become increasingly congested over the past week and her parents suspect that she has developed a respiratory infection when she becomes febrile with a temperature of 37.9° C (100.2° F). They phone her pediatrician, who recommends that she be admitted to the children's hospital 20 miles away. The pediatrician calls the hospital and informs the chief respiratory resident physician of Erin's history, chief complaints at present, and impending arrival. Sputum cultures, complete blood count, serum electrolyte panel, chest x-ray, and pulmonary function diagnostics are prescribed. Erin's last admission for pulmonary clean-out was 6 months ago. Erin is admitted and her diagnostic results include hemoglobin, 18 g/dL; hematocrit, 51%; white blood cell count, 15,000 cells/mm^3; platelets, 250,000 cells/mm^3; red blood cell count, 5.1 million cells/mm^3; serum glucose, 130 mg/dL; potassium, 4.0 mmol/L; sodium, 130 mmol/L; chloride, 90 mmol/L; blood urea nitrogen (BUN), 26 mg/dL; and creatinine, 0.7 mg/dL. Her chest X-ray shows consolidation in her right lower and middle lobes and her oxygen saturation is 89%. Erin's pulmonary function is determined to be 45% and as you are compiling Erin's history, her mother tells you that Erin has been on the lung transplant list for 9 months. Erin weighs 44 lb on admission.

Questions and Suggested Answers

1. **Discuss your impressions about Erin's diagnostic values.** Erin's platelet count is normal (150,000–450,000 cells/mm^3); however, her hemoglobin and hematocrit levels are elevated (11–16 g/dL and 31% to 41%, normals, respectively for children 1–10 years of age) as is her red blood cell count (4.5–4.8 million/mm^3, normals). This may indicate dehydration, which can occur in children with cystic fibrosis (CF) especially during late spring and summer months owing to increased perspiration. Her blood urea nitrogen (BUN) level also is elevated (5–18 mg/dL) and considering her creatinine level is not elevated, this is indicative of dehydration. Her white blood cell count is elevated (4,400–10,800 cell/mm^3 normal values), usually indicating the presence of infection. Her elevated temperature is consistent with infection. Her blood glucose level is elevated (60–100 mg/dL), which is consistent with impaired pancreatic function characteristic of severe CF. Erin's potassium level is within normal limits (3.4–4.7 mEq/L); however, both her sodium and chloride levels are decreased (138–145 mEq/L and 98–106 mmol/L, normals respectively), also consistent with CF. Her oxygen saturation (normal is 95% to 100%) indicates hypo-oxygenation, which can result from both CF and respiratory infection. The chest x-ray further substantiates the presence of a lung infection. Erin's lab results indicate infection, dehydration, and worsening CF.
2. **Discuss what risks Erin has for developing a pulmonary infection.** Risk factors include living with preschool and toddler siblings, who are common sources of infection, especially respiratory infections which are the most common infections in children (80% of all infections in children). Erin also is potentially exposed at

school because of the close proximity of other children in the classroom. Her greatest risk, however, is her CF. In CF, the exocrine glands secrete a thick tenacious mucus that is an excellent medium for bacteria. Because of the thickness of those secretions, expelling them through coughing is impaired.

3. **What pertinent information is missing?** Breath sounds and pulmonary function tests would provide more complete information concerning her respiratory status. Although the sputum cultures are prescribed, results of these cultures would indicate the presence and identification of microorganisms in the respiratory tract. Arterial blood gases would provide information concerning her acid–base status that also would be necessary if her condition worsened and she needed a lung transplant. An electrocardiogram would demonstrate the condition of her cardiac electrical conduction. Urinalysis and culture and sensitivity testing would not only show evidence of urinary function but also rule out the urine as the source of the infection.

4. **Identify the common microorganisms that cause respiratory infections in a child with CF.** The most common microorganisms responsible for respiratory infections in a child with CF are *Streptococcus aureus, Pneumococcus,* and *Pseudomonas.*

5. **What is the relationship between Erin's condition and her oxygen saturation level?** The thick tenacious mucus interferes with alveolar gas exchange. In addition, over time the mucus and repeated respiratory infections result in fibrosis (scar tissue) of the lung tissue and in the alveolar beds. Scar tissue is not functional in exchanging gases. Also, the presence of consolidation resulting from her current infection interferes with alveolar function. This results in reduced oxygenation of the blood and hypo-oxygenation and can lead to hypoxia.

6. **The health care provider prescribes ceftazidime 1 g IV every 8 hours; gentamicin 50 mg IV every 8 hours; and vancomycin 265 mg IV every 8 hours. Discuss why these drugs are prescribed for Erin.** A triple antimicrobial protocol is the standard of care for CF respiratory clean-out. Ceftazidime is the drug of choice for infections caused by *Pseudomonas,* a common causative microorganism. This fourth-generation cephalosporin has a predominantly gram-negative action. Gentamicin is an aminoglycoside that is used to treat severe respiratory infections and is a common adjunct to ceftazidime in treating respiratory infections in children with CF. Vancomycin hydrochloride is a tricyclic glycopeptide used to treat gram-positive bacterial infections of the lower respiratory tract that do not respond or are resistant to antibiotic-resistant microorganisms. Because of the presence of repeated respiratory infections in children with CF, antibiotic resistance can occur.

7. **Discuss the safety and efficacy of the doses of the antimicrobial agents prescribed for Erin.** All three of these antimicrobials are prescribed per kilogram of body weight. Erin weighs 44 lb, so the first step is to convert Erin's weight to kilograms. Dividing 44 lb by 2.2 kg (2.2 kg equal 1 lb) gives 20 kg. Facilities that specialize in the treatment of children with CF and the associated respiratory infections that occur with this disease use doses that are higher than the standard dosage ranges due to the severity and recurrence of these infections. The safe dosage range for ceftazidime in pseudomonal lung infection in CF is 30–50 mg/kg every 8 hours (Gahart and Nazareno, 2005, p. 258). Erin's dose, based on her weight, should be 600–1,000 mg every 8 hours. The safe dosage range of gentamicin sulfate is 2–2.5 mg/kg every 8 hours (Gahart and Nazareno, 2005, p. 593). Erin can receive 50 mg every 8 hours. The safe dosage range for vancomycin is 40 mg/kg every 24 hours and 13.33 mg/kg per dose if administered every 8 hours (Gahart and Nazareno, 2005, pp. 1145–1146). Peak and trough levels should be drawn for both the gentamicin sulfate and vancomycin and children receiving these agents should be monitored for ototoxicity and renal toxicity respectively.

8. **What are the criteria established for lung transplant candidates?** According to the Scientific Registry of Transplant Recipients, "A lung transplant is only offered to people who have irreversible lung failure. These people will not live longer than 1 to 2 years unless they receive a lung transplant." Among the common causes of lung failure are cystic fibrosis, emphysema, pulmonary fibrosis, pulmonary hypertension, and alpha-1-antitrypsin deficiency. The recipient receives a psychological examination to detect any problems that would interfere with compliance with the long-term and complex post-transplant therapies. The presence

of certain conditions including most cancers; infections that cannot be completely treated; and severe heart, liver, or renal problems contraindicate for lung transplantation for these individuals.

9. **Erin's condition worsens, and when no cadaver lungs become available, Erin's mother states that she wants to donate part or all of one of her lungs to Erin. After testing her mother for compatibility, the surgeon decides to proceed with the transplant the following day. Identify the priority client problems for Erin following the transplant.**
   a. Impaired gas exchange related to acute pain secondary to incision and chest tubes, atelectasis secondary to thoracic surgery
   b. High risk for infection related to immunosuppression, invasive lines and tubes, donor organ
   c. Risk for injury rejection related to organ transplantation
   d. Acute pain related to chest-tube placement, tissue trauma, and surgical incision
   e. Deficient knowledge related to postoperative standards of care

10. **Discuss the common immunosuppressant agents used to prevent organ rejection.** The most common immunosuppressant agents used for lung transplantation are cyclosporine, mycophenolate mofetil (CellCept), azathioprine (Imuran), methylprednisolone, prednisolone, prednisone, tacrolimus (Prograf, FK 507), sirolimus, and rapamycin (Rapamune).

11. **Erin receives a single lung transplant. Discuss what the risks are for her CF recurring in her transplanted lung.** Once the diseased lungs are removed and a healthy lung is transplanted into Erin, her CF will not affect the transplanted lung. CF is an inherited disease of the exocrine glands. The transplanted lung does not have exocrine glands affected by CF, so a lung transplant is a cure for the lung involvement of CF. It is not a cure for CF, as the other exocrine glands in the pancreatic ducts and reproductive glands are still affected by the disease.

12. **Erin and her mother recover from the surgery. Discuss the teaching priorities you will address with Erin and her parents prior to Erin's discharge.**
   a. Assess Erin's and her parent's current level of knowledge regarding caring for her after her transplant.
   b. Discuss risk factors for infection and the signs and symptoms to monitor.
   c. Discuss how to take Erin's temperature and advise that it should be done according to the schedule specified by her health care provider.
   d. Impress the importance of compliance with Erin's medication regimen including correct dosages, schedule of administration, and adverse effects.
   e. Dietary modifications as prescribed should be reviewed.
   f. Provide Erin's rehabilitation schedule and stress the importance of compliance with it.
   g. Discuss signs and symptoms to report immediately and provide contact numbers.
   h. Stress the importance of handwashing and teach the proper technique.
   i. Discuss the importance of follow-up visits with the health care provider and the need to discuss appropriate immunizations for Erin and modifications necessary because of her immunosuppression.
   j. Provide information concerning appropriate referrals that have been made to assist the family with her home adjustment.
   k. Provide these instructions both verbally and in writing, and have the family view a video of care after lung transplantation, if available. NOTE: These are frequently available at facilities that specialize in organ transplantation

13. **What are the current statistics for successful lung transplants?** In 2003, approximately 1,100 lung transplants were performed in the United States. According to the Organ Procurement and Transplantation Network, 1-year survival for children 6–10 years of age is 84.6% and 3 year survival for the same age group is 49.5%. For all ages current survival rates are as high as 80% at 1 year following transplantation and 60% at 4 years. Both 1-year and 3-year survival is highest in the 18- to 34-year-old age group.

References

American Society of Transplantation. *http://www.a-s-t.org*

Broyles, B.E. (2005). *Medical-surgical clinical companion.* Durham, NC: Carolina Academic Press.

Daniels, R. (2002). *Delmar's manual of laboratory and diagnostic tests.* Clifton Park, NY: Thomson Delmar Learning.

Gahart, B.L. and Nazareno, A.R. (2005). *2005 Intravenous medications* (21st ed.). St. Louis: Mosby.

National Heart, Lung, and Blood Institute of the National Institutes of Health. *http://www.nlm.nih.org*

North American Nursing Diagnosis Association. (2005). *Nursing diagnoses: Definitions & classifications, 2005–2006.* Philadelphia: NANDA.

Organ Procurement and Transplantation Network. *http://www.optn.org*

Potts, N. and Mandleco, B. (2002). *Pediatric nursing: Caring for children and their families.* Clifton Park, NY: Thomson Delmar Learning.

Scientific Registry of Transplant Recipients. *http://www.ustransplant.org*

Spratto, G.R. and Woods, A.L. (2005). *2005 Edition PDR: Nurse's drug handbook.* Clifton Park, NY: Thomson Delmar Learning.

United Network for Organ Sharing. *http://www.transplantliving.org*

CASE STUDY 5

Anna

GENDER

F

AGE

4

SETTING

- Hospital

ETHNICITY

- White American

CULTURAL CONSIDERATIONS

PREEXISTING CONDITIONS

- Autism

COEXISTING CONDITIONS

SIGNIFICANT HISTORY

COMMUNICATION

- Child is nonverbal

DISABILITY

SOCIOECONOMIC

SPIRITUAL

PHARMACOLOGIC

PSYCHOSOCIAL

- Anxiety
- Caregiver stress

LEGAL

ETHICAL

ALTERNATIVE THERAPY

- Vitamins

PRIORITIZATION

- Yes

DELEGATION

- Yes

MODERATE

THE RESPIRATORY SYSTEM

Level of difficulty: Moderate

Overview: This case requires knowledge of autism, the role of alternative therapy in this child's care, tonsillitis growth and development, as well as an understanding of the client's background, personal situation, and parent-child relationship.

Client Profile

Anna is a 4-year-old autistic preschooler who lives at home with her parents and three older siblings. Anna is nonverbal although she intermittently cries out while playing and can be disruptive at home. She attends a Head Start educational program in town and, according to her teacher, her behavior at school has gradually become less disruptive. Over the past year, she has experienced three episodes of tonsillitis. With each episode she was treated with antibiotics that seemed to effectively treat the problem until the next episode occurred. Following treatment for her last episode a month ago, her pediatrician recommended a tonsillectomy. Her parents are quite anxious at the thought of Anna having surgery and being hospitalized. The surgery is scheduled for the following week.

Case Study

During her preoperative visit Anna is very quiet and clings to her mother. Her parents speak and understand sufficient English to communicate with the nurse. They express their concerns about Anna having surgery and state that they have given her daily vitamins since she was just a baby to help prevent her from getting "these kinds of infections." Further, they have avoided talking about Anna's situation at home because they don't want to increase the child's anxiety. They state she would be very afraid if surrounded by strangers. They explain to the nurse that Anna has autism and express their concerns about the child's response to hospitalization because her behavior worsens when she is in an unfamiliar environment. Anna weighs 35 lb.

Questions and Suggested Answers

1. **What is autism and what is its incidence and etiology?** According to the National Institutes of Health, "Autism is a complex disorder that usually emerges during the first three years of life and affects the ability to communicate, reason and interact with others. Some type of autism is diagnosed in one in 166 individuals, according to the U.S. Centers for Disease Control and Prevention. According to the Autism Society of America, rates are soaring and could rise from 1.5 million Americans to 4 million in the next decade." The cause of autism is unknown, however, it has been linked to an intestinal virus. In addition, the National Alliance for Autism Research "has launched the NAAR Autism Genome Project, the largest study ever conducted to find the genes associated with inherited risk for autism. Over the next 6 months, about 170 of the world's leading genetics researchers will pool their resources and use a promising new technology, the DNA microarray, to scan the human genome in the search for the genetic causes of this devastating disorder, which continue to elude the medical field as prevalence rises" (*naar.org*).

2. **Discuss the potential impact Anna's autism may have on her hospital experience.** Anna's parents noted that Anna's behavior worsens when she is not in her familiar environment of either home or school. This may create an additional concern postoperatively that she could worsen her risk for bleeding in the operative area if she strains her throat by crying out. She will need to rest postoperatively to allow for healing. Her autism may interfere with her compliance in drinking cool liquids postoperatively to maintain hydration. Dehydration is the leading cause for readmission to the hospital following a T & A.

3. **Discuss the parents' comment about giving Anna vitamins to prevent "these kinds of infections."** The nurse's first responsibility is to assess what vitamins Anna's parents have been giving her—multivitamins, specific megavitamins, and what brand of vitamins. Many parents believe that giving their children multivitamins will "miraculously" prevent infections. Some parents may take megavitamin supplements and assume that these are safe for children. The key to good health is good nutrition, however, even the best nutrition may not prevent "normal" childhood infections when the child is exposed to massive numbers of microorganisms. Much study has been done on the benefits of certain vitamin supplements and their positive influence on health; however, these studies do not include children and the vitamins are not recommended as safe in megadoses for children. The parents need to understand that the purpose of

multivitamins for children is to supplement, not to replace adequate nutritional intake. Much assessment needs to be done regarding this issue.

4. **How can the nurse interact to address the family's anxiety?** First, the nurse needs to determine what the health care provider has told Anna's parents. This will provide a baseline for continuity of communication about Anna's surgery. Next the nurse should arrange for Anna and her family to tour the facility where the surgery is to be performed, including plans to allow them to stay with Anna in the surgical hold area where her pre-anesthetic medications will be administered. That way Anna will be relaxed and her parents will be the last people she sees before surgery. They can be present in the post-anesthesia care unit so that they are the first people she sees when she awakens from anesthesia. Inform them that the health care provider or representative will come out to see them as soon as the surgery is complete, and that if the surgery takes longer than the surgeon anticipates they will be kept informed at all times. Reinforce the fact that T & A's are simple procedures and that most children are discharged home within hours of the surgery. Preoperative and preprocedural teaching should begin, using the guideline of 1 day/year of age, although Anna's autism may create a challenge for this. The teaching is a joint responsibility of the health care provider, the nurse, and the family. The nurse should address this with Anna's parents, explaining that the teaching is done based on the child's level of growth and development. For instance, telling Anna 4 days before surgery that she and her parents are going to a place that will fix her sore throat is appropriate for Anna's age. Detailed preoperative teaching that is provided for adults is inappropriate for children and in Anna's case would increase her anxiety. The nurse should encourage the parents to ask questions and answer their questions before they return home. Also, contact numbers should be made available for them in case they have other questions. The most important aspect of this is that the nurse provide a calm, caring environment for the teaching.

5. **Discuss the incidence and causes of tonsillitis.** Tonsillitis is very common in childhood with the peak incidence in children 5-10 years of age. As a result of tonsillectomies no longer routinely performed before children go to school, young adults also experience tonsillitis and may require a T & A during adolescence or young adulthood. The most common causative organism for tonsillitis is beta-hemolytic *streptococcus;* however, *Haemophilus influenzae* and *Pneumococcus* also can cause the condition.

6. **What diagnostic studies should be performed prior to Anna's surgery?**
   a. Complete blood count to determine if white blood cells are elevated, indicating infection
   b. Throat culture
   c. Inspection of the tonsils
   d. Rapid Strep Test to determine if infection by strep is present
   e. Serum chemistry
   f. Urinalysis and culture/sensitivity

7. **Anna is admitted to the same-day surgical unit and is accompanied by her parents. When approached, her parents verbalize that Anna is afraid that the people are going to hurt her. How should the nurse respond to Anna and her parents?** The nurse should begin by sitting in a chair at eye level with Anna. Smiling at Anna and talking to her calmly, the nurse should explain to her in language appropriate for her level of growth and development that:
   a. She will not be getting any "shots."
   b. A small tube will be put in her arm after applying "magic medicine" (eutectic mixture of local anaesthetics [EMLA]) that will make sure it doesn't hurt.
   c. While her tonsils are being taken out, she will be asleep so she won't hurt.
   d. Mommy and daddy will be with her before she falls asleep and will be there when she wakes up.
   e. When she wakes up after her tonsils are out, we have medicine for her (acetaminophen with codeine or oxycodone elixir) that will make her throat feel better.
   f. She will get all of the ice water, Kool-aid, and Popsicles she likes and these will make her throat feel better and better. The nurse must carefully assess Anna for nonverbal indications of whether she understands what is being said to her. A caring attitude is important to instill confidence in Anna's parents, who can then help calm their daughter.

8. **What are the nursing priorities for Anna's postoperative care?**
   a. Risk for injury, bleeding related to vessel and tissue trauma secondary to surgery
   b. Risk for ineffective airway clearance related to blood and oral secretions secondary to surgery
   c. Acute pain related to tissue trauma secondary to surgery
   d. Risk for deficient fluid volume related to decreased oral intake secondary to postoperative pain
   e. Deficient knowledge related to Anna's postoperative needs and home care

9. **Discuss the appropriate priority nursing interventions for Anna.**
   a. Risk for bleeding
      (1) Place in prone or side-lying position with head of bed elevated 15-30°.
      (2) Assess for continuous drooling of bright red secretions from mouth.
      (3) Assess for frequent swallowing.
      (4) Assess vital signs according to facility postoperative protocol and as needed.
      (5) Notify health care provider if bleeding occurs.
      (6) When child is responsive, offer cool clear liquids to help with vasoconstriction.
      (7) Monitor closely for nausea and medicate as prescribed to prevent vomiting.
   b. Risk for ineffective airway clearance
      (1) Position to maintain patent airway.
      (2) Avoid suctioning of the throat.
      (3) Gently suction mouth to remove secretions if child is unable to.
      (4) Monitor postoperative vital signs according to facility protocol and as needed.
   c. Acute pain
      (1) Assess pain hourly using appropriate pain assessment scale.
      (2) Administer the prescribed analgesic as soon as child can swallow for proactive pain control.
      (3) Administer morphine sulfate intravenously as prescribed if the child is unable to swallow.
      (4) Encourage parents to remain at Anna's bedside to decrease her anxiety, which can intensify pain perception.
   d. Risk for deficient fluid volume
      (1) Maintain strict intake and output.
      (2) Assess mucous membranes and skin for signs of dehydration.
      (3) Maintain intravenous fluid administration until adequate oral intake has been established.
      (4) Provide proactive pain management to encourage oral intake.
      (5) Ask about the child's favorite cold beverages and provide these.
      (6) Encourage parents to actively participate in getting the child to take oral fluids.
   e. Deficient knowledge
      (1) Explain all procedures and equipment.
      (2) Allow the child to touch and handle equipment if awake.
      (3) Explain to parents what Anna's needs are and how to meet them.
      (4) Prepare for discharge teaching.

10. **Anna refuses to take fluids following her surgery and her urine output has decreased. She is then transferred to the pediatric surgical unit for an overnight stay. What is the rationale for this action? What is the expected urine output for Anna, who weighs 15.9 kg (35 lb)?** Decreased urine output is a critical manifestation of dehydration. The fluid and electrolyte balance in children is more fragile than for adults because children have a higher water content in their bodies. Anna was NPO for at least 4 hours prior to surgery. Although she is receiving intravenous fluids, she must take oral fluids prior to discharge. The normal urine output for Anna should be 15.9-31.8 mL/hour. (35 pounds divided by 2.2 kg = 15.9 kg times 1-2 cc/kg per hour). The most common reason for children to be readmitted to the hospital after T & A is dehydration.

11. **Anna cries and becomes withdrawn when visiting hours on the unit are over as her parents prepare to go home to check on their other children. Discuss Anna's reaction, relating it to her growth and development and the**

impact hospitalization has on a child Anna's age. Three hospital stressors affect hospitalized children: (1) separation anxiety, (2) fear of injury and pain, and (3) loss of control. It is normal for Anna to want her parents to remain with her because she believes they will keep her safe. A unique characteristic of preschoolers is their fear of mutilation. As a result of their limited cognition and their imagination, they perceive what adults tell them at face value. For instance, if the nurse tells the preschooler that she is going to remove her blood for a test, the preschooler believes that the nurse is going to remove all of her blood. To feel safe, Anna needs to have familiar people and objects with her. In addition, her autism is probably magnifying Anna's response.

12. **What could the nurse do to decrease Anna's anxiety and minimize the stressors of hospitalization?** The best thing the nurse could do is to encourage one of Anna's parents to remain with her overnight. The nurse must be sensitive to the parents' need to check their other children. Preschool children are extremely anxious about staying in an unfamiliar environment without at least one of their parents. Most facilities that provide pediatric services are equipped with couch beds or recliners for parents who wish to stay with their children. Parent visitation should not be interrupted or limited to general visiting hours. The child is in a strange place with people she doesn't trust yet; she needs one of her parents to stay with her if possible. If neither of Anna's parents can stay with her, the nurse should be sure to maintain Anna's home routine as much as possible, for instance, reading to her before she goes to sleep and provide continuity of care for her so she can develop trust. The reading can be delegated to ancillary personnel.

13. **Anna's mother spends the night with her, and the following morning Anna is drinking and her urine output is within normal limits, so she is to be discharged. Discuss the discharge teaching for Anna and her parents.**
    - **a.** Assess their current level of knowledge about Anna's care.
    - **b.** Include Anna in the discharge planning, focusing on her fluid intake.
    - **c.** Provide verbal and written instructions regarding:
        - **(1)** Signs of bleeding to be reported immediately
        - **(2)** Signs of infection, ensuring that the parents know the proper technique for monitoring Anna's temperature
        - **(3)** Medication administration and the importance of proactively treating Anna's discomfort
        - **(4)** Signs and symptoms of adverse effects of pain medications (constipation) and how to avoid them
        - **(5)** Special postoperative instructions by the health care provider
        - **(6)** Importance of Anna drinking adequate fluids including the appropriate parameters and how to achieve them, for instance, using a 1-ounce cup and having Anna drink a full cup every half hour
        - **(7)** Contact numbers to report any of the above signs and symptoms
        - **(8)** Importance of follow-up visit with health care provider
    - **d.** Provide sufficient time for Anna and her parents to ask questions, answering them honestly.
    - **e.** Document teaching and Anna and her parents' response.

References

Autism Society of America. *http://www.autism-society.org*

Centers for Disease Control and Prevention. *http://www.cdc.gov*

Daniels, R. (2002). *Delmar's manual of laboratory and diagnostic tests.* Clifton Park, NY: Thomson Delmar Learning.

Gahart, B.L. and Nazareno, A.R. (2005). *2005 Intravenous medications* (21st ed.). St. Louis: Mosby.

Intravenous Therapy. *http://www.nursewise.com*

National Alliance for Autism Research. *http://www.naar.org*

North American Nursing Diagnosis Association. (2005). *Nursing diagnoses: Definitions & classifications, 2005-2006.* Philadelphia: NANDA.

Potts, N. and Mandleco, B. (2002). *Pediatric nursing: Caring for children and their families.* Clifton Park, NY: Thomson Delmar Learning, pp. 703-705

Tonsillitis. *http://www.mayoclinic.com*

Wong, D.L., Perry, S.E., and Hockenberry, M.J. (2002). *Maternal child nursing care* (2nd ed.). St. Louis: Mosby, pp. 1195-1197.

CASE STUDY 6

Dwight

EASY

GENDER

M

AGE

4

SETTING

- Hospital

ETHNICITY

- White American

CULTURAL CONSIDERATIONS

PREEXISTING CONDITIONS

- Recurrent otitis media

COEXISTING CONDITIONS

SIGNIFICANT HISTORY

COMMUNICATION

DISABILITY

SOCIOECONOMIC

- Middle class

SPIRITUAL

PHARMACOLOGIC

- EMLA

PSYCHOSOCIAL

- Client fear and anxiety

LEGAL

- Informed consent

ETHICAL

ALTERNATIVE THERAPY

PRIORITIZATION

- Yes

DELEGATION

THE RESPIRATORY SYSTEM

Level of difficulty: Easy

Overview: This case requires knowledge of surgical preparation, growth and development, as well as an understanding of the client's background, personal situation, and family–child relationship.

Client Profile

Dwight is a 4-year-old who lives with his parents and 18-month-old sister. Dwight's parents decided to send him to preschool when he turned 3 years old to provide him with contact and interactions with other preschoolers. Dwight loves going to "school"; however, over the past year Dwight has experienced recurrent episodes of otitis media (OM) secondary to respiratory infections. Following his last episode of OM, his pediatrician suggested to his parents that Dwight should have "tubes put in his ears."

Case Study

On a follow-up visit, Dwight's parents discuss the surgery and decide to have it performed. Dwight's surgery is scheduled in 5 days.

Questions and Suggested Answers

1. **Discuss who is responsible for preparing Dwight psychosocially for his hospitalization and surgery.** This is a joint responsibility shared by the health care provider, the nurse, and Dwight's parents. A 4-year-old has a short attention span (20 minutes) and needs reinforcement of coming events. If the health care provider explains to Dwight that he is to have surgery in 5 days, Dwight will forget this before he reaches home with his parents. His parents need to reinforce his upcoming experience each day prior to the event. Most 4-year-olds understand the time concepts of tomorrow, afternoon, and next week (next Thursday, next Friday, etc.); however, owing to their short attention span, they frequently forget scheduled events from one day to the next.

2. **When should the preoperative teaching begin for Dwight and what topics should be addressed?** The usual formula used by professionals is 1 day of preparation for each year of life, so for Dwight, his preoperative teaching should begin 4 days prior to his hospitalization. His teaching must be consistent with his level of growth and development and understanding. Most preschoolers learn by observing and imitating, making the type of preoperative teaching that nurses perform with adults inappropriate. He should be told that he will be going to a building called a hospital to have tiny tubes (showing him the length) put into his ears so he doesn't keep getting sick. When he arrives, he should be told about any equipment in his environment, and if electronic equipment is used to obtain his vital signs he should be encouraged to touch the machine so he can tell that it won't hurt him. A simple explanation should be given before any procedure or assessment is performed. Dwight should also be told that his parents will remain with him until he goes to sleep and that they will be waiting for him when he wakes up.

3. **Dwight is admitted to the hospital in the morning and his surgery is scheduled for 2:00 P.M. Discuss the stressors for the preschooler who is hospitalized in terms of their priority.** There are three primary hospital stressors for children: (1) separation anxiety, (2) fear of injury and pain, and (3) loss of control. For the preschooler the most powerful stressor is the fear of mutilation. Preschoolers are very literal in their understanding of what is said to them, especially in a foreign environment such as the hospital. Their imaginations are very active during this time and can be their best friends, but they can also be their worst enemies in stressful situations. If you tell a preschooler that you are going to take some of his blood, he believes that his blood will be lost forever. One part of their psychosocial development tasks is initiative and the opposing side is guilt. Preschoolers believe things happen because of a thought they had or something they said.

4. **What are the priorities of care for Dwight on admission?**
   a. Fear of mutilation related to an unfamiliar environment and people, hospital stressors, and level of growth and development
   b. Anxiety (on the part of Dwight and his parents) related to his need to have surgery and undergo anesthesia

c. Risk for acute pain related to invasive procedure, such as venipuncture
d. Deficient knowledge related to the entire process of preoperative, intraoperative, and postoperative events and how to care for him at home following surgery

5. **Describe therapeutic nursing interventions that can lessen Dwight's stressors.**
   a. Encourage parents to remain with Dwight during this experience.
   b. Explain all equipment, procedures, and events at his level of understanding.
   c. Let him touch equipment, if this can be done safely.
   d. When talking to him, sit down at his level so you can have eye contact.
   e. Do not attempt to physically separate him from his parents.
   f. Encourage his parents to assist in his preoperative preparation if they are comfortable with this.
   g. Establishing trust with a preschooler during the short preoperative contact is very difficult for the nurse, but can be accomplished adequately to help decrease his anxiety and that of his parents. His anxiety level can be decreased or increased according to the anxiety he senses in his parents, so keep them informed at all times.

6. **The nurse discusses with Dwight's parents that he needs to have an intravenous access initiated. Dwight is visibly upset and begins to cry, telling his mother, "Don't let them hurt me!!" What measures should the nurse take prior to performing Dwight's venipuncture?** Prior to any planned venipuncture, eutectic mixture of local anesthetics (EMLA®) cream or patch should be applied for 1–2 hours. This blocks the local nerves, providing anesthesia to the site of the venipuncture. More than one site should be identified and prepared with EMLA in the event attempt at the first site is unsuccessful. EMLA is a prescription medication, so the nurse must collaborate with the health care provider to obtain the prescription unless the pediatric unit has a written protocol that EMLA is to be used prior to venipuncture. Because of the availability of EMLA, venipuncture should not be a painful experience for a child. The nurse might refer to EMLA as "magic cream" or "magic patch" that prevents Dwight from being hurt from the venipuncture. Hopefully, Dwight and his parents are familiar with EMLA because it was prescribed for him prior to his immunizations. If not, nurses need to encourage the use of EMLA prior to all finger sticks, immunizations, and venipuncture.

7. **Discuss the difference between the parents' informed consent and Dwight's assent for surgery.** Parental informed consent is written consent by the child's parent or legal guardian giving the medical staff permission to perform the said procedure on the child and stating that the parent understands what the procedure is and potential risks of the procedure. A child's assent is a verbal or nonverbal consent by the child to the proposed procedure.

8. **Discuss the importance of including Dwight in the surgical preparation process.** By including the child in the surgical preparation process, the child is more likely to be compliant with the preoperative and postoperative events associated with surgery. Involving the child also helps decrease the child's anxiety level and helps conserve that energy for the healing process. In addition, involving the child is a way of nurturing his feelings and those of his parents.

9. **How can a health care facility address a child's separation anxiety as the child is being transferred to the preoperative hold area and in the PICU following surgery?** Most health care facilities that specialize in treating children have policies in place that allow a child's parent(s) to accompany the child to the preoperative holding area where anti-anxiety preoperative medications are administered. This usually induces drowsiness so that by the time the child is transferred to the operating suite, the child is asleep and unaware that his parents are not present. In addition, these facilities provide for the parents to be present in the postanesthesia care unit when the child wakes up, thus creating an environment in which the parents are the last people the child sees before he goes to sleep and the first people he sees when he awakens from anesthesia. This dramatically reduces the separation anxiety stressor for hospitalized children.

10. **Discuss the nursing priorities of care for Dwight following his surgical procedure.** Dwight's priorities are the same as for any child (or adult) following surgery that involves general anesthesia. The first priority is assessing the ABCs (airway–breathing–circulation) and maintaining a patent airway. Maintain adequate ventilation

including the use of oxygen to maintain oxygen saturation within normal limits. The child's vital signs must be monitored at least every 15 minutes to assess their stability. The intravenous access must be maintained patent and the intravenous fluids administered as prescribed. Intake and output must be monitored, as well as bowel sounds. A continuous nursing assessment should be performed and the health care provider must be notified of any adverse client responses.

References

Delaune, S.C. and Ladner, P.K. (2002). *Fundamentals of nursing: Standards & practice* (2nd ed.). Clifton Park, NY: Thomson Delmar Learning, pp. 750–770.

Intravenous Therapy. *http://www.nursewise.com*

Josephson, D.L. (2004). *Intravenous infusion therapy for nurses: Principles & practice* (2nd ed.). Clifton Park, NY: Thomson Delmar Learning.

North American Nursing Diagnosis Association. (2005). *Nursing diagnoses: Definitions & classifications, 2005–2006.* Philadelphia: NANDA.

Potts, N. and Mandleco, B. (2002). *Pediatric nursing: Caring for children and their families.* Clifton Park, NY: Thomson Delmar Learning, pp. 265–267.

Wong, D.L., Perry, S.E., and Hockenberry, M.J. (2002). *Maternal child nursing care* (2nd ed.). St. Louis: Mosby, pp. 1128–1133.

CASE STUDY 7

Helen

GENDER

F

AGE

10 months old

SETTING

- Clinic

ETHNICITY

- White American

CULTURAL CONSIDERATIONS

PREEXISTING CONDITIONS

COEXISTING CONDITIONS

SIGNIFICANT HISTORY

COMMUNICATION

DISABILITY

SOCIOECONOMIC

- Middle class

SPIRITUAL

PHARMACOLOGIC

- Amoxicillin (Amoxil)
- Amoxicillin and Clavulanate potassium (Augmentin)

PSYCHOSOCIAL

Growth and development

LEGAL

ETHICAL

ALTERNATIVE THERAPY

PRIORITIZATION

DELEGATION

MODERATE

THE RESPIRATORY SYSTEM

Level of difficulty: Moderate

Overview: This case requires knowledge of tobacco addiction, otitis media, growth and development, as well as an understanding of the client's background, personal situation, and family relationship.

Client Profile

Helen is a 10-month-old girl who lives with her parents and two siblings. Her mother has just returned to work after being at home for 3 years as a "stay-at-home mom." For financial reasons, her mother has decided to resume her career as a nurse. Helen, her 2-year-old brother Hunter, and 3-year-old sister Emily are now attending a daycare center near their home while their parents are at work. All were breastfed and weaned to the bottle at 7 months of age. Helen is now being bottlefed. The family lives in a middle-class neighborhood, and the father is a heavy smoker, having smoked cigarettes for 10 years.

Case Study

Last week Helen developed an upper respiratory infection after being exposed to an infected child at the daycare center. Five days later her mother took her to the pediatrician's office for fever of 38.3° C (101° F), fussiness, decreased appetite, pulling on her right ear, and crying. During the visit the nurse practitioner examines Helen and on otoscopic exam notes that Helen's right tympanic membrane is bulging, red, and opaque with a small amount of purulent drainage in the ear canal. Helen weighs 19.8 lb and is placed on amoxicillin 250 mg t.i.d. for 10 days. Nine days into the regimen of amoxicillin, Helen's mother brings her back to the pediatrician's office with symptoms similar to those that began 2 days ago, including crying, diarrhea, vomiting, and pulling at her right ear. This morning Helen was experiencing a fever of 38.3° C (101° F) that prompted her mother to return to the office. Helen is prescribed Augmentin (amoxicillin and clavulanate potassium) 400 mg q8h in a suspension containing 400 mg/5 mL for 10 days.

Questions and Suggested Answers

1. **Discuss your impressions about the above situation.** The student should discuss Helen's clinical manifestations and relate these to the diagnosis of otitis media. Otitis media is an infection of the middle ear frequently associated with upper respiratory infections and other risk factors (see Fig. A-8). Clinical manifestations of otitis media include earache that is noted in children Helen's age by the child pulling on the ear affected. Other symptoms are irritability; sleep disturbances; persistent crying; fever; vomiting; anorexia; diarrhea; otorrhea; and a tympanic membrane that appears bulging, opaque, and usually red. The student should further discuss the pathophysiology of otitis media to provide rationale for these manifestations.
2. **What risk factors does Helen have for developing acute otitis media (OM)?** Risk factors that predispose children to develop otitis media include prior respiratory infections, the immature immune system of a child Helen's age, the physiological characteristics of an infant's Eustachian tube, exposure to other children who may have an upper respiratory infection or otitis media, bottle-feeding (especially if child lies down with a bottle), and exposure to second-hand smoke.
3. **Discuss the difference between acute OM and chronic OM.** Acute otitis media commonly follows an upper respiratory infection, with an incidence of more than 24 million cases in the United States annually. Acute otitis media has a rapid onset and a short duration. Chronic otitis media is an inflammation of the middle ear that persists beyond 3 months and poses a higher risk of conductive hearing loss. The symptoms of both are similar and consistent with the symptoms Helen presents in the case study.
4. **Discuss the relationship between Helen's recent enrollment in daycare and her condition.** At the time a child initially becomes exposed to other children, the child's immune system has not developed antibodies to resist microorganism invasion, especially given the number of children and the confined area of a daycare center (see Fig. A-9). The close contact with other children, some of whom may be harboring infectious microorganisms, places the child at risk for infections, especially upper respiratory infections that are passed

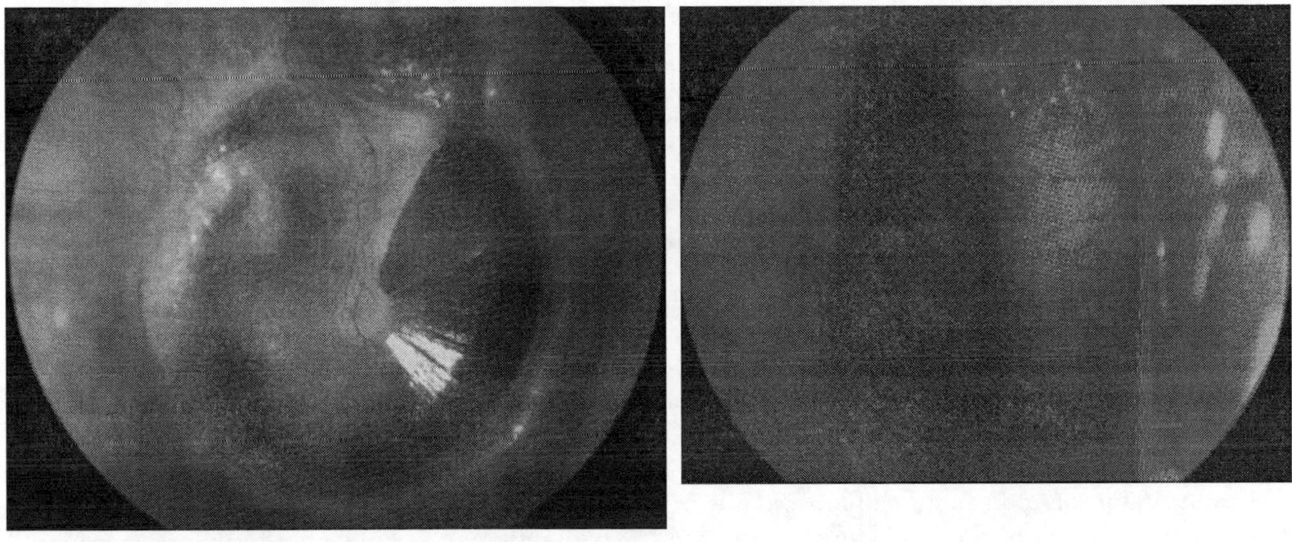
A. B.

Figure A-8 *Comparison of A. Normal tympanic membrane and B. Acute otitis media.*

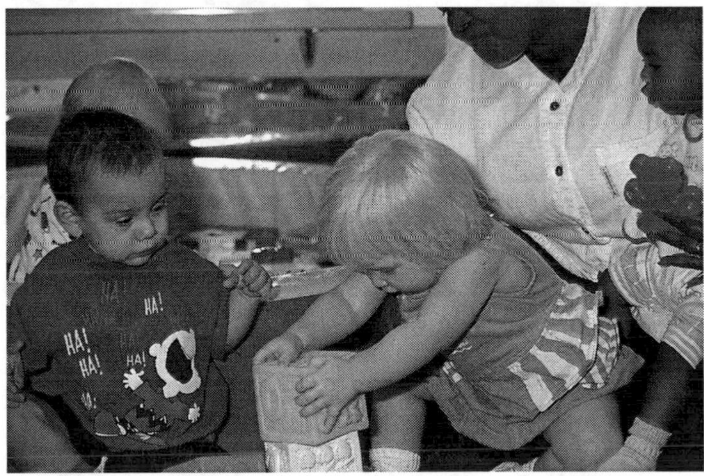

Figure A-9 *Children in daycare.*

by droplets during coughing, sneezing, and nasal drainage. The close physical proximity among children in a daycare setting provides an opportunity for cross-contamination.

5. **What is the relationship between upper respiratory infections and the development of OM?** The immune systems of children are immature, making them targets for infections, 80% of which occur in the respiratory system. The Eustachian tubes of young children are shorter, narrower, and more horizontal than in older children and adults. As a result, they do not drain efficiently. They also lack adequate cartilage support, causing the immature Eustachian tubes to collapse easily, inhibiting drainage of the middle ear. Mucosal edema that accompanies upper respiratory infections and enlarged adenoids frequently obstruct the tube. This blocks drainage and does not allow for ventilation to the middle ear. Negative pressure builds up in the middle ear space, creating an excellent medium for bacterial growth. If the Eustachian tube remains blocked for more than several days, the drainage thickens, becoming almost glue-like. Repeated episodes place the child at risk for conductive hearing loss.

6. **OM is the leading cause of what sensory deficit? Discuss this process.** Otitis media is the leading cause of conductive hearing loss. In the presence of recurrent otitis media, scar tissue develops on the structures of the middle ear, causing a blockage in the transmission of sound through these structures. This interrupts the conduction of sound causing it to be muffled. This creates a safety risk as the children cannot hear sounds such as automobiles or warnings of danger.

7. **How does passive cigarette smoke increase Helen's risk for OM?** Passive cigarette smoke irritates the Eustachian tube, leading to an inflammatory response. This causes edema and increased fluid in the ear. It further irritates the cilia in the ear canal, causing them to stiffen, decreasing the airflow in the ear. For children with allergies, this response is even more pronounced. Increased fluid and decreased airflow place the child at risk for otitis media.

8. **Discuss how you could approach Helen's father about his smoking and the risks it poses to his family.** The nurse needs to approach the father in a nonjudgmental and understanding way. Smoking is an extremely difficult addiction to resolve. Many smokers have tried multiple times to stop smoking, understanding the health risks involved in continued tobacco use.

   The nurse can provide literature to assist the father in quitting smoking as well as support groups, if available. The nurse also can suggest that the father smoke outdoors or refrain from smoking in the same room where the children are playing or eating.

9. **Discuss the relationship between amoxicillin suspension and Augmentin including the pediatrician's reasons for changing antibiotics before the course of amoxicillin was completed.** Amoxicillin is a semisynthetic broad-spectrum penicillin that is effective in the treatment of otitis media caused by gram-positive streptococcae including *Streptococcus faecalis* and *Streptococcus pneumoniae.* It is also used to treat infections caused by *Hemophilus influenzae, Proteus mirabilis, Escherichia coli,* and *Neisseria gonorrhoeae.* Because most upper respiratory infections in children are caused by streptococcae or secondary to influenzae, amoxicillin remains the drug of choice to treat otitis media in children. It is better absorbed than ampicillin sodium. With recurrent use, amoxicillin-resistant microorganisms develop resulting in the drug being ineffective in treating otitis media. Augmentin is a combination agent containing both amoxicillin and potassium clavulanate. Potassium clavulanate acts by inactivating the enzymes (lactamase) that are responsible for the development of resistance to penicillins. Usually when amoxicillin is effectively used, symptoms begin to subside in 24–48 hours so when Helen returned to the pediatrician with symptoms of otitis media returning after 7 days of amoxicillin therapy, the pediatrician could conclude that the microbe causing Helen's infection was amoxicillin-resistant and thus prescribed Augmentin.

10. **The safe dose of Augmentin (amoxicillin and clavulanate potassium) is 90 mg/kg per day. What is the safe range for Helen and is the prescribed dose safe for her?** Helen weighs 19.8 lb. Her weight needs to be converted to kilograms. Dividing 19.8 lb by 2.2 kg gives 9 kg. Multiply 9 kg times 90 mg = 810 mg per day. This needs to be divided by 2 because she receives a dose every 12 hours. Her safe individual dose is 405 mg. Her prescribed dose is safe, and with the suspension provided by the pharmacy of 400 mg/5 mL, she should receive 5 mL/dose. The safe dose of Augmentin is based on 400 mg and 57 mg of potassium clavulanate in each 5 mL.

11. **Develop the priority nursing diagnoses that apply to Helen related to her OM.**
    a. Acute pain related to inflammation and pressure in the middle ear
    b. Ineffective protection related to the presence of pathogenic microorganisms
    c. Risk for hyperthermia related to inflammatory and infection processes
    d. Risk for deficient fluid volume related to elevated temperature, decreased intake, nausea and vomiting
    e. Deficient knowledge, parental, related to disease process, risk factors, and treatment

References

Centers for Disease Control and Prevention. *http://www.cdc.gov*

Drugs @ FDA. *http://www.fda.gov*

North American Nursing Diagnosis Association. (2005). *Nursing diagnoses: Definitions & classifications, 2005–2006.* Philadelphia: NANDA.

Potts, N. and Mandleco, B. (2002). *Pediatric nursing: Caring for children and their families.* Clifton Park, NY: Thomson Delmar Learning.

Spratto, G.R. and Woods, A.L. (2005). *2005 PDR nurse's drug handbook.* Clifton Park, NY: Thomson Delmar Learning, pp. 58–59.

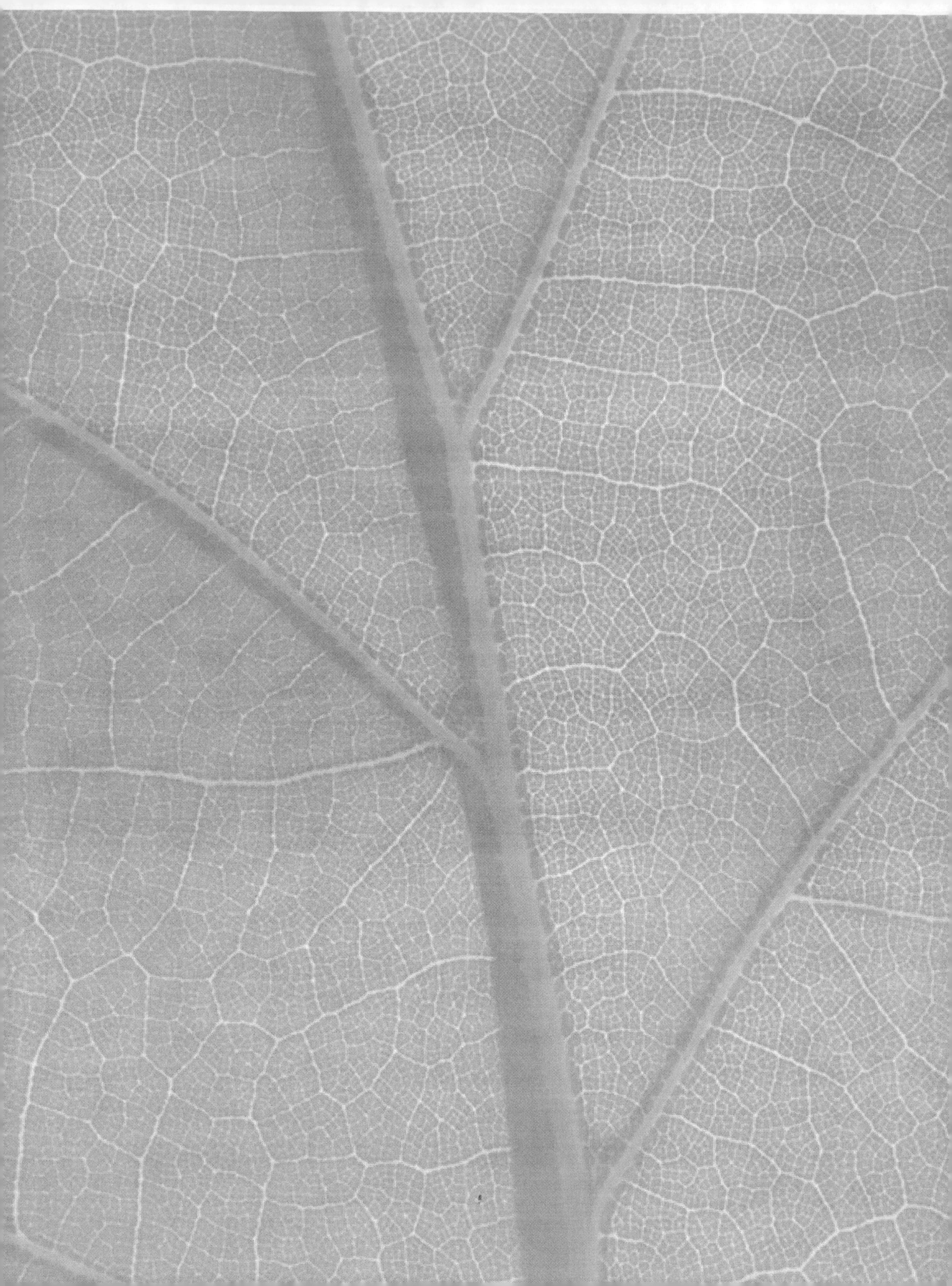

PART THREE

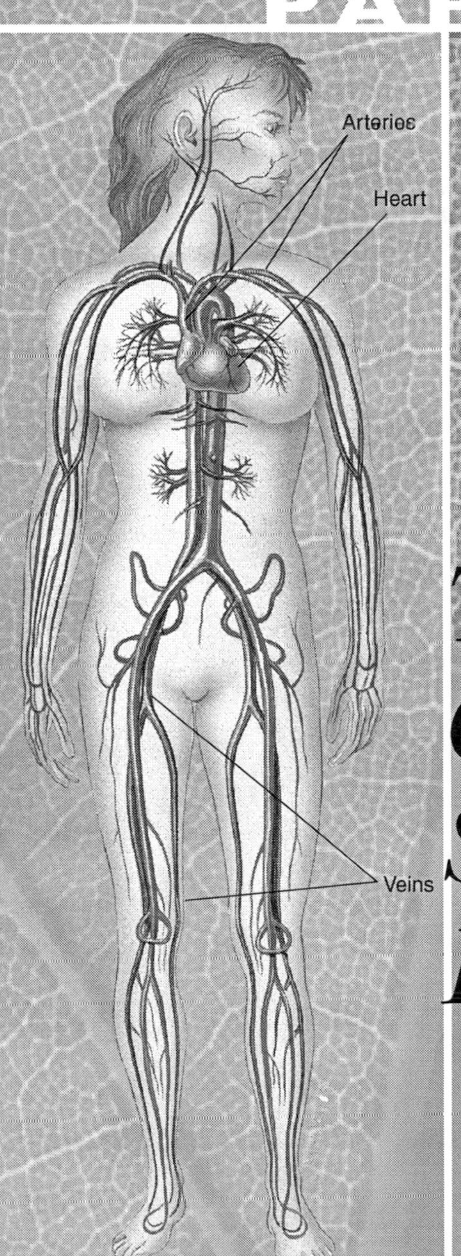

Circulatory system Heart, arteries, veins, capillaries and blood.

The Cardiovascular System and the Blood

CASE STUDY 1

Nisha

GENDER

F

AGE

14

SETTING

- Hospital

ETHNICITY

- Black American

CULTURAL CONSIDERATIONS

PREEXISTING CONDITIONS

COEXISTING CONDITIONS

- Sickle cell anemia

SIGNIFICANT HISTORY

COMMUNICATION

DISABILITY

SOCIOECONOMIC

SPIRITUAL

PHARMACOLOGIC

- Morphine sulfate (Duramorph)
- Acetaminophen (Tylenol)

PSYCHOSOCIAL

- Client anxiety
- Parent anxiety

LEGAL

ETHICAL

ALTERNATIVE THERAPY

PRIORITIZATION

- Yes

DELEGATION

- Client teaching

THE CIRCULATORY SYSTEM

Level of difficulty: Easy

Overview: This case requires knowledge of sickle cell disease, growth and development, as well as an understanding of the client's background, personal situation, and mother–child attachment relationship.

Client Profile

Nisha is a 14-year-old with sickle cell anemia. She lives with her mother and grandmother in a rural neighborhood. Nisha has experienced several "sickle cell crises"; however, they seem to have become more frequent since she became an adolescent. Nisha is enjoying her summer break from school. She is active in softball and enjoys shopping with her girlfriends.

Case Study

Nisha's mother brings her to the hematology clinic at the hospital with complaints of severe generalized pain following a softball game in which she pitched seven innings. She is admitted to the medical pediatric unit. Her vital signs are: temperature, 37.6° C (99.7° F); pulse, 110 beats/minute; respirations, 30 breaths/minute; and blood pressure, 96/70. She weighs 110 lb. Her complete blood count reveals: hemoglobin, 9 g/dL; hematocrit, 24%; white blood cell count, 12,000 cells/mm^3; and platelet count, 140,000 cells/mm^3. Her oxygen saturation is 89%.

Questions and Suggested Answers

1. **Discuss your impressions of Nisha's clinical manifestations.** Nisha is experiencing vaso-occlusive crisis secondary to her sickle cell anemia. This crisis is common during summer months, especially if the child is active outdoors, because of the risk of dehydration. She is 14 years old and probably experiencing menses as well, which adds another physiological stressor. Her hemoglobin and hematocrit levels reveal anemia and her temperature is elevated, perhaps indicating an infection, dehydration, or vaso-occlusive crisis. Children with sickle cell disease (SCD) experience more frequent infections than other children. Most of Nisha's clinical manifestations indicate vaso-occlusive crisis and include pain in the joints, pain distal to the occlusions, fever, abdominal pain, dyspnea, and tachycardia. Other manifestations are decreased range of motion, cerebrovascular accident (CVA), palpitations, pallor, weakness, and visual difficulties. Her oxygen saturation indicates ineffective tissue perfusion.

2. **Discuss the pathophysiology of sickle cell anemia.** Sickle cell disease is an autosomal codominant recessive genetic blood disorder characterized by the production of a sickle-shaped hemoglobin, hemoglobin S (see Fig. A-10). The mutant gene causes a change in a single amino acid in the beta-chain of hemoglobin, resulting in hemoglobin S (HbS) molecules instead of hemoglobin A. The S shape interferes with the red blood cell (RBC) uptake of oxygen, resulting in the RBC assuming a sickle shape rather than the normal round shape. Precipitating factors that can result in decreased oxygen concentration include dehydration, infection, stress, hypoxia, trauma, and acidosis. Because of their sickled shape, the RBCs aggregate or clump together and are not as flexible as normal RBCs. They thus cannot flow through small blood vessels. This leads to vaso-occlusive crisis. The cells are very responsive to reoxygenation and most return to the normal round shape. With repeated sickling episodes, the cells become permanently sickle shaped. The permanently altered cells have a shorter life span than normal round RBCs. Normal red blood cells have a life span of 120 days compared to the 12-day life span of the permanently sickled cells. This causes the spleen to become engorged with these short-lived cells, resulting in malfunction of the spleen. This is why people with SCD experience more infections than normal. Bacterial infections are a significant cause of morbidity and mortality in people with SCD. The brain and lungs are the other two organs most affected by the sickled cells. Cerebrovascular accidents can occur when the sickled cells cause infarctions in the brain. Acute chest syndrome results from sickled cells becoming trapped in the lungs, impairing gas exchange and causing chest pain, coughing, fever, and dyspnea. Because of the small vessels in the eye, the congestion of sickled cells in the vessels can lead to retinopathy (Broyles, 2005).

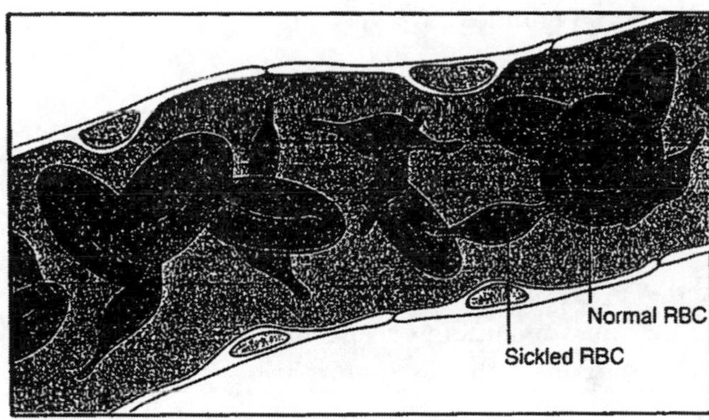

Figure A-10 *Regular and sickled RBCs.*

3. **What causes sickle cell anemia and how common is it?** Sickle cell disease is an autosomal codominant recessive genetic blood disorder that affects mainly African-Americans. Approximately 1 in 400 African-American infants is born with sickle cell disease and about 8% of African-Americans are born with the trait. Carriers' blood contains about 55% hemoglobin A and 45% hemoglobin S. Carriers are usually asymptomatic (Broyles, 2005, p. 768).

4. **What is sickle cell crisis?** Sickle cell crisis and painful crisis are terms usually used by nonprofessionals to describe the symptoms of vaso-occlusive crisis. When the RBCs clump together they interrupt blood and oxygen supply to the distal tissues. This results in tissue ischemia and pain. Eventually it can lead to organ damage.

5. **What other assessment data would be helpful for the nurse to have to prepare Nisha's care plan?**
   a. Pain assessment to determine location, characteristics, and level of pain
   b. Date of Nisha's last hospitalization
   c. The number of vaso-occlusive crises Nisha has experienced
   d. Nisha's fluid intake and urinary output
   e. Neurological assessment
   f. Breath and heart sounds
   g. Bowel sounds
   h. Skin assessment
   i. Chest x-ray

6. **What are the priorities of care for Nisha on admission?**
   a. Ineffective tissue perfusion related to clumping of sickled cells in the vessels
   b. Acute pain related to tissue ischemia
   c. Risk for infection related to compromised state
   d. Risk for injury, CVA, and organ damage related to recurrent crises
   e. Deficient knowledge related to predisposing factors for vaso-occlusive crisis

7. **The health care provider prescribes the following for Nisha:**

   Vital signs q4h. Notify health care provider of temperature >38° C (100.4° F)

   Regular diet

   Strict bedrest

   CBC with differential in A.M.

   Urine for urinalysis (U/A) and culture and sensitivity (C/S)

   Chest x-ray

   IV fluids of 5% dextrose in water with .45% normal saline to infuse at 175 ml/hour

PCA morphine sulfate 1.5 mg continuous and 1 mg every 8 minutes PCA dose

Acetaminophen 650 mg q4h po for temperature >38° C

Oxygen at 2 L per nasal cannula titrating to maintain oxygen saturation >94%

Discuss these prescriptions and if the nurse should question any of them. The standards of care for vaso-occlusive crisis are rehydration, reoxygenation, and pain management during the crisis. Intravenous fluids are prescribed at one and one half the normal rate to rehydrate the client. Supplemental oxygen is prescribed and titrated to maintain the normal saturation level of 95% to 100%. Because of the severity of the pain in vaso-occlusive crisis, continuous IV infusion and PCA dosing of morphine sulfate is the standard of care. All the other prescriptions are also appropriate for Nisha's treatment except the strict bedrest activity level. Nisha should be on bedrest with bathroom privileges because of the discomfort involved in placing her on a bedpan. The nurse should collaborate with the health care provider to have this prescription modified. Clients in vaso-occlusive crisis are generally bedfast by choice because of the pain of crisis, however, most would rather get up to go to the bathroom than to use a bedpan and there is no physiological reason for strict bedrest. Acetaminophen is the antipyretic of choice and the safe dosage range is 10–15 mg/kg per dose (Spratto and Woods, 2005, p. 7). Nisha can safely receive 500–750 mg per dose and be within the safe parameters. Some resources suggest that adolescents with the weight of an adult be given the usual adult dose of 650 mg. Sometimes the transfusion of blood products is prescribed to provide additional normal round RBCs. Because of the risks involved in transfusing blood products, these are prescribed only when necessary.

8. What nursing interventions would be appropriate in meeting Nisha's needs?

a. Tissue perfusion

- **(1)** Assess oxygen saturation continuously via pulse oximetry.
- **(2)** Administer oxygen as prescribed, titrating to maintain saturation >94% and per client response.
- **(3)** Assess capillary refill and cardiovascular status with vital signs.
- **(4)** Maintain a quiet restful environment to conserve energy and oxygenation.
- **(5)** Change bed linens when the client is in the bathroom attending to toileting needs.
- **(6)** Assess vital signs every 4 hours and as needed.
- **(7)** Elevate the head of the bed.
- **(8)** Encourage use of incentive spirometry, turning, and deep breathing.
- **(9)** Monitor laboratory test results.

b. Acute pain

- **(1)** Establish and maintain patency of intravenous access, monitoring hourly.
- **(2)** Assess pain hourly, using a growth and development appropriate pain assessment tool.
- **(3)** Instruct Nisha about use of patient-controlled analgesia to augment the continuous infusion and importance of dosing proactively.
- **(4)** Stress the importance of communicating effectiveness or ineffectiveness of analgesia.
- **(5)** Collaborate with the health care provider for increase in dosing or change of analgesic agent if pain not effectively managed with prescribed opioid analgesic.
- **(6)** Collaborate with health care provider if bolus doses of morphine are needed for break-through pain.
- **(7)** Position for comfort, maintaining proper alignment to avoid stress to joints and tissues.
- **(8)** Move Nisha slowly during position changes to avoid increasing her pain.
- **(9)** If Nisha or her mother have concerns about addiction to morphine, reassure that addiction is very uncommon especially when used short term and the usual duration for pain management is 3–5 days. Once the cells have been rehydrated and reoxygenated adequately, the pain resolves.
- **(10)** Collaborate with the health care provider for moist heat (K-pad) for comfort.
- **(11)** Encourage to ask for assistance to bathroom and back to bed.
- **(12)** Straighten or change bed linens while the client is in the bathroom to avoid discomfort of occupied bed linen change.

c. Risk for infection
   (1) Monitor vital signs every 4 hours and as needed during hospitalization.
   (2) Avoid invasive procedures including IM injections.
   (3) Maintain strict asepsis during any invasive procedures.
   (4) Maintain standard (universal) precautions at all times.
   (5) Assess breath sounds every 8 hours and as needed.
   (6) Administer antibiotics, antipyretics as prescribed.
   (7) Encourage use of incentive spirometry, deep breathing.
d. Risk for injury
   (1) Assess heart sounds and neurological status every 8 hours.
   (2) Stress the importance of maintaining adequate hydration.
   (3) Monitor diagnostic tests results.
   (4) Maintain facility protocols when administering blood and blood products.

9. **After 4 days of treatment, Nisha's intravenous fluids and medication are discontinued and her pain assessment reveals a pain level of 1/10. When the nurse enters Nisha's room, Nisha is sitting quietly in a chair at the bedside and she seems sad. Discuss your impressions of Nisha's condition based on her level of growth and development.** Nisha is a 14-year-old adolescent who has been away from friends and activities for 4 days. For an adolescent, this is a very long time. Now that her pain is resolved, she does not want to remain in the hospital. Nisha is probably very anxious to get back to her activities, especially softball and shopping with her friends. Adolescents are very social individuals with their peers, who provide them with their greatest sense of belonging. Nisha is now eager to spend more time with her friends.

10. **Discuss the teaching priorities for Nisha prior to her discharge from the hospital after her crisis is resolved.**
   a. Assess Nisha and her mother's current level of knowledge.
   b. Provide verbal and written information regarding:
      (1) Risk factors for developing infection and provide instructions as needed to avoid risk factors, for instance, being compliant with prophylactic antibiotic therapy (if prescribed); being vaccinated against pneumonia and influenza; and avoiding contact with friends, family, or others with known communicable diseases
      (2) Medication administration including importance of compliance with the prescribed medication regimen
      (3) Signs and symptoms of adverse effects of medications (constipation with opioid analgesics and hypersensitivity response with antibiotics)
      (4) Signs and symptoms of vaso-occlusive crisis
      (5) Contact phone numbers to report signs and symptoms
      (6) Importance of regular handwashing and appropriate technique
      (7) Importance of follow-up with health care provider
      (8) Referral information as needed
   c. Allow for sufficient time for Nisha and her mother to ask questions, answering them honestly.
   d. Document teaching and Nisha and her mother's response.

References

Broyles, B.E. (2005). *Medical-surgical nursing clinical companion.* Durham, NC: Carolina Academic Press.
Centers for Disease Control and Prevention. *http://www.cdc.gov*
Daniels, R. (2002). *Delmar's manual of laboratory and diagnostic tests.* Clifton Park, NY: Thomson Delmar Learning.
Gahart, B.L. and Nazareno, A.R. (2005). *2005 Intravenous medications* (21st ed.). St. Louis: Mosby.
Intravenous Therapy. *http://www.nursewise.com*
Medline Plus from the National Library of Medicine: Sickle Cell Disease: *http://www.nlm.nih.gov*

North American Nursing Diagnosis Association. (2005). *Nursing diagnoses: Definitions & classifications, 2005–2006.* Philadelphia: NANDA.

Potts, N. and Mandleco, B. (2002). *Pediatric nursing: Caring for children and their families.* Clifton Park, NY: Thomson Delmar Learning, pp. 818–824.

Sickle Cell Disease Association of America. *http://www.sicklecelldisease.org*

Spratto, G.R. and Woods, A.L. (2005). *2005 Edition PDR: Nurse's drug handbook.* Cifton Park, NY: Thomson Delmar Learning.

Wong, D.L., Perry, S.E., and Hockenberry, M.J. (2002). *Maternal child nursing care* (2nd ed.). St. Louis: Mosby, pp. 1359–1364.

CASE STUDY 2

Brandon

MODERATE

GENDER

M

AGE

8

SETTING

- Clinic/hospital

ETHNICITY

- White American

CULTURAL CONSIDERATIONS

PREEXISTING CONDITIONS

- Hemophilia A

COEXISTING CONDITIONS

- Hemophilia A

SIGNIFICANT HISTORY

COMMUNICATION

DISABILITY

SOCIOECONOMIC

- Middle class

SPIRITUAL

PHARMACOLOGIC

- Acetaminophen (Tylenol)

PSYCHOSOCIAL

- Parental and client anxiety

LEGAL

ETHICAL

ALTERNATIVE THERAPY

PRIORITIZATION

- Hourly assessments

DELEGATION

- Nursing assessment
- Yes

THE BLOOD

Level of difficulty: Moderate

Overview: This case requires knowledge of hemophilia, growth and development, as well as an understanding of the client's background, personal situation, and parent–client relationship.

Client Profile

Brandon is an 8-year-old with a history of hemophilia A, diagnosed when he was 13 months old. He lives with his parents and 10-year-old and 6-year-old sisters. He attends the local grade school with his sisters and routinely receives factor replacement at the hematology clinic. The family has adjusted well to Brandon's diagnosis although he has required hospitalization for hemarthrosis twice since he was a preschooler.

Case Study

Brandon experiences an abrasion and some contusions while playing on the playground at school. It has been 6 months since his last factor replacement, and when the abrasions continue to bleed and the contusions increase in size, his parents take him to the clinic.

Questions and Suggested Answers

1. **Discuss hemophilia and its incidence.** According to the National Heart, Lung, and Blood Institute of the National Institutes of Health, "Hemophilia is the oldest known hereditary blood disorder." It is diagnosed during childhood and affects more than 20,000 children and adults in the United States and occurs at an incidence of 1 out of every 5,000 births. Approximately 70% have less than 1% of the normal level of factor. There are two types, hemophilia A and hemophilia B. The difference between the two is that those with hemophilia A lack appropriate levels of the clotting factor VIII; those with hemophilia B, also called Christmas disease, lack factor IX. According to the National Library of Medicine, hemophilia C also exists, although it is very rare. It further states, "Hemophilia A and B occur almost always in boys. Generally, hemophilia A and B pass from mother to son through one of the mother's genes. Everyone has two sex chromosomes, one from each parent. Females inherit an X chromosome from their mother and an X chromosome from their father. Males inherit an X chromosome from their mother and a Y chromosome from their father. The gene that causes hemophilia A or B is located on the X chromosome. This is why men can't pass along the gene that causes hemophilia to their sons. Most women who have the defective gene are simply carriers and exhibit no signs or symptoms of hemophilia. It's also possible for hemophilia A or B to occur through spontaneous gene mutation. Hemophilia C can occur in both boys and girls. The defective gene that causes hemophilia C can also be passed on to children by mothers and fathers, but it follows an inheritance pattern different from that which occurs with hemophilia A and B." Hemophilia A is the most common, accounting for 75% to 80% of all cases. The obvious complication with this disease is uncontrolled bleeding that can occur with or without injury and can be life-threatening. It is treated with specific factor replacement that is extremely expensive, costing more than one dollar per unit, with required doses as high as 2,500 units and over.

2. **Discuss how factor replacement is administered in a clinic setting and the specific nursing responsibilities associated with factor replacement.** Depending on the severity of the child's condition, a venous access must be established to administer the factor replacement. The child may have a central venous access if he experiences frequent bleeding episodes. For most children, the factor is administered either through venipuncture or the establishment of a temporary peripheral venous access. In most facilities, the pharmacy mixes the factor as soon as it receives the prescription. The nurse must coordinate the administration with the pharmacy because factor has a very short shelf life. It is also very expensive and must be handled with great care to avoid breakage if it is processed in a glass bottle for infusion. Care must also be taken to prevent contamination. Prior to establishing the venous access, a eutectic mixture of local anesthetics (EMLA) should be applied to the child 1–2 hours before the venipuncture. Having the parent apply this before coming to the clinic would decrease the amount of time the child and parent must be in the clinic, however, the nurse needs to be sure that the parents have a prescription for EMLA. Nurses usually draw serum factor levels

before and after the factor replacement, as prescribed, and set up the follow-up visit to recheck the level. The nurse must be familiar with growth and development and the use of therapeutic communication with both the parents and the child.

3. **Discuss the risks of HIV or hepatitis transmission and transfusion reactions as a result of factor replacement.** Most factor products, especially for factor VIII replacement, are plasma derived or recombinant and are considered very safe. Because clotting factors do not contain antibodies, transfusion reactions have not been a concern; however, when blood transfusions were the standard of care, this was a real problem. Blood transfusions are used only in the presence of need for blood replacement as a result of ineffective tissue perfusion secondary to blood loss. In the past two decades, viral activation and removal steps in manufacturing factor effectively have been preventing transmission of hepatitis B, hepatitis C, or human immunodeficiency virus (HIV) from plasma-derived products. The first recombinant antihemophilic factor was approved by the Food and Drug Administration (FDA) in 1992. According to the FDA, however, until 2003, "all recombinant factor VIII products still were made with the use of blood-derived additives of human or animal origin, such as albumin." On July 25, 2003, the FDA "licensed a new recombinant DNA-derived clotting factor to treat people with hemophilia A. This new antihemophilic human factor VIII product is the first one produced without using additives derived from human or animal blood in the manufacturing process." It is plasma/albumin free, which adds an additional reassurance for those with hemophilia concerned about blood transmission of disease. This information should be communicated to the clients in collaboration with the health care provider.

4. **For the past 2 months, Brandon has not had any other injuries; however, his mother notices that his right knee is slightly swollen and he is starting to limp when he walks. What is your impression of Brandon's current condition as it relates to his level of growth and development?** These are early clinical manifestations of hemarthrosis, a condition involving bleeding into a joint. The knee is the most common joint affected; however, hemarthrosis can occur in the ankles, elbows, wrists, or shoulders. Brandon is a school-age child and children at this level of growth and development are very active in sports, running games, and climbing. By following rules of the games, the school-age child develops a sense of industry through accomplishment. Whenever a person runs, the knee absorbs 40 times the stress as the hips and ankles, so internal stress on the knee can trigger bleeding into the joint as a result of the normal activities for this age group. School-age boys are the most frequently hospitalized with hemarthrosis because of this activity.

5. **Brandon and his mother return to the hematology clinic and his health care provider determines that he should be admitted to the hospital. Why do you think Brandon's health care provider makes the decision to admit Brandon for treatment now?** If hemarthrosis is not treated, joint contractures and permanent joint problems can occur. The joint must be rested and maintained in extension and replacement factor must be prescribed.

6. **What are the priorities of care for Brandon?**
   a. Risk for injury, bleeding, related to lack of clotting factor VIII
   b. Impaired physical mobility related to edema and soreness
   c. Risk for delayed development related to risk for bleeding and impaired physical mobility
   d. Deficient knowledge related to injury prevention and growth and development needs

7. **Brandon is admitted to the pediatric unit and prescribed the following:**
   a. Draw serum factor VIII now
   b. Placed in 15 lb of traction
   c. Diet as tolerated
   d. Vital signs routine
   e. Establish peripheral intravenous access and medlock
   f. Urinalysis now
   g. Hemoccult all stools
   h. Acetaminophen 325 mg PO every 4 hours as needed for pain

Discuss the above prescriptions. Would the nurse question any of them? What about Brandon's activity level? The above prescriptions are appropriate. The standard of care for hemarthrosis is placement in skin traction to maintain limb alignment, rest, and factor replacement. The child needs to have a peripheral venous access for the administration of replacement factor that also is a standard of care for hemarthrosis. No dietary restrictions are needed for hemarthrosis and the nurse should encourage family members to bring in Brandon's favorite foods, especially because inactivity negatively impacts on appetite. Vital signs should be monitored every 4 hours for at least 24 hours following admission to check for changes indicating increased bleeding. The urine and stool should be monitored for the presence of blood as mucous membranes are the most fragile tissues in the body and the most prone to bleed if compromised. The nurse should collaborate with the health care provider for a prescription for a stool softener because inactivity decreases bowel activity, placing the client at risk for constipation. Once the child is placed in traction and the stress removed from the affected joint, hemarthrosis usually does not require medications stronger than non-opioid analgesics to maintain comfort level. The health care provider also should be consulted about the need for referrals for recreation therapy and hospital school. Because Brandon is placed in traction, his activity is strict bedrest because traction must stay in place continuously to be effective.

8. **Brandon has just been placed in traction at the shift change on the pediatric unit. His nurse should make what routine (hourly) assessments on Brandon?** Brandon's nurse must make assessments of the traction to ensure that it is properly functioning. Those assessments include:
   a. Proper weight and as prescribed
   b. Pulleys are correctly placed.
   c. Weight(s) are hanging free, not touching the floor or the bed
   d. The child's position in bed is correct. (Many children will slide to the bottom of the bed as a result of the weights and frequently must be pulled up in bed to maintain traction.)
   e. Color and edema of affected joint
   f. Pain assessment (hourly)
   g. Neurovascular assessment of the limb in traction
   h. Intake and output per facility protocol

9. **The nurse is assigned a nursing assistant to work with her in providing care for her four pediatric clients. What aspects of Brandon's care can the nurse delegate to the nursing assistant?** The nurse must make Brandon's assessments; however, the nursing assistant can be delegated to obtain Brandon's vital signs, empty his urinal and maintain intake and output records, provide for Brandon's hygiene needs unless Brandon prefers to have his mother help him, ensure that he receives a diet tray and liquids, and be involved in growth and development activities with Brandon (as long as the nurse makes sure the nursing assistant is familiar with Brandon's growth and development needs.) The nurse must ensure communication between the nursing assistant and nursing staff.

10. **Brandon's factor result is 2 mg/100 mL. Explain the significance of this result.** The normal factor VIII level is 50–100 mg/100 mL. Hemophilia is categorized as mild, moderate, or severe based on factor level. Mild status is characterized as a factor level of 6% to 49% of the normal level; the client can bleed if significantly injured or as a result of surgery or injections, may never experience a bleeding problem, and seldom has joint problems. Moderate hemophilia is characterized by a factor level of 1% to 5% of the norm; the client bleeds with only slight injury, experiences bleeding episodes monthly or more frequently depending on the level of growth and development, and can experience joint problems if joint bleeds are not treated. Finally, the person with severe hemophilia has a factor level of <1%, can bleed spontaneously, has bleeding episodes as frequently as two times per week, and usually experiences joint problems if the bleeds are not treated. Brandon's level is 4% of the lowest normal value.

11. **Brandon's mother, who remains at Brandon's bedside throughout his hospitalization, tells the nurse that Brandon is complaining of being "stiff" and "so bored." How should the nurse respond to Brandon and his mother?** Being in traction can be a very boring situation for a child. Also, if the child remains in a constant

position, the muscles and joints not affected by hemarthrosis can become stiff. The nurse should explain what types of activities Brandon can do while in traction and facilitate scheduling these activities. Range of motion of the three uninvolved extremities can be accomplished by making range-of-motion exercises a matching word game—match the word with the activity. Throwing wads of paper or a soft foam ball into a trash basket also provides exercise for the upper extremities. Playing computer games exercises the fine motor skills, challenges the child, and can give him a sense of accomplishment. If the facility has a playroom, the child can be taken in his bed to play with other children. Card games or board games can be brought from home and family encouraged to play with him. If hospitalized during school, hospital school should be involved.

12. After 2 weeks of hospitalization, Brandon is preparing to be discharged. Discuss the client and family teaching the nurse should perform prior to Brandon's discharge.

- **a.** Assess client and family's current level of knowledge.
- **b.** rovide verbal and written information regarding:
  - **(1)** Risk factors for injuries, including instructions as needed to prevent injuries
  - **(2)** Signs and symptoms of bleeding and how to apply pressure for minor topical injuries
  - **(3)** Importance of seeking medical attention immediately if more severe injury occurs
  - **(4)** Referrals as needed after collaboration with hospital, school, and social services
  - **(5)** Play activities for Brandon according to his level of growth and development
  - **(6)** Importance of compliance with medications
  - **(7)** Signs and symptoms of worsening of condition
  - **(8)** Contact phone numbers to report signs and symptoms
  - **(9)** Importance of follow-up with health care provider
- **c.** llow sufficient time for client and family questions, answering them honestly and providing referrals as needed
- **d.** Document teaching and client and family response

References

Broyles, B.E. (2005). *Medical-surgical nursing clinical companion.* Durham, NC: Carolina Academic Press.

Daniels, R. (2002). *Delmar's manual of laboratory and diagnostic tests.* Clifton Park, NY: Thomson Delmar Learning.

Food and Drug Administration. *http://www.fda.gov*

Gahart, B.L. and Nazareno, A.R. (2005). *2005 Intravenous medications* (21st ed.). St. Louis: Mosby.

Josephson, D.L. (2004). *Intravenous infusion therapy for nurses: Principles & practice* (2nd ed.). Clifton Park, NY: Thomson Delmar Learning.

National Hemophilia Foundation. *http://www.hemophilia.org*

National Heart, Lung, and Blood Institute. *http://www.nhlb.nih.gov*

North American Nursing Diagnosis Association. (2005). *Nursing diagnoses: Definitions & classifications, 2005–2006.* Philadelphia: NANDA.

Reiss, B.S., Evans, M.E. and Broyles, B.E. (2002). *Pharmacological aspects of nursing care* (6th ed.). Clifton Park, NY: Thomson Delmar Learning, pp. 760–797.

U.S. National Library of Medicine. *http://www.nlm.nih.gov*

CASE STUDY 3

Ryan

GENDER

M

AGE

11 months old

SETTING

- Hospital

ETHNICITY

- White American

CULTURAL CONSIDERATIONS

PREEXISTING CONDITIONS

COEXISTING CONDITIONS

- Atrial septal defect

SIGNIFICANT HISTORY

- With parents

COMMUNICATION

DISABILITY

- Down syndrome

SOCIOECONOMIC STATUS

- Middle class

SPIRITUAL

PHARMACOLOGIC

- Digoxin (Lanoxin)
- Furosemide (Lasix)

PSYCHOSOCIAL

- Parental anxiety

LEGAL

ETHICAL

ALTERNATIVE THERAPY

PRIORITIZATION

- Yes

DELEGATION

- Client teaching

THE CARDIOVASCULAR SYSTEM

Level of difficulty: Difficult

Overview: This case requires knowledge of normal and abnormal heart function; understanding of the client's background, personal situation, and parent–child relationship; and management of client pain.

Client Profile

Ryan is an 11-month-old infant who was born with Down syndrome and lives with his parents in a middle-class neighborhood. Ryan weighed 3.2 kg (7 lb) at birth and a heart murmur was heard. Ryan was breast fed for 4 months. His mother says that at the time, he became "disinterested" in the breastfeeding, but when she was able to get him to nurse, he would fall asleep after having nursed for only 5 minutes. Because he was not gaining weight appropriately, his pediatrician prescribed infant formula with iron and suggested that his mother begin feeding Ryan rice cereal twice a day. At 4 months of age Ryan was diagnosed with an atrial septal defect that has been monitored since the diagnosis. Ryan sits unsupported but, according to his mother, does not crawl or attempt to stand because "he gets out of breath when he tries to crawl so we bought a walker that he moves around in." Since he was 5 months old, Ryan has been receiving digoxin 200 μg and furosemide 10 mg every day.

Case Study

Ryan's parents bring Ryan in to see his cardiologist because he has been lethargic and has had diarrhea for the past 24 hours. When the nurse assesses Ryan, she finds he weighs 7 kg (15.4 lb) and his vital signs are:

Temperature: 36.5° C (97.7° F)

Pulse: 80 beats/minute

Respirations: 35 breaths/minute

His laboratory results are:

Potassium level: 2.9 mmol/L

Digoxin level: 2.5 ng/mL

Questions and Suggested Answers

1. **Discuss the pathophysiology of atrial septal defect.** Atrial septal defect is a left-to-right shunt between the upper chambers of the heart. The defect is acyanotic and often results from the foramen ovale remaining patent after birth instead of closing (see Fig. A-11). With an opening between the two atria, a portion of the blood from the left atria is shunted back to the right atria because the pressure is higher in the left side of the heart and fluid moves from an area of greater pressure to one of lesser pressure. This increases the amount of blood in the right atria, resulting in increased pressure in the systemic system. This leads to decreased venous return and systemic congestion. It further causes an increased workload on the right side of the heart that eventually leads to hypertrophy of the right ventricle. The goal of treatment is to prevent the progression to hypertrophy of the ventricle.

2. **What is the incidence and etiology of this congenital heart defect?** Congenital heart defects occur at an annual incidence of 10 per 1,000 live births, and atrial septal defects account for approximately 8% of these defects. As with most congenital heart defects, the exact cause is unknown; however, a higher incidence occurs in neonates who have mothers with (1) rubella, (2) alcoholism, (3) type 1 diabetes, or (4) age >40 years during pregnancy. Infants born with Down syndrome have a 40% higher incidence of congenital heart defects than other infants.

3. **What is the relationship between Ryan's current weight and his heart defect?** The primary manifestation of congenital heart defect that warrants treatment is dyspnea on exertion. This represents an increased workload on the heart to meet metabolic needs. Because eating is the most energy-consuming activity for a neonate and young infant, these infants are unable to take in adequate nutrition to meet the growth needs of doubling their birth weight by 6 months of age and tripling it by 1 year of age. Ryan was 3.2 kg (7 lb) at birth and at his present age should be approaching 9.5 kg (21 lb); however, he weighs only 7 kg (15.4 lb).

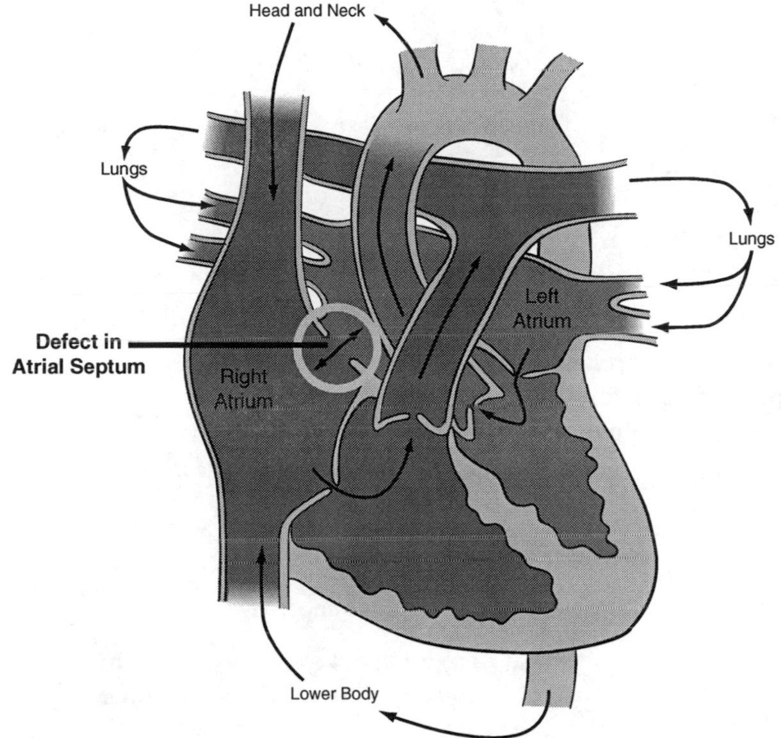

Figure A-11 *Atrial septal defect.*

4. **What other assessment data indicate an impact on Ryan's growth and development?** At 11 months, Ryan should be crawling to get from one place to another. He also should be standing, supporting himself with one hand. His sitting unsupported represents the developmental stage of an infant 8–9 months old. His fatigue and dyspnea on exertion have prevented him from progressing with his gross motor skills.

5. **Discuss the rationale for the medication regimen for Ryan.** Digoxin is a cardiac glycoside with a positive inotropic effect of increasing cardiac output by slowing and strengthening the force of contractions. Furosemide is a potent loop diuretic used to increase excretion of fluid and decrease edema that in Ryan occurred as a result of systemic congestion.

6. **What is your impression of Ryan's assessment data at his cardiologist's office?** The assessment date represents digoxin toxicity. Diarrhea, fatigue, dyspnea on exertion, the client's pulse rate of 80 beats/minute, and his serum digoxin level indicate toxicity. Bradycardia is a common sign of digoxin toxicity as the drug slows the heart rate beyond the therapeutic range. The normal digoxin level is 0.5–2.0 ng/mL (Spratto and Woods, 2005, p. 360). Ryan's level is toxic. In addition, although Ryan's dose is at the lower end of the safe dosage range for his weight (0.025–0.035 mg/kg per day) (Spratto and Woods, 2005, p. 363), he is experiencing hypokalemia, probably due to the furosemide, which increases the serum level of digoxin. Both the digoxin toxicity and hypokalemia must be resolved, especially if Ryan has to have surgical repair of his defect.

7. **Ryan's cardiologist determines that Ryan's atrial septal defect (ASD) should be surgically repaired. What preoperative assessment data are required prior to Ryan's surgery?**
   a. Electrocardiogram
   b. Serum cardiac enzymes
   c. Serum electrolyte levels
   d. Complete blood count
   e. Coagulation studies
   f. Chest x-ray

g. Echocardiogram
h. Cardiac catheterization
i. Pulmonary function test
j. Urinalysis

8. **What are the priorities for Ryan's preoperative care?**
   a. Altered cardiac output related to congenital heart defect and adverse effects of digoxin
   b. Deficient fluid volume related to adverse effects of furosemide therapy
   c. Imbalanced nutrition: less than body requirements related to inadequate intake secondary to fatigue
   d. Deficient knowledge, parental, related to surgical treatment, postoperative care, and home care

9. **Discuss the potential complications associated with open heart surgery performed on an infant.**
   a. Cardiac dysrhythmias secondary to stopping the heart so that repair can be done
   b. Hypothermia secondary to the decrease in environmental temperature to decrease metabolic demands
   c. Respiratory failure related to imposed atelectasis secondary to surgical opening of the thoracic cavity
   d. Hemorrhage secondary to tissue trauma in the heart resulting from surgical assault
   e. Organ failure secondary to impaired tissue perfusion
   f. CVA secondary to damaged red blood cells from passage through cardiopulmonary bypass machine
   g. Pleural effusion secondary to fluid accumulation in the pleural cavity due to inactivity

10. **Ryan's parents are very anxious about his surgery and expressing concern about what they are going to see when they get to visit him in the pediatric critical care unit after his surgery. How can the nurse intervene to help Ryan's parents prepare for their visit?** The nurse should explain what equipment they will see in the PICU. These include cardiac, arterial blood gas, pulse oximetry, and central venous pressure monitoring devices as well as the tubes in and around Ryan. Initially he will have an endotracheal tube and will be on mechanical ventilation until he warms up and is able to exchange gases on his own. This usually takes only 6–8 hours. He will have a nasogastric tube for gastric decompression so he will not develop an ileus secondary to surgery. He will have a central venous access for intravenous fluids and central venous pressure (CVP) monitoring. Ryan will have an indwelling catheter to monitor his urine output, an indicator of cardiac output. Further he will have an arterial line to monitor his blood pH. He will have chest tubes including a pericardial chest tube, all connected to wall suction through a water-sealed system. He will have pacemaker wires in case he develops dysrhythmias during the immediate postoperative period. Ryan's parents should be aware that the critical care area will be very active and that the nurse–client ratio is one nurse to one client in the pediatric critical care unit.

11. **His parents express great concern about Ryan's pain management following surgery. They've heard "some doctors don't think infants feel that much pain and what they do feel they don't remember." They have talked to Ryan's surgeon, who has attempted to reassure them that Ryan will be adequately medicated to control his pain after surgery. What should the nurse do in response to their concerns?** The nurse can reassure Ryan's parents by explaining that he will still be experiencing the analgesic effects of anesthesia for 24 hours following surgery. He also will be medicated (usually fentanyl) while he is on mechanical ventilation, and this medication is a potent analgesic. The nurse then needs to determine what analgesia Ryan's surgeon will be prescribing. If the surgeon does not prescribe an opioid analgesic (morphine sulfate is the agent of choice for moderate to severe pain in children), the nurse needs to collaborate with the surgeon to obtain this prescription. At this point the nurse can provide the parents with information backed by years of research indicating that morphine sulfate is both safe and effective for postoperative pain and the agent of choice in children.

12. **Ryan successfully undergoes open heart surgery to repair his ASD. Discuss the reason and purpose of the chest tubes placed in Ryan.** The pericardial chest tube removes drainage from the pericardial sac to prevent cardiac tamponade. Cardiac tamponade occurs when the pressure within the pericardial sac exceeds the pressure within the heart, rendering the heart unable to contract and maintain cardiac output and tissue perfusion. The chest tubes (see Fig. A-12) serve to help reinflate the lungs, which collapsed when the thoracic cavity

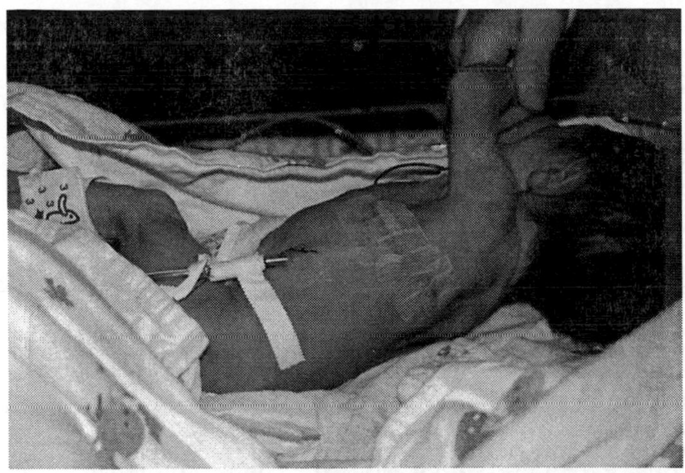

Figure A-12 *Thoracotomy incision with a chest tube in an infact after repair of ASD.*

was entered and environmental pressure exceeded thoracic pressure. The closed drainage system provides suction to remove air that entered the pleural cavity during surgery and to remove drainage that resulted from the trauma to the lung capillaries when the lungs collapsed. As the water seal system suctions drainage and air from the pleural cavity, the lungs are able to reinflate as the pressure within the pleural cavity becomes less than the pressure within the lungs.

13. What are the nursing responsibilities associated with the care of Ryan's chest tubes? The nurse is responsible for maintaining the closed water seal system, maintaining the prescribed suction to remove air and fluid for the pleural cavity and pericardial sac, and monitoring the chest tube drainage. If the drainage exceeds 25 mL/hour for the first 4 hours postoperatively, it represents hemorrhage that can progress to shock and death. The nurse needs to maintain an occlusive dressing over the chest tube insertion sites and tapes the connections between the chest tubes and the drainage system to prevent air leaks that break the integrity of the water-seal system. The drainage systems must remain below the level of the chest and be properly anchored to the floor to prevent them from tipping over, which would result in inaccurate drainage reading. Breath sounds must be auscultated, and the child prepared for chest radiology to determine the progress of lung reinflation.

14. What are the priorities of care for Ryan during his postoperative stay in the pediatric critical care unit?

- **a.** Ineffective tissue perfusion related to hypothermia secondary to cardiac surgery
- **b.** Impaired gas exchange related to atelectasis secondary to thoracic surgery
- **c.** Risk for altered cardiac output related to cardiac dysrhythmias secondary to surgery
- **d.** Risk for ineffective tissue perfusion related to blood loss during and following surgery
- **e.** Acute pain related to tissue trauma secondary to surgery
- **f.** Risk for injury, thrombosis formation related to erythrocyte damage secondary to cardiopulmonary bypass machine
- **g.** Risk for infection related to impaired skin integrity and multiple invasive lines
- **h.** Disturbed sleep pattern related to critical care environment activity and sounds
- **i.** Deficient knowledge related to postoperative care and course

15. Discuss nursing interventions to meet the goals of care for Ryan.

- **a.** Tissue perfusion
  - **(1)** Maintain hemodynamic monitoring and evaluate tissue perfusion.
  - **(2)** Assess neurological status continuously during warming period and every 4 hours during postcritical care period.
  - **(3)** Monitor body temperature continuously using skin probe.

(4) Maintain heating blankets and mattress (if used) until body temperature returns to within normal limits (WNL).
(5) Maintain warming control on mechanical ventilation.
(6) Monitor chest tube drainage hourly and report if drainage exceeds 25 mL/hour.
(7) Maintain patency of intravenous access, monitoring hourly.
(8) Maintain hydration with intravenous fluids as prescribed.
(9) Monitor urinary output hourly.
(10) Administer medications prescribed to support tissue perfusion.
(11) Administer blood transfusions as prescribed and indicated by lab values.
(12) Administer oxygen through ventilator and then by nasal cannula after mechanical ventilation discontinued, titrating to pulse oximetry as prescribed and according to respiratory status.
(13) Provide as calm and relaxed an environment as possible to decrease oxygen demand.

b. Gas exchange/airway clearance
(1) Assess breath sounds for endotracheal tube placement every hour while the client is on mechanical ventilation.
(2) Maintain mechanical ventilation settings and titrate according to facility protocols and health care provider's guidelines, coordinating care with the respiratory therapist.
(3) Monitor pulse oximetry and respiratory status continuously.
(4) Assess breath sounds hourly during mechanical ventilation and report adventitious breath sounds.
(5) Suction according to facility procedure and established standards for endotracheal suctioning of pediatric client as needed while the client is on mechanical ventilation NOTE: Avoid oversuctioning that can result in bronchospasms, stimulate secretion of mucus, and damage to airway tissues.
(6) Maintain chest tube drainage system as prescribed according to facility protocol and manufacturer's instructions.

c. Cardiac output
(1) Maintain continuous hemodynamic monitoring and pulse oximetry and evaluate continuously.
(2) Assess mediastinal chest tube drainage and report drainage >25 mL/hour during first 4 hours.
(3) Monitor for cardiac tamponade.
(4) Monitor urine output hourly.
(5) Assess for manifestations of fluid overload.
(6) Assess breath sounds hourly.
(7) Administer diuretics and cardiac agents to reduce afterload as prescribed.
(8) Palpate liver every shift.
(9) Administer humidified oxygen, titrating to pulse oximetry and respiratory status.

d. Acute pain
(1) Assess for nonverbal cues of pain hourly.
(2) Collaborate with health care provider to ensure client has adequate pain control.
(3) Assess family's attitude about pain medications and provide accurate information to dispel fears of addiction.
(4) Stress to parents the need to use pain medication routinely throughout hospitalization and as needed after Ryan returns home.

e. Risk for injury, thrombus formation
(1) Maintain hemodynamic monitoring.
(2) Assess for signs of altered tissue perfusion due to emboli (difficulty breathing, changes in neurologic status).
(3) Administer heparin sodium as prescribed.

f. Risk for infection
(1) Monitor body temperature during hospitalization.
(2) Assess incisions for redness, swelling, drainage, and approximation of incision borders.
(3) Provide incision care according to facility protocol.
(4) Administer antibiotics if prescribed.

g. Disturbed sleep pattern
   (1) Monitor Ryan's sleep pattern.
   (2) Encourage Ryan's parents to stay with Ryan as much as they wish within the constraints of the critical care unit and without constraints once he is transferred out of critical care.
   (3) Maintain a calm, quiet environment within the constraints of the critical care unit.
   (4) Provide 3- to 4-hour periods of undisturbed sleep during the night coordinating vital signs, medication administration, and feedings to minimize sleep disturbances.
   (5) Coordinate respiratory therapy, physical therapy, and nursing care during the day to provide for periods of undisturbed rest.
   (6) Control nursing unit noise.

h. Deficient knowledge, parental
   (1) Refer to Answer to question #10.
   (2) Explain all care and equipment used in care of client.
   (3) Encourage verbalization of feelings.
   (4) Encourage parents to ask questions and provide honest answers, referring questions to appropriate sources as needed.

16. Ryan is transferred from the pediatric critical care unit to the pediatric surgical unit. Five days later his parents are preparing to take him home. Discuss the teaching priorities for Ryan's parents prior to his discharge.

a. Assess the parents' current level of knowledge regarding home care.

b. Provide verbal and written instruction regarding:
   (1) Gradual return of activity
   (2) Incision care
   (3) Medication administration and compliance
   (4) Importance of telling other health care providers and dentists about open heart surgery history before they provide care
   (5) Importance of receiving antibiotics prior to any dental procedures
   (6) Signs and symptoms to report to health care provider
   (7) Importance of follow-up care with cardiac surgeon

c. Collaborate with other members of the health care team to initiate referrals as needed.

d. Allow sufficient time for Ryan's parents to ask questions, answering them honestly.

e. Document teaching and parent's response and interactions with Ryan

References

American Heart Association. *http://www.americanheart.org*

Broyles, B.E. (2005). *Medical-Surgical nursing clinical companion.* Durham, NC: Carolina Academic Press.

Congenital Heart Defects. *http://www.kidhealth.org*

Congenital Heart Information Network. *http://www.tchin.org*

Daniels, R. (2002). *Delmar's manual of laboratory and diagnostic tests.* Clifton Park, NY: Thomson Delmar Learning.

North American Nursing Diagnosis Association. (2005). *Nursing diagnoses: Definitions & classifications, 2005–2006.* Philadelphia: NANDA.

Potts, N. and Mandleco, B. (2002). *Pediatric nursing: Caring for children and their families.* Clifton Park, NY: Thomson Delmar Learning, pp. 759–761.

Reiss, B.S., Evans, M.E., and Broyles, B.E. (2002). *Pharmacological aspects of nursing care.* (6th ed.). Clifton Park, NY: Thomson Delmar Learning.

Spratto, G.R. and Woods, A.L. (2005). *2005 Edition PDR: Nurse's drug handbook.* Clifton Park, NY: Thomson Delmar Learning.

Wong, D.L., Perry, S.E., and Hockenberry, M.J. (2002). *Maternal child nursing care* (2nd ed.). St. Louis: Mosby, p. 1310.

CASE STUDY 4

Sean

GENDER

M

AGE

1 month old

SETTING

- Hospital

ETHNICITY

- White American

CULTURAL CONSIDERATIONS

PREEXISTING CONDITIONS

COEXISTING CONDITIONS

SIGNIFICANT HISTORY

COMMUNICATION

DISABILITY

SOCIOECONOMIC

- Middle class

SPIRITUAL

PHARMACOLOGIC

- Antibiotics during pregnancy

PSYCHOSOCIAL

- Parental anxiety

LEGAL

ETHICAL

ALTERNATIVE THERAPY

PRIORITIZATION

- Yes

DELEGATION

- Yes

THE CARDIOVASCULAR SYSTEM

Level of difficulty: Difficult

Overview: This case requires knowledge of organ transplantation, immunosuppressant therapy, growth and development, as well as parent–child attachment relationship.

Client Profile

Sean is the first child for John and Jenny, a 27-year-old couple who live in a suburb of a large city. Jenny's pregnancy was uneventful until the eighth month of Sean's gestation, when Jenny developed a severe respiratory infection that required 10 days of antibiotic therapy. At 40 weeks' gestation Sean was born weighing 3 kg (6 lb, 8 oz) and was 47.5 (19 in.) long. Jenny planned to breast feed and had quit her part-time job to stay home with her baby. Sean's Apgar scores at 1 minute and 5 minutes were 4 and 6, respectively, so he was admitted to the neonatal intensive care unit.

Case Study

Sean is stabilized but unable to maintain his oxygen saturation >50% unless receiving 100% oxygen. This treatment sustains an 90% oxygen saturation. Following diagnostic evaluation, Sean is diagnosed with severe hypoplastic left heart syndrome (HLHS). When the pediatric cardiologist explains Sean's heart defect, she explains that she would like to place Sean on an extracorporeal membrane oxygenator (ECMO) and keep him in the hospital until he is 1 month old, if possible, and then perform surgery to repair his heart. After the surgeon leaves, Jenny says to the nurse, "I know this is my fault because of the antibiotics I took last month. I didn't mean to hurt my baby." She begins to cry as John attempts to comfort her.

Questions and Suggested Answers

1. **Describe hypoplastic left heart syndrome (HLHS).** HLHS is a complex congenital heart defect in neonates characterized by severely underdeveloped structures in the left side of the heart. The mitral and aortic valves may be completely closed or have a very small opening. The left ventricle is very small (as opposed to the normal ventricle that is the largest heart chamber) and the aorta is abnormally short. This results in the inability of the left ventricle to maintain cardiac output and tissue perfusion because the ventricle cannot pump a sufficient amount of oxygenated blood into systemic circulation.

2. **What is the appropriate response for the nurse concerning Sean's parents' feelings of guilt?** As with most congenital heart defects, the cause is unknown. In addition, the defect occurs during heart development early in gestation. Fetal circulation is established during the 6th week of gestation and heart development is complete by the 8th week. Antibiotic therapy during the 8th month of pregnancy would not impact on Sean's heart defect development as it was already present at that time. The nurse needs to be compassionate and understand that Sean's parents are experiencing the grief response, which for parents is a common reaction to health alterations in their newborns.

3. **Discuss the clinical manifestations of HLHS.** Cyanosis, as indicated by Sean's Apgar scores, usually is the first sign of HLHS and results in decreased cardiac output of oxygenated blood. Respiratory distress is common as a result from increased blood flow in the lungs that impairs pulmonary function. As with most cardiac defects, a murmur can be heard and represents a leak or shunting of blood. This occurs because the right ventricle's workload is increased to pump more blood into the lungs and out of the ductus arteriosus, which remains patent. The presence of an atrial septal defect also is common with HLHS. The stenosis of the mitral and aortic valves allows only leaking of blood through them and the small lumen and length of the aorta also cause an audible murmur. Sean will be unable to eat because of the energy expenditure required to compensate for decreased cardiac output and respiratory distress. HLHS affects 2–4 out of every 10,000 live births and occurs slightly more often in males than in females. HLHS accounts for 2% to 3% of all congenital heart defects.

4. **How is HLHS diagnosed?**
   a. Cardiac auscultation
   b. Chest x-ray

c. Echocardiogram
d. Cardiac catheterization
Echocardiography is the most common test used to diagnose hypoplastic left heart syndrome.

5. **Discuss nursing interventions specific to the diagnostic tests Sean will undergo.** Other than explaining the procedure for cardiac auscultation, no specific nursing interventions are required. For chest x-ray, the procedure is explained and the nurse holds the neonate very still while he or she wears a lead apron to protect the nurse from the radiation beams. The nurse may be required to help the neonate lie still while echoes are created by the deflection of high-frequency sound waves off the cardiac structures. The parents need to be reassured that the echocardiogram is noninvasive and does not cause any discomfort to their child. If a cardiac catheterization is prescribed, the nurse must maintain the neonate as NPO for at least 4–6 hours prior to the procedure. The parents must sign an informed consent explained by the health care provider. A eutectic mixture of local anesthetics (EMLA) should be applied to both groins 2 hours before the procedure (the right one is usually used; however, if difficulty with it arises, the health care provider may need to use the left groin). The parents should be reassured that the use of EMLA has been shown to be safe and effective on neonates over 36 weeks of gestation. Following the procedure, the nurse must provide post-procedure assessments including vital signs, groin dressing, groin pulse, peripheral pulses, temperature, and color of feet and toes of affected limb every 15 minutes for at least an hour according to facility protocol. The affected leg must be maintained straight to prevent bleeding and hematoma formation. The dressing should be assessed for any evidence of bleeding; even a small spot represents bleeding because the dressing is so thick. These assessments continue for 24 hours with decreasing frequency.

6. **Describe the most commonly used surgical treatment for HLHS.** The most commonly used treatment for HLHS is the surgical creation of a partial internal bypass of blood from the body through lungs. This is accomplished by a three-step procedure called "the Norwood" because the first repair procedure is called the Norwood Procedure, and is usually performed within the first few days of life. The second procedure, performed at 4–6 months of age, is the hemi-Fontan, which sends half of the blood returning from the body to the lungs through a device called a modified Blalock–Taussig shunt, reducing the workload on the right ventricle. This procedure is part of the preparation to convert the hypoplastic left heart into a two-chamber pumping heart that will function to pump blood to the body. The third operation is the Fontan operation that diverts the other half of the blood returning from the body through the lungs instead of the heart. The Fontan is usually performed on children older than 2 or 3 years of age. Following each of these procedures, the infant is closely monitored and may require medication including digoxin and furosemide at least until after the Fontan procedure is completed.

7. **Sean undergoes unsuccessful reconstructive surgery for his HLHS and the decision is made that he needs a heart transplant. How common are heart transplants in children younger than 1 year of age?** Congenital heart disease accounts for 7% to 8% of heart transplants, and the average number performed per year for children younger than 1 year of age is 77, with 72 performed in 2004.

8. **Discuss the complications associated with heart transplants in children.**
   a. Cardiac dysrhythmias
   b. Life-threatening infection
   c. Organ rejection
   d. Fluctuations in blood pressure
   e. Respiratory dysfunction
   f. Gastrointestinal dysfunction
   g. Increased risk of renal failure
   h. Psychosocial maladjustment
   i. Related to lack of sympathetic and parasympathetic stimulation

9. **A donor for Sean was located and plans went into action for Sean to receive his transplant. Discuss the process of matching the donor heart prior to the transplantation into Sean.** The donor heart is harvested from a person who has been declared brain dead, is on life support equipment, has no cardiac pathology, is free of infectious diseases, and is histologically compatible with the recipient. The blood type and tissue must match to prevent rejection of the donor heart. The donor heart must be transplanted into the recipient within 6–8 hours after it has been harvested.

10. **The heart transplant procedure was successful. What is the standard of care to prevent rejection of Sean's transplanted heart?** The standard of care is administering immunosuppressant agents. The most common of these agents include cyclosporine (Sandimmune), azathioprine (Imuran), mycophenolate mofetil hydrochloride (CellCept), muromonab-CD-3 (Orthoclone OKT3), and tacrolimus (Prograf, FK 506). Prednisone is used in conjunction with these agents and cytomegalovirus immune globulin (CMV-IGIV) may be given to prevent potentially serious CMV infection. The immunosuppressant agents suppress the recipient child's immune system so that it will not build up antibodies against the donor heart and are administered on a life-long basis. Unfortunately, the immunosuppressants present the child with a high risk of infection that can be life threatening. Infection is the leading cause of death following heart transplantation (Broyles, 2005).

11. **Discuss the priorities of care for Sean following his heart transplant.**
    a. Risk for decreased cardiac output
        (1) Maintain continuous cardiac monitoring, pulse oximetry, and arterial blood gas monitoring.
        (2) Monitor cardiac output.
        (3) Follow facility protocol for postoperative cardiac transplantation and pediatric critical care.
        (4) Administer medications as prescribed, titrating to prescribed parameters.
        (5) Report any abnormal findings to the transplant team.
        (6) Implement seizure precautions when high-dose steroids are prescribed.
        (7) Wean drips to maintain specific hemodynamic parameters.
        (8) Maintain patency of intravenous access device, monitoring hourly and as needed.
        (9) Administer intravenous volume expanders and blood replacement as prescribed.
        (10) Monitor laboratory values.
        (11) Auscultate heart sounds hourly during the critical period and at least every 4 hours thereafter.
        (12) Monitor peripheral pulses and vital signs according to facility and unit protocol.
        (13) Monitor hourly urine output.
        (14) Maintain a calm and restful environment.
        (15) Encourage parental visitation within the constraints of pediatric critical care.
    b. High risk for infections
        (1) Monitor temperature at least every 4 hours (q 4h).
        (2) Monitor the surgical incision for redness and drainage.
        (3) Maintain compromised host or reverse isolation precautions according to facility protocol.
        (4) Implement neutropenic precautions.
        (5) Limit the number of visitors in Sean's room to two at a time.
        (6) Instruct parents about protective precautions including proper handwashing.
        (7) Notify the health care provider if the temperature exceeds 37.5° C (99.4° F).
        (8) Provide wound care as prescribed.
    c. Risk for injury, complications following transplant
        (1) Monitor for infection (see above).
        (2) Monitor for hypertension and hypotension.
        (3) Monitor respiratory function.
        (4) Monitor renal function.
        (5) Maintain strict intake and output.
        (6) Monitor gastrointestinal function.

(7) Monitor for cardiac changes secondary to lack of sympathetic and parasympathetic stimulation.
(8) Monitor for adverse effects of immunosuppressant therapy including:
   (a) Monitor for infection.
   (b) Do not administer vaccines containing live viruses.
   (c) Monitor intake and output and body weight if Sean is receiving azathioprine.
   (d) Assess Sean for jaundice, fever, fatigue, and bleeding tendencies which are adverse effects of cyclosporine therapy.
   (e) Instruct Sean's parents on effective oral hygiene to minimize gum hyperplasia.
   (f) Monitor complete blood count, white blood cell differential, and platelet counts.
   (g) Monitor urine output.

12. **Discuss the priorities of teaching for Sean's parents during his hospitalization. When should the teaching begin? How can the nurse evaluate the effectiveness of the teaching?** Jenny and John's teaching should commence from the very beginning and should include explanation of all procedures, medications, and care that Sean receives. They should be encouraged to actively participate in his care, and the nurse should encourage and assist Jenny in pumping her breast if she still desires that Sean receive breast milk. Jenny and John should be encouraged to administer Sean's medications as soon as he is taking oral or enteral medications. The nurse should evaluate their ability to administer the medications. Jenny and John should be instructed on infant care including bathing, diaper changing, feeding, and the importance of holding and touching Sean. Provide written as well as verbal information to them about Sean's medications including what the medications are, why they are prescribed for Sean, the medication dosages, and the adverse effects, primarily the high risk for infection. They need to be taught how to monitor Sean's temperature and ways to avoid Sean's exposure to infection risks including limiting visitors, screening visitors for communicable diseases, and sterilization of Sean's bottles. Information concerning follow-up visits after Sean is discharged should be given, including that Sean will undergo follow-up echocardiograms, laboratory studies, and heart biopsy (usually done every 7–10 days for the first month after transplant and every 14 days during the second month while Sean is hospitalized), monthly during months 3–6, and then once every 3 months for an indefinite period. As with all teaching, Jenny and John should have sufficient time for questions and feedback on their care of Sean. They should be active participants in referrals prescribed. Social Services is usually required for financial assistance although most insurance plans pay the majority of the cost of the transplant (may be >$25,000); the life-long immunosuppressant therapy and follow-up will exceed most insurance plans that have a maximum lifetime benefit.

References

Broyles, B.E. (2005). *Medical-surgical nursing clinical companion.* Durham, NC: Carolina Academic Press, p. 403.

Centers for Disease Control and Prevention. *http://www.cdc.gov*

Daniels, R. (2002). *Delmar's manual of laboratory and diagnostic tests.* Clifton Park, NY: Thomson Delmar Learning.

Gahart, B.L. and Nazareno, A.R. (2005). *2005 Intravenous medications* (21st ed.). St. Louis: Mosby.

Hypoplastic Left Heart Syndrome *http://www.cincinnatichildrens.org*

Hypoplastic Left Heart Syndrome Website. *http://www.hlhs.org*

Littleton, L.Y. and Engebretson, J.C. (2002). *Maternal, neonatal, and women's health nursing.* Clifton Park, NY: Thomson Delmar Learning, p. 593.

North American Nursing Diagnosis Association. (2005). *Nursing diagnoses: Definitions & classifications, 2005–2006.* Philadelphia: NANDA.

Organ Procurement and Transplantation Network. *http://www.optn.org*

Potts, N. and Mandleco, B. (2002). *Pediatric nursing: Caring for children and their families.* Clifton Park, NY: Thomson Delmar Learning, pp. 775–777.

CASE STUDY 5

Cassie

GENDER

F

AGE

9

SETTING

- Hospital

ETHNICITY

- Black American

CULTURAL CONSIDERATIONS

PREEXISTING CONDITIONS

COEXISTING CONDITIONS

SIGNIFICANT HISTORY

COMMUNICATION

DISABILITY

SOCIOECONOMIC

- Middle class

SPIRITUAL

PHARMACOLOGIC

PSYCHOSOCIAL

- Mother died 6 years ago
- Parent anxiety
- Client anxiety
- Grieving

LEGAL

ETHICAL

- Do not resuscitate order

ALTERNATIVE THERAPY

PRIORITIZATION

- Yes

DELEGATION

- Client referrals

THE BLOOD

Level of difficulty: Difficult

Overview: This case requires knowledge and understanding of aplastic anemia, the grief response; additional care measures for the grieving family; as well as an understanding of the client's background, personal situation, and father–child relationship.

DIFFICULT

Client Profile

Cassie is a 9-year-old fourth grader who lives in a small community with her father, grandmother, and two older siblings. Cassie's mother died when Cassie was 3 years old and her father and grandmother are raising the children. They are very attentive to all of them, helping the children with their homework and attending their school activities. Cassie's father owns an automobile repair shop and her grandmother is active in the community. During the past 2 months, Cassie, who was always a healthy and active child, has become increasingly more fatigued; her appetite has become poor, and she is no longer interested in school, complaining each school day morning that she is too tired to go to school even though she sleeps 10 hours each night. Previously an A–B student, she is now doing poorly. Both her father and grandmother have noticed that Cassie is bruising easily, coughing frequently, and has a temperature. They are concerned about Cassie and her father makes an appointment with her pediatrician.

Case Study

After visiting her pediatrician, Cassie is admitted to the local hospital for tests to rule out aplastic anemia. Her admission vital signs are:

Temperature: 38° C (100.4° F)
Pulse: 120 beats/minute
Respirations: 30 breaths/minute
Blood pressure: 100/62

Cassie's admission complete blood count is:

Hemoglobin: 8 g/dL
Hematocrit: 25%
Erythrocyte count: 3.1 million/mm^3
Platelet count: 80,000/mm^3
White blood cell count: 900 cells/mm^3
Neutrophils: 630 cells/mm^3
Lymphocytes: 180 cells/mm^3
Monocytes: 63 cells/mm^3
Eosinophils: 18 cells/mm^3
Basophils: 9 cells/mm^3

Questions and Suggested Answers

1. **What other information would help you gain a full impression about Cassie's situation?**
   - **a.** Cassie's assessment information from the nurse who admitted her
   - **b.** Her oxygen saturation
   - **c.** Iron level
   - **d.** Bone marrow aspiration—the definitive diagnostic test for aplastic anemia
   - **e.** Chest x-ray
   - **f.** Urinalysis and culture and sensitivity
2. **What is the significance of Cassie's lab values and vital signs?** All of Cassie's lab values are abnormally low. The normal hemoglobin for a child her age is 11–16 g/dL. The normal hematocrit is 31% to 41%. The normal

red blood cell (RBC) count is 4.5–4.8 million cells/mm^3; normal platelet count is 150,000–450,000 cells/mm^3; and the normal white blood cell count is 4,100–10,800 cells/mm^3 (Daniels, 2002). Her lab values suggest anemia, thrombocytopenia, and leukopenia. These are consistent with aplastic anemia, which is a condition of bone marrow depression causing a dramatic reduction in the manufacturing of cells (erythrocytes, platelets, and leukocytes). The white blood cell differential is consistent in percentage with the normal percentages of these granulocytes.

The normal temperature for a child Cassie's age is 36.7–36.8° C (98°–98.2° F); normal pulse rate is 70–110 beats/minute; normal respiratory rate is 16–20 breaths/minute; and minimum normal blood pressure is 109/71. Cassie is febrile, suggesting the presence of an infection; her pulse rate indicates tachycardia, which is a compensatory mechanism in the presence of ineffective tissue perfusion. She is tachypneic, which accompanies the tachycardia, and she is hypotensive, which is consistent with what you would expect given her hemoglobin, hematocrit, and erythrocyte count.

3. **Discuss the three types of aplastic anemia.** Aplastic anemia is (1) congenital, (2) acquired, or (3) idiopathic. The pathophysiology of all types is the same. The congenital type is inherited and is referred to as Fanconi's anemia; the acquired type may occur from contact with chemotherapy, other chemicals, and/or radiation therapy. Cassie has no history to indicate contracting aplastic anemia by contact with these agents. Idiopathic aplastic anemia is the most common type and is so named because the cause of this type is unknown.

4. **Discuss the incidence of and prognosis for aplastic anemia.** Aplastic anemia has a low incidence, occurring in four persons/million. Thirty percent of childhood cases are congenital in origin. Thirty percent of acquired cases result from chemical or radiation exposure and 70% of acquired cases are idiopathic. The mortality rate for aplastic anemia is high, with fewer than 10% of acquired cases recovering spontaneously and only 10% to 20% of all cases recovering at all.

5. **Identify the priorities of care for Cassie.**
   a. Risk for infection related to decreased white blood cell count secondary to bone marrow depression
   b. Risk for injury and bleeding related to decreased platelets secondary to thrombocytopenia
   c. Ineffective tissue perfusion related to decreased erythrocytes secondary to bone marrow depression
   d. Anticipatory grieving related to the poor prognosis of this disease
   e. Deficient knowledge related to child's condition, treatment, prognosis, and home care

6. **Discuss the treatment you anticipate for Cassie.** The focus of medical management is to determine the cause, if possible, and eliminate it. As most cases are idiopathic, removing the cause is not possible. The immediate focus is to treat the infection with antimicrobials, specific to the location of the infection and usually involving broad-spectrum antibiotics because of the decreased white blood cells. To replace red blood cells and platelets, transfusion of packed red blood cells and units of platelets is standard. "The use of immunosuppressant therapy with antithymocyte globulin (ATG), a horse serum polyclonal antibodies against human T-cells, and cyclosporine has dramatically improved outcomes." (Broyles, 2005). The success of this therapy is related to aplastic anemia being an immune-mediated condition. The use of epoetin alfa recombinant may be indicated in the supportive management of aplastic anemia to increase red blood cells and improve tissue perfusion. Oxygen therapy will help tissue perfusion, as well. Further lab testing is needed to determine the effectiveness of therapy or to indicate a decline in Cassie's condition. Intravenous fluids of isotonic volume expanders will help increase vascular volume. In serious cases, medications to maintain Cassie's blood pressure may be required. Finally, bone marrow transplantation may be a last resort as long as a human leukocyte antigen-matched donor can be found.

7. **Discuss the nursing responsibilities prior to and during Cassie's blood products administration.** The following are standards of care; however, the exact procedure is based on facility protocol: The nurse must be sure that Cassie's blood is typed and cross-matched and that these lab results are current according to facility protocols. Many children are premedicated with diphenhydramine and acetaminophen prior to the transfusion. The nurse must be sure that Cassie's intravenous access is adequate for infusion of blood. The equipment

must be collected including a volumetric intravenous infusion pump and blood administration tubing. The tubing must be primed with 0.9% normal saline. Dextrose solutions will cause the blood for transfusion to coagulate. Once the intravenous access has been established, the primed intravenous tubing placed in the volumetric pump, and the nurse has verified that the access is patent, the nurse needs to delegate to another staff member (clerk, nursing assistant, licensed practical nurse) to retrieve the unit of packed red blood cells and bring it immediately to Cassie's room. Vital signs must be taken prior to initiating the transfusion. They may be obtained by the nurse or may be delegated to an appropriately trained staff member. The nurse must then verify the blood products, client identification, blood expiration date, blood type, and blood unit number with another licensed professional. The vital signs and verification must be documented on the appropriate facility forms. At this time the unit of red blood cells is started. In children, the initial rate of infusion is one third to one half the estimated hourly rate for the first 15–30 minutes of the transfusion to decrease the severity of a transfusion reaction. All clients receiving blood transfusions must be monitored continuously during the initial 15–30 minutes of the transfusion, as this is the most likely period during which a transfusion reaction will occur. If reaction occurs, the nurse immediately stops the transfusion while maintaining patency of intravenous access with 0.9% normal saline and notifies the health care provider. Any unit containing RBCs must be infused within 4 hours after hanging the unit, so the rate of administration needs to be based on this guideline. If the infusion is not complete within 4 hours, the remaining blood must be discontinued. Children must be monitored for fluid overload, and following the blood infusion, post-transfusion vital signs must be obtained and documented. Follow-up lab values are prescribed after blood has been transfused and it is the nurse's responsibility to ensure that these tests are completed. Platelets are administered at a much more liberal rate and without the risk of the transfusion reaction associated with red blood cell transfusion because platelets do not carry antibodies. If multiple transfusion of platelets is prescribed, all the units can be obtained at the same time and infused one right after the other. Follow-up platelet count is required to evaluate the effectiveness of treatment.

8. **Cassie does not respond to treatment and after a bone marrow transplant fails, her condition worsens as her lab values decline. How can you respond to her father and grandmother when they ask if she is going to die?** The nurse needs to clarify their question and follow-up with their reasons for believing that Cassie is going to die. The nurse needs to encourage the father and grandmother to express their feelings. Further, she needs to collaborate with the health care provider to discuss Cassie's prognosis with them. This follow-up needs to be timely so that the father and grandmother are not left with unanswered questions. When the health care provider addresses his or her concerns with them, the nurse needs to be present as a liaison and client/family advocate and to be aware of what the health care provider and Cassie's family discuss.

9. **Cassie's health care provider tells her father and grandmother that Cassie's condition is terminal. They say they want to take her home to die, but the health care provider is reluctant. How might you feel in a similar situation if Cassie was your child?** Each student will have a personal answer. Most will express that they also might want to gain some control over this situation by taking the child back to her familiar home environment. Some may express that they would want the child to remain in the hospital rather than face the emotional stress of the child dying at home. There is not a right or wrong answer here as long as the student provides a rationale for the answer. The legal implications also must be addressed. With a "do not resuscitate" status agreed upon between the health care provider and the child's father, the hospital and health care provider would avoid potential liability of letting the father take the child home.

10. **Cassie's father and grandmother prepare to take Cassie home. What referrals might benefit this family and what is the nurse's role as client advocate?** With a "do not resuscitate" order, the most appropriate referral would be to Hospice. For Hospice to become an active option, the family must decide that they do not anticipate pursuing any aggressive treatment for Cassie. Hospice believes that all clients have the right to die without pain and with dignity. They actively work with the family to assist in the grieving process and provide services to help the family care for Cassie at home. Once Hospice is involved, they assume care responsibility in collaboration with the family. Following the child's death, Hospice continues to follow up with the family

to assist them with the grieving process. Encouraging the family to seek support for their spiritual needs is an important nursing responsibility, as is involving Social Services to help the family with financial concerns so they can focus their energy on caring for the child. If Hospice is determined not to be an appropriate referral at this time, Social Services can help the family with needed equipment to care for Cassie at home.

References

Broyles, B.E. (2005). *Medical-surgical nursing clinical companion.* Durham, NC: Carolina Academic Press.

Centers for Disease Control and Prevention. *http://www.cdc.gov*

Daniels, R. (2002). *Delmar's manual of laboratory and diagnostic tests.* Clifton Park, NY: Thomson Delmar Learning.

Gahart, B.L. and Nazareno, A.R. (2005). *2005 Intravenous medications* (21st ed.). St. Louis: Mosby.

Hospice Foundation of America. *http://www.hospicefoundation.org*

Intravenous Therapy. *http://www.nursewise.com*

Josephson, D.L. (2004). *Intravenous infusion therapy for nurses: Principles & practice* (2nd ed.). Clifton Park, NY: Thomson Delmar Learning.

North American Nursing Diagnosis Association. (2005). *Nursing diagnoses: Definitions & classifications, 2005–2006.* Philadelphia: NANDA.

Potts, N. and Mandleco, B. (2002). *Pediatric nursing: Caring for children and their families.* Clifton Park, NY: Thomson Delmar Learning, pp. 826–829.

Wong, D.L., Perry, S.E., and Hockenberry, M.J. (2002). *Maternal child nursing care* (2nd ed.). St. Louis: Mosby, pp. 1365–1366.

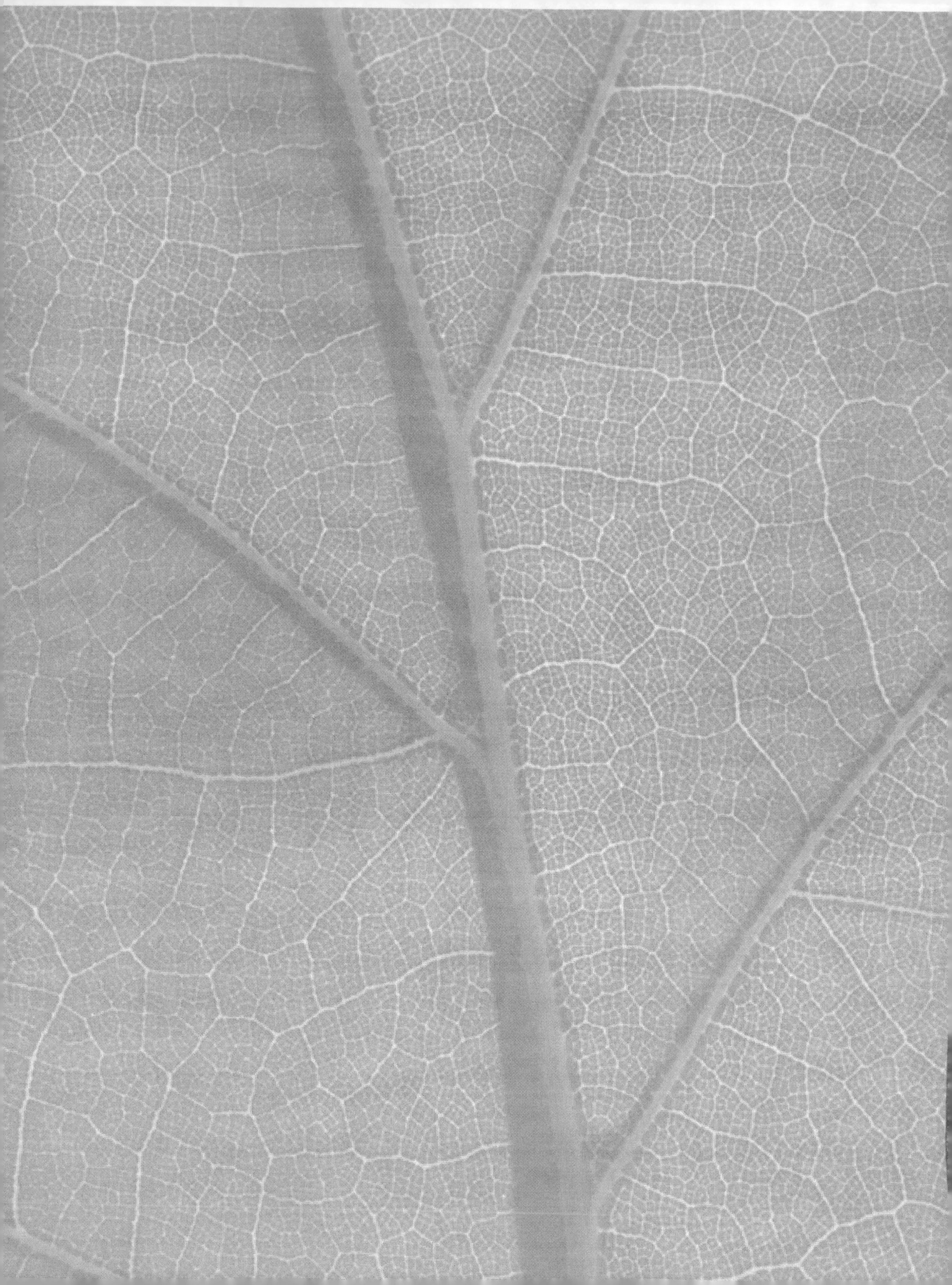

PART FOUR

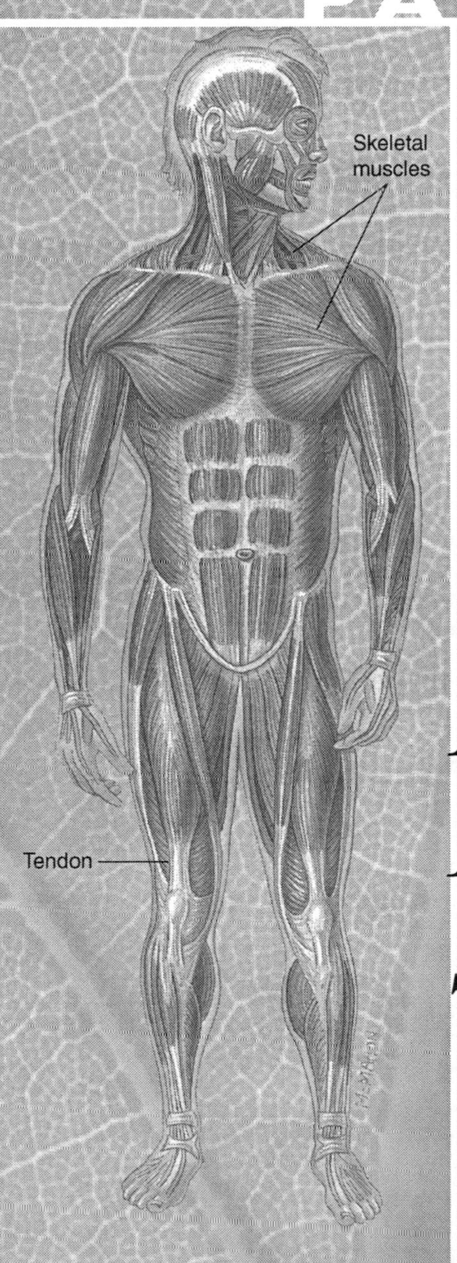

The Skeletal, Muscular, and Integumentary Systems

CASE STUDY 1

Julie

GENDER

F

AGE

5

SETTING

- Hospital

ETHNICITY

- Asian American

CULTURAL CONSIDERATIONS

PREEXISTING CONDITIONS

- Burns

COEXISTING CONDITIONS

SIGNIFICANT HISTORY

COMMUNICATION

DISABILITY

SOCIOECONOMIC

- Middle class

SPIRITUAL

PHARMACOLOGIC

- Fentanyl (Sublimaze)

PSYCHOSOCIAL

- Family anxiety
- Grief

LEGAL

ETHICAL

ALTERNATIVE THERAPY

PRIORITIZATION

- Yes

DELEGATION

- Yes

THE INTEGUMENTARY SYSTEMS

Level of difficulty: Difficult

Overview: This case requires knowledge of burns and related care, the grief response, the client's background and personal situation, as well as the mother–child attachment relationship.

Client Profile

Julie is a 5-year-old girl who lives in North Carolina with her parents and two siblings, a 3-year old brother and an 18-month-old sister. Her father works at a brokerage firm in Raleigh and her mother stays at home to care for the children. Julie has never had any health problems other than occasional episodes of the common cold.

Case Study

Julie and her parents were returning home from a family visit 4 weeks ago when they were involved in a motor vehicle accident resulting in an explosion that caused their car to become engulfed in flames. Julie's mother, who was sitting in the back seat with the children, perished in the fire while trying to save the children. Her father and two younger siblings escaped serious injury; however, Julie sustained third-degree burns over 80% of her body and was admitted to the Jaycee Burn Center. She was intubated and placed on mechanical ventilation. Currently she is no longer on mechanical ventilation and has a tracheostomy from which the nursing staff suctions thick green-yellow secretions every 2–3 hours. Julie is receiving total parenteral nutrition (TPN) and intralipids (IL) through a central venous access. Julie has severe wounds to her face, neck, left arm (necessitating the amputation of her left hand), left leg (necessitating a below-the-knee amputation), and back requiring extensive wound and graft care. She is premedicated with intravenous fentanyl prior to each dressing change, and this provides adequate pain management for these procedures.

Julie's father visits frequently. Julie is aware of the death of her mother and tends to be withdrawn and has had episodes of crying during which time she could not be consoled.

Questions and Suggested Answers

1. **Discuss the classifications and types of burns and how burns are measured to determine the percentage of body surface area involved.** Burns are classified according to depth of penetration. These include:
   - **a.** *First-degree (superficial)* involving the destruction of the epidermis although physiological functions may remain intact
   - **b.** *Second-degree (partial thickness)* involving the destruction of the epidermis and some (superficial) or all (deep) of the dermis resulting in loss of function
   - **c.** *Third-degree (full-thickness)* characterized by destruction of the epidermis, dermis, and underlying tissue including the fascia and into the muscle
   - **d.** *Fourth-degree (full-thickness)* that include destruction through the muscle and also may include tendons and bone injuries (see Fig. A-13).

   According to the "Estimation of the Extent of Burns in Children" chart used by many burn centers and the Shriners' facilities in particular, Kyla's burn percentage of total body surface area (TBSA) was estimated by:

   Right buttocks = 2½%
   Left buttocks = 2½%
   Genitalia = 1%
   Right thigh = 5½%
   Left thigh = 5½%
   Right leg = 5%
   Left leg = 5%
   Right foot = 3½%
   Left foot = 3½%

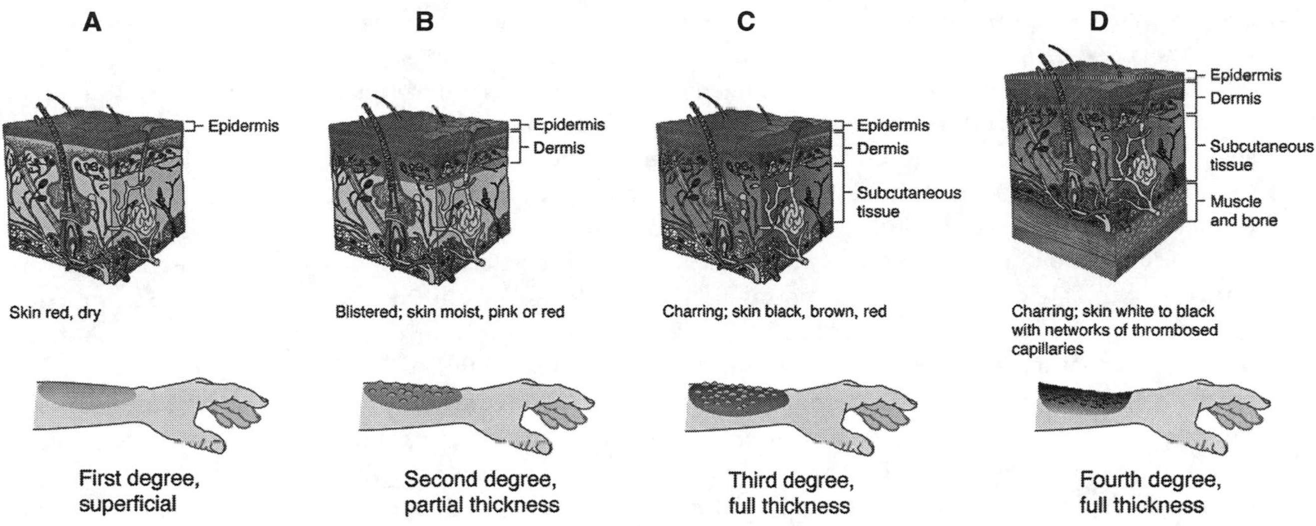

Figure A-13 *Skin layers involved in burn injuries: A, First-degree burn; B, Second–degree burn; C, Third-degree burn; D, Fourth-degree burn.*

2. Identify the negative and positive factors affecting Julie's prognosis and her chances of survival.

Negative factors:

- **a.** Third-degree burns over 80% of her body that result in fluid and electrolyte imbalances
- **b.** Receiving total parenteral nutrition, which indicates she is unable to take foods and fluids orally
- **c.** Her growth and development level (preschooler)
- **d.** Inactivity/immobility
- **e.** The emotional impact of her mother's death

Positive factors:

- **a.** Her health status prior to sustaining her injuries
- **b.** Being cared for at a facility that specializes in the care of burn victims where she is receiving meticulous skin care and rehabilitation
- **c.** Surviving the first 3 weeks post-burn

Julie continues to have a high risk for life-threatening infections and fluid and electrolyte imbalances. Of the more than 20,000 victims of major burns, 10,000 die annually of burn-related infections. According to the Centers for Disease Control and Prevention, children older than 5 years of age have the same mortality statistics as adults; however, children under 5 years old have a higher mortality than adults. Since 1998, more than 50% of all individuals with burns over 80% of their total body surface have survived (*http://www.ameriburn.org*). Hypertrophic scarring (raised areas of skin) is more severe in children, requiring the use of pressure garments 24 hours a day for at least a year.

3. Why is Julie at high risk for developing an infection? Julie has lost skin integrity over 80% of her body, resulting in loss of the major protection the body has against microorganism invasion—intact skin. The major cause of death from burns after the first 24–48 hours is infection. Julie has a tracheostomy that increases her risk of microorganisms entering her respiratory tract. Her condition places her at risk for complications of inactivity including hypostatic pneumonia. In addition, she has a central venous access and is receiving total parenteral nutrition (TPN) and intralipids. The major complication of each of these is infection. The central venous access involves a break in skin integrity and a catheter entering systemic circulation. Because the base solution for TPN usually is 50% but in burn victims may be as high as 70%, this creates an excellent medium for bacteria. In addition, the amino acids in the TPN favor growth of microorganisms. To closely monitor her fluid balance, a Foley catheter is a standard of care for children, which further increases her risk of infection. Finally, being in a health care facility poses the risk of nosocomial infections.

4. **Discuss Julie's needs regarding her tracheostomy.** Julie requires tracheal suctioning following assessment of respiratory indications that suctioning is necessary. These indications include increased respiratory rate, decrease in oxygen saturation (per pulse oximetry) to below prescribed parameters, and auditory evidence of mucus in the tracheostomy tube. Suctioning should be accomplished using sterile technique and approved suctioning guidelines for children (each catheter pass should not exceed 5–10 seconds). Between each pass of the catheter, the catheter should be rinsed with sterile normal saline. Tracheostomy care should be performed according to facility protocol at every shift and as indicated by client assessment. Tracheostomy site care is established by each facility and addressed in either a procedure or protocol format. The usual site care involves donning clean gloves and removing fenestrated dressing from the tracheostomy site. The prepackaged tracheostomy care kit is then opened and hydrogen peroxide is poured into a sterile container and normal saline is poured into another sterile container. Sterile cotton-tipped applicators are moistened in the normal saline and sterile gloves are donned. The skin around the tracheostomy is cleaned and the swabs discarded. If the tracheostomy consists of an inner cannula and an outer cannula, the inner cannula is gently removed and placed in the hydrogen peroxide. At this time the inner cannula is cleaned and then rinsed in the sterile normal saline. Facility procedures vary at this point as to whether the inner cannula is dried with sterile pipe cleaners and gauze or replaced in the outer cannula without drying (allowing for ease in replacing the inner cannula). A fenestrated dressing is applied to keep the skin around the tracheostomy clean and the ties are changed if needed. Many facilities now are using Velcro fasteners on the tracheostomy collars, replacing the fabric ties. Sterile gloves are removed and the nurse's hands washed.

5. **Discuss TPN, including general care and special nutritional needs of children with burn injuries.** TPN solution is changed every 24 hours, at which time all tubing also should changed. This process should be done using sterile technique. TPN and intralipid solutions are prescribed each day and the nurse must check each container of TPN with the prescribed solution. The usual dose of TPN for children is 1.5–3 g of amino acid products every 24 hours and dextrose ranging from 100–300 kcal/kg per day. Children with burn injuries require higher levels of amino acids and dextrose in their TPN solutions because of the increased metabolism present. Nutritional requirements for a client with major burns are two to three times the normal nutritional intake. TPN and intralipids require administration via a central venous access because of the high concentration of dextrose (>10%) and tubing containing a filter. TPN can be administered without intralipids; however, intralipids must not be infused without TPN because of the high risk of fat embolism formation. Multiple lab studies are monitored before, during, and after TPN. Among these are blood urea nitrogen (BUN); complete blood count (CBC); platelet count; creatinine; electrolytes (sodium, potassium, chloride, magnesium, calcium, glucose); triglycerides; cholesterol; albumin; bilirubin; and liver function tests (especially ammonia levels in children). Julie must be weighed daily at the same time under similar conditions. Urine checks for glucose or blood capillary testing should be done every 6 hours throughout the course of TPN. Central venous catheter (CVAD) care (dressing changes) should be performed using aseptic technique and is recommended every 48–72 hours. The nurse should follow the facility guidelines for care (flushing of CVAD, blood draws) and dressing changes. Enteral feedings are preferred over TPN and intralipids; however, children with major burns such as Julie's require TPN because nutritional needs during the acute phase of a major burn exceed what can be tolerated enterally. Enteral feedings, however, should be started as soon as possible so Julie can be weaned from the TPN and intralipids. This will remove one factor that increases her risk for infection.

6. **What is the relationship between Julie's fluid and electrolyte balance and her burn status?** Intact skin helps prevent fluid loss from evaporation and with 80% of the body experiencing third-degree burns, she loses fluids, electrolytes, and plasma protein. Plasma protein is required to maintain vascular osmotic pressure so that adequate fluids remain in vascular volume to provide tissue perfusion. This placed Julie at risk of burn shock (a form of hypovolemic shock) due to loss of interstitial and vascular fluids that stimulate the inflammatory response, resulting in more body fluids being sent to the injured area. As more body fluids rush to the injury, more are lost through evaporation through the damaged skin. Aggressive fluid resuscitation is necessary to maintain fluid balance and urine output of 0.5–1.0 mL/kg of body weight per hour (for severe burns).

7. **Discuss why fentanyl has been chosen for pain management for Julie's dressing changes.** Dressing changes following burns cause severe pain. Morphine sulfate and fentanyl are opioid analgesics and are standards of care for pain control in burn clients. Fentanyl is 100 times more effective for acute pain than morphine; however, it carries a much higher risk for respiratory depression than morphine. If adequate pain management is not maintained for Julie, midazolam hydrochloride (Versed) may be used in conjunction with morphine sulfate to produce conscious sedation for dressing changes. Julie must be monitored continuously during dressing changes for altered respiratory function whether fentanyl or midazolam HCl is used.

8. **Discuss how Julie's level of growth and development could affect her ability to cope with her mother's death.** According to Erikson, Julie's growth and development level is that of a preschooler. He identified the developmental task of Julie's age group as initiative versus guilt. The two major driving forces for preschoolers are socialization and imagination. Imagination is a positive trait of preschoolers, as it allows for imaginary playmates to provide socialization opportunities in the absence of other children, pets, or social interactions.

   Imagination in the preschooler also is the root of potential guilt feelings. They believe if something "bad" happens, it is the direct result of something they said, thought, or did. Julie may be experiencing feelings of guilt about her mother's death even though she had nothing to do with the accident. Nurses need to be familiar with growth and development for Julie to reassure her that she was in no way responsible for her mother's death.

9. **What nursing interventions could help Julie cope with her hospitalization?**
   a. Use measures to ensure pain control.
      (1) Monitor pain level hourly and more often as needed.
      (2) Collaborate with the health care provider to provide adequate pain management according to nurse's assessment of Julie. REMEMBER: Pain is what the client says it is.
      (3) Position for comfort, gently changing positions every 1–2 hours.
      (4) Gently perform passive range-of-motion exercises to prevent painful contractures.
      (5) Provide guided imagery, relaxation techniques, and diversional activities in collaboration with pediatric recreational therapists.
   b. Reassure Julie, using terminology appropriate for her level of growth and development.
   c. Maintain surgical asepsis during dressing changes, tracheostomy suctioning and care, CVAD care, also maintain strict infection control.
   d. Encourage the father to visit as often as possible and participate in Julie's care.
   e. Provide positive feedback to Julie and her father.
   f. Ensure that nursing interactions include spending time with Julie to promote her growth and development and provide support.
   g. Document pertinent observations about Julie's coping.
   h. Collaborate with the health care provider for referral for the child psychologist and pastoral care as appropriate.
   i. Sibling visitation should be limited because of the risk of exposure to communicable diseases in 18-month-olds and 3-year-olds. The 18-month-old would probably not understand what is happening and the 3-year-old with the active preschool imagination may become very traumatized.

10. **Discuss how you might feel in this situation if you were Julie's father.** Most individuals in a similar situation would have feelings of guilt because a loved one died and a child is critically injured. Julie's father may feel that he should have perished instead of his wife because Julie needs her mother more than she needs her father. These feelings are probably compounded because of Julie's perilous condition and the fact that he can't visit as often as he feels he should because he has to work and take care of his 18-month-old daughter. He also must make arrangements for childcare while he is working or visiting Julie in the hospital. This is a very stressful situation for any parent and he probably needs guidance in activating his support systems. The father also may not have health insurance and may be experiencing financial stressors related to Julie's hospitalization.

References

American Burn Association. *http://www.ameriburn.org*

Centers for Disease Control. *http://www.cdc.gov*

Cinicnnati Shriners Hospital, 3229 Burnet Avenue, Cincinnati, OH 45229-3095. (513) 872-6000; FAX (513) 872-6999.

Daniels, R. (2002). *Delmar's manual of laboratory and diagnostic tests.* Clifton Park, NY: Thomson Delmar Learning.

Gahart, B.L. and Nazareno, A.R. (2005). *2005 Intravenous medications.* (21st ed.). St. Louis: Mosby.

Intravenous Therapy. *http://www.nursewise.com*

Jaycee Burn Center at The University of North Carolina Hospitals. *http://viper.med.unc.edu*

Josephson, D.L. (2004). *Intravenous infusion therapy for nurses: Principles & practice* (2nd ed.). Clifton Park, NY: Thomson Delmar Learning.

Lucchesi, M. (2002). Burns, thermal. *eMedicine Journal.* 3(5). *http://author.emedicine.com*

North American Nursing Diagnosis Association. (2005). *Nursing diagnoses: Definitions & classifications, 2005–2006.* Philadelphia: NANDA.

Potts, N. and Mandleco, B. (2002). *Pediatric nursing: Caring for children and their families.* Clifton Park, NY: Thomson Delmar Learning.

Shriners' Hospital for Children. *http://shrinershq.org*

EASY

CASE STUDY 2

Lauren

GENDER

F

AGE

Neonate

SETTING

- Hospital/clinic

ETHNICITY

- White American

CULTURAL CONSIDERATIONS

PREEXISTING CONDITIONS

COEXISTING CONDITIONS

SIGNIFICANT HISTORY

COMMUNICATION

DISABILITY

SOCIOECONOMIC

- Middle class

SPIRITUAL

PHARMACOLOGIC

PSYCHOSOCIAL

- New parent anxiety

LEGAL

ETHICAL

ALTERNATIVE THERAPY

PRIORITIZATION

- Yes

DELEGATION

- Yes

THE SKELETAL SYSTEM

Level of difficulty: Easy

Overview: This case requires knowledge of congenital hip dysplagia, normal growth and development, as well as an understanding of the client's personal situation and mother–child attachment relationship.

Client Profile

Lauren is a neonate admitted into the newborn nursery after her breech vaginal delivery. She is the first child of a 25-year-old couple who have been anxiously awaiting Lauren's birth. Lauren's mother successfully breastfed her immediately after Lauren was born.

Case Study

On admission to the nursery, Lauren is weighed and measured. She weighs 4.5 kg (9 lb, 14 oz) and measures 55 cm (22 in.) in length. Her vital signs are within normal ranges; her skin color is pink and she is crying. The nurse notes no murmur when he listens to her heart and her bowel sounds are present. As the assessment continues, the nurse notes asymmetry of Jessica's thigh and gluteal folds and limited right hip abduction. Her right upper leg appears shorter than her left.

Questions and Suggested Answers

1. **Discuss the significance of Lauren's clinical manifestations.** Lauren's musculoskeletal manifestations are typical of developmental dysplasia of the hip or congenital hip dysplasia. The asymmetry of the thigh and gluteal folds and the limited abduction indicate that her hips are displaced from the normal positioning. That her right leg appears shorter indicates that the most significant dysplasia is in the right hip (see Fig. A-14).
2. **Discuss the potential causes for Lauren's musculoskeletal manifestations.** Prenatal factors influence the development of hip dysplasia in the neonate and include maternal secretion of estrogen and mechanical factors in utero. Lauren's size at 4.1 kg (9 lb, 2 oz) is above the normal weight of 2.5 kg (5 lb, 8 oz) to 4.0 kg (8 lb, 13 oz) for a neonate. The normal length is 45.7–53.0 cm (18–20.9 in.) and she is 55.8 cm (22 in.). The fact that she was in a breech position prenatally and during delivery indicates she was probably unable to assume a cephalic position because of her size. The breech position places the hips in very tight adduction to accommodate the mother's pelvis and birth canal.
3. **What other assessment data would be helpful for the nurse to have to prepare Lauren's care plan?** Radiographic studies usually are not accurate in neonates because the highly cartilaginous nature of their bones makes the bones difficult to visualize. Ultrasonography is helpful and can definitively diagnose congenital hip dysplasia and determine which type it is.
4. **Lauren is diagnosed with developmental dysplasia of the hip (DDH). Describe this condition, including the different types.** Developmental dysplasia of the hip (DDH) is a condition in which the head of the femur is not properly situated in the acetabulum of the hip socket. DDH occurs in three degrees. The first is unstable hip or preluzation in which the femoral head is situated in the acetabulum but can be partially or completely dislocated with manual manipulation. This is due to incomplete gestational development of the acetabular roof. The cartilage part of the roof, however, is intact. The second degree of DDH is subluxation and occurs when the head of the femur is partially dislocated or positioned under the edge of the acetabular roof. This is the most common degree of DDH. The third and most severe degree is dislocation, in which the femoral head is positioned completely outside the acetabulum.
5. **What is the incidence of DDH?** DDH occurs in 1 in 1,000 live births and is more common in Caucasians than in other races/cultures. It also affects more females than males at a 7:1 ratio. According to *The Course Book Preparation for the NCLEX-RN Exam* (Kaplan Nursing Review, p.159), "some cultures carry their children straddled against the hip joint, causing a decreased incidence (Far Eastern and African); cultures that wrap infants tightly in blankets or strap to boards have high incidence (Navajo Indian)." The Far Eastern and African cultures, by

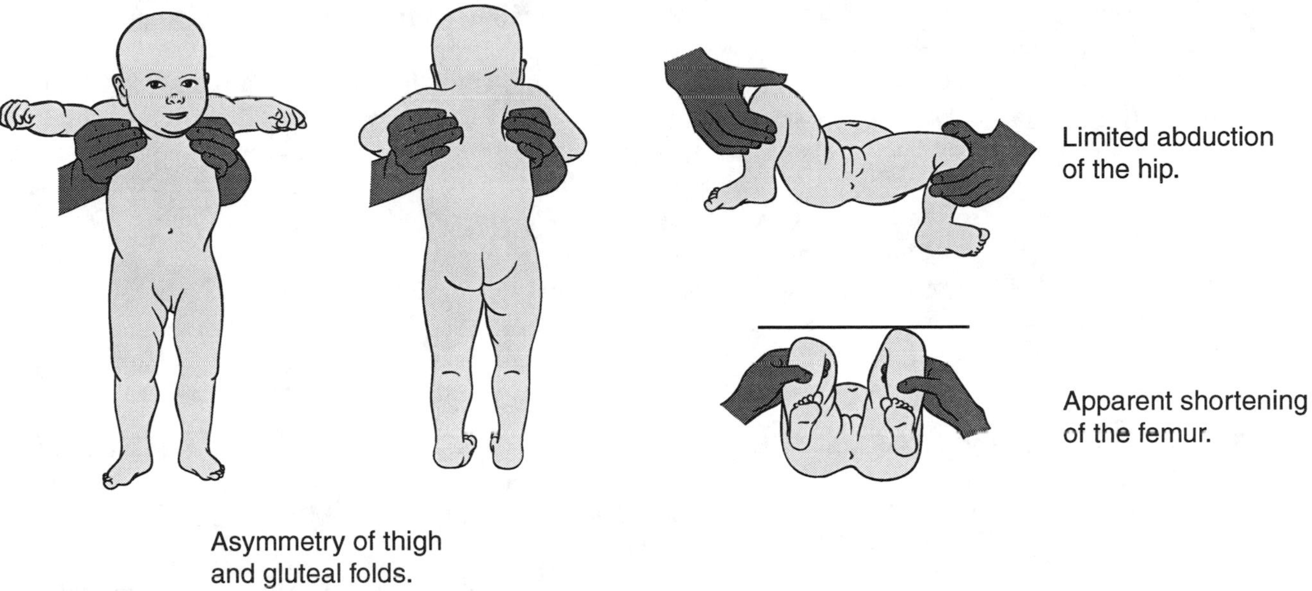

Figure A-14 *Signs of developmental dysplasia of the hip.*

carrying their children straddled against the hip joint, simulate the anatomical positioning and has an effect similar to the Pavlik Harness, abducting the legs better positions the head of femur into the acetabulum. Cultures that wrap the infants tightly in blankets create a physical positioning that abducts the child's legs together, thereby increasing the potential for the head of femur to be less secured within the acetabulum.

6. **Lauren has subluxation DDH. What are the priorities of care for Lauren prior to discharge?**
   a. Impaired physical mobility related to the improper placement of the femoral head in the hip joint
   b. Deficient knowledge, parental, related to Lauren's condition, treatment, and home care
7. **Lauren is referred to a pediatric orthopedist who recommends medical treatment for Lauren. She is fitted for an orthopedic device. What is this device and how does it work?** The device is a Pavlik harness and is the most common device used to splint the hip joint and maintain the femoral head in the acetabulum. The harness must be worn continuously until the clinical and radiographic confirmation that the hip is stable, which usually takes 3–6 months.
8. **What are the priorities of care for Lauren after she is fitted with the device?**
   a. Risk for impaired skin integrity related to possible chafing of the skin by the harness
   b. Risk for altered tissue perfusion in the lower extremities related to impaired circulation by the harness
   c. Risk for injury related to difficult positioning of the infant in infant-carrying devices and car seats
   d. Deficient knowledge, parental, related to the application of the harness, skin care, neurovascular checks, and placement of Lauren in infant-carrying devices
9. **Lauren's mother asks if she will still be able to breast feed Lauren after the harness is placed. What is the nurse's best response to this question?** The harness should not interfere with breastfeeding. Lauren may require pillow support to assume a nursing position; however, this is an easy obstacle to overcome. Her mother may need to do some trial-and-error positioning to come up with one that works for them. The nurse must be supportive and assist Lauren's mother with positioning; however, the nurse must stress that the harness cannot be removed for breastfeeding. Infants with DDH need high-calorie, high-calcium, high-protein, and high-fluid intake, and breastfeeding will provide this nutrition.
10. **Discuss the teaching necessary for Lauren's mother before she takes Lauren home with the device.**
    a. The Pavlik harness must be secure enough to keep the hips flexed, but not so tight that it interferes with circulation.

b. The harness must be worn at all times except during bathing; however, Lauren's hips and buttocks must be well supported during her bath.
c. Lauren's diaper must be changed without removing the harness and this technique must be taught, allowing sufficient time for her parents to repeat the demonstration to ensure they are comfortable with it.
d. The parents must be instructed about how to inspect Lauren's skin for irritation from the harness and how to assess the circulation status of her lower extremities.
e. The nurse should provide information concerning age-appropriate activities for Lauren to encourage and maintain her level of growth and development.
f. The parents should be given the phone numbers of contact persons so they can ask questions as they arise and obtain answers. Stress that these also are support persons.
g. Follow-up care should be emphasized, ensuring that the parents have the information on Lauren's next appointment.

11. **Discuss the impact of Lauren's condition on her growth and development.** The primary negative impact her condition and treatment will have on her growth and development is the delay in developing lower limb gross motor skills. By 4–5 months of age, most infants are able to bear weight when held in a standing position, play with their feet, turn from abdomen to back, and place their feet in their mouths. This will not be possible for Lauren in the Pavlik harness. Also, most infants sit leaning forward and turn from back to abdomen by 6–7 months of age. These skills can be accomplished, however, once her DDH is resolved. The primary task of infancy is trust versus mistrust, so as long as her needs for food, comfort, and love are met, trust will develop regardless of the harness. The nurse might suggest the use of an exercise ball for abdominal strengthening when the infant is old enough to perform this activity.

References

American Academy of Orthopaedic Surgeons. *http://www.aaos.org*

Centers for Disease Control and Prevention. *http://www.cdc.gov*

North American Nursing Diagnosis Association. (2005). *Nursing diagnoses: Definitions & classifications, 2005–2006.* Philadelphia: NANDA.

Potts, N. and Mandleco, B. (2002). *Pediatric nursing: Caring for children and their families.* Clifton Park, NY: Thomson Delmar Learning, pp. 1154–1156.

Wong, D.L., Perry, S.E., and Hockenberry, M.J. (2002). *Maternal child nursing care* (2nd ed.). St. Louis: Mosby, pp. 1560–1563.

CASE STUDY 3

Jason

GENDER

M

AGE

13

SETTING

- Emergency department

ETHNICITY

- White American

CULTURAL CONSIDERATIONS

PREEXISTING CONDITIONS

COEXISTING CONDITIONS

SIGNIFICANT HISTORY

COMMUNICATION

DISABILITY

SOCIOECONOMIC

- Middle class

SPIRITUAL

PHARMACOLOGIC

PSYCHOSOCIAL

- Possible abuse

LEGAL

- Mandatory reporting

ETHICAL

- Child abuse
- Possible nurse bias

ALTERNATIVE THERAPY

PRIORITIZATION

DELEGATION

- Yes

MODERATE

THE SKELETAL SYSTEM

Level of difficulty: Moderate

Overview: This case requires knowledge of growth and development, as well as an understanding of the client's background, personal situation, and parent–child attachment relationship, child abuse, and legal and ethical implications for nursing.

Client Profile

Jason is a 13-year-old adolescent who lives with his mother, father, 10-year-old sister, and 5-year-old brother in a middle-class rural neighborhood. Jason attends middle school and has been an average student, although he has demonstrated both attendance and behavior problems beginning 3 months ago. Teachers have suspected his difficulties stem from problems at home, but Jason denies this. They have noted that Jason appears in pain when sitting in class, especially on Mondays, that he is regularly absent, and that most of his absences occur on Mondays. He has been suspended twice this school year for being involved in altercations with other students on school property. Jason's mother attends all parent conferences and when these observations were communicated to her, she responded that Jason and his father were "not getting along very well." When teachers suggested that it would be beneficial to speak to both his mother and father, Mrs. King responded that her husband was "frequently gone in the afternoons and evenings and that any communications from the school should be made directly with her."

Case Study

Mrs. King brings Jason to the emergency room at 0100 after "he fell down the stairs at home." His breathing suggests a patent airway; however, he is bleeding from both nares. When the nurse attempts to apply pressure to Jason's nose to stop the bleeding, Jason grimaces and rates his pain level at 10/10, complaining of pain in his right arm as well as the bridge of his nose. During his triage assessment, the nurse notes the following:

Vital signs:

- Temperature: 37° C (98.6° F)
- Pulse: 98 beats/minute
- Respirations: 30 breaths/minute
- Blood pressure: 128/88

Breath sounds clear to auscultation

Heart sounds regular with no audible dysrhythmias or murmurs

Areas of ecchymosis on upper arms bilaterally

Displacement of the bridge of the nose to the right and bleeding from the nares

Guarding of his right forearm

Neurological assessment reveals no apparent deficits.

Skin assessment revealed multiple horizontal lacerations across Jason's back from the thoracic area extending down to and including his buttocks bilaterally. In addition, 2.5-cm (1-in.) wide horizontal scars were also noted in this area. Jason states that he had awakened at "about midnight" and fell when he was walking to the bathroom in his home. Although both Jason and his mother are cooperative during the history-taking, the nurse notes that neither makes eye contact with the nurse, but rather keep looking at each other during the interview. As Jason is in no acute distress, the nurse leaves the triage room to report his findings to the health care provider on call in the emergency room.

Questions and Suggested Answers

1. **Discuss your impressions about the above situation.** Jason may be a victim of child abuse. His injuries, including past injuries, are not consistent with a fall. The bones of an adolescent should be strong enough to withstand a fall, especially if he fell on a carpeted floor. It is common in adolescence to be at odds with the same-sex parent as the child is striving for identity and is involved in behaviors that conflict with parental guidelines and authority. According to the U.S. Department of Health and Human Services Administration

for Children & Families, children 12–15 years of age are victims of child maltreatment at a rate of 10.6 per 1,000 children. The highest rate occurs in children 0–3 years of age at a rate of 16 per 1,000 children. Of the cases reported in 2002, 54.2% involved Caucasian children and parents. Fathers are identified as the abusers in 19.1% of the cases.

2. What data obtained by the nurse are most pertinent regarding the client's present condition?

- **a.** Vital sign findings (pulse, respirations, and blood pressure) are elevated compared to normal values for Jason's age group.
- **b.** Displacement of the bridge of the nose to the right is evidence of trauma to the face that may be the result of his fall or may indicate he was struck by a right-handed person.
- **c.** Epistaxis is common in nasal injuries, but can be a source of major blood loss.
- **d.** Guarding of his right forearm may indicate bone injury from attempting to catch himself as he fell or it may be a defensive wound as he tried to protect himself from being hit by another person.
- **e.** Jason is neurologically intact and participates in the interview.
- **f.** Bruising on the upper arms bilaterally is inconsistent with a single fall.
- **g.** The multiple laceration wounds on his back are inconsistent with a fall and more indicative of physical abuse.
- **h.** One-inch wide horizontal scars may indicate that this is not the first time he has sustained physical abuse.
- **i.** Jason and his mother's inability to make eye contact with the interviewer may indicate their concern that each other's story is consistent.
- **j.** Jason's father is absent in the emergency department.

3. What additional data would be helpful in determining the extent of Jason's injuries?

- **a.** Complete blood count with focus on hemoglobin and hematocrit to gain perspective on Jason's blood loss secondary to the epistaxis and lacerations
- **b.** Radiologic examination of Jason's arm and head to determine the presence of bone fractures
- **c.** Serum electrolytes
- **d.** Abdominal computed tomography to determine the presence of abdominal trauma

4. Jason is diagnosed with a complete closed fracture of the right ulna and nasal septum, and multiple skin lacerations. Identify four priority goals of care for Jason during triage.

- **a.** Risk for impaired tissue perfusion related to blood loss secondary to his injuries
- **b.** Acute pain related to tissue trauma secondary to his injuries
- **c.** Impaired skin integrity related to lacerations
- **d.** Deficient knowledge related to Jason's present condition, resources available to the family

These are the priorities, although a number of others may be identified, including:

- **e.** Risk for infection related to impaired skin integrity
- **f.** Anxiety related to injuries, cause of injuries, potential repercussions
- **g.** Fear
- **h.** Risk for post-traumatic stress syndrome

5. Discuss interventions to achieve the identified priority goals.

- **a.** Risk for impaired tissue perfusion related to blood loss secondary to his injuries
  - **(1)** Monitor vital signs frequently.
  - **(2)** Apply pressure to nose to stop bleeding and monitor continuously.
  - **(3)** Measure oxygen saturation via pulse oximetry.
  - **(4)** Apply gentle pressure using gauze soaked in cooled sterile normal saline to any back lacerations that are bleeding.
  - **(5)** Monitor hemoglobin and hematocrit levels, reporting abnormal findings to health care provider.
  - **(6)** Maintain calm, nonjudgmental affect, encouraging Jason and his mother to express their feelings.
  - **(7)** Monitor for changes in neurological status.
  - **(8)** Prepare to initiate intravenous fluid infusion.

b. Acute pain related to tissue trauma secondary to his injuries
   (1) Assess pain hourly, remembering that "pain is what the client says it is."
   (2) Collaborate with health care provider for prescription for morphine sulfate 1–2 mg IV every 1–2 hours.
   (3) Avoid moving client's arm, maintaining it in guarded position.
   (4) Apply cool sterile gauze soaked in normal saline soaked to lacerations on back.
   (5) If lacerations are not suitable for suturing, apply antibiotic cream/ointment as prescribed.
   (6) Provide a calm, relaxing environment within the constraints of the emergency department.
c. Impaired skin integrity related to lacerations
   (1) Monitor lacerations for manifestations of infection.
   (2) Apply antibiotic cream/ointment as prescribed.
   (3) Avoid abrasive tape when applying dressings.
   (4) Ensure that Jason is medicated prior to applying antibiotic cream/ointment and dressings.
   (5) Use surgical asepsis when applying medication and dressings to wounds.
d. Deficient knowledge related to Jason's condition, resources available to family
   (1) Assess Jason and his mother's current level of knowledge.
   (2) Provide verbal and written information concerning:
      (a) Dressing changes and application of antibiotic cream/ointment
      (b) Oral antibiotic administration if prescribed including the importance of completing entire prescription
      (c) Taking prescribed pain medication on regular intervals for the first 24–48 hours and then as needed to control discomfort; stress importance of proactively treating pain
      (d) Signs and symptoms of infection
      (e) Notifying health care provider of temperature elevation; redness and/or purulent drainage from laceration wounds; numbness, tingling, change in color or temperature of fingers of right hand; discoloration or heat noted on cast; increased pain or pain not controlled
      (f) Phone numbers of hospital and health care provider
      (g) Importance of keeping follow-up appointments to monitor lacerations and fracture
      (h) Information concerning referrals
   (3) Allow sufficient time for Jason and his mother to ask questions and provide honest answers.
   (4) Document teaching and client/family response.

6. **What referrals should be implemented in this situation and why are they appropriate?** The nurse should collaborate with the health care provider for the following referrals:
   a. Social Services/social worker
   b. Psychologist
   c. Local law enforcement (to report suspected child abuse) and ensure environment is safe prior to child's discharge from the hospital
   d. Facility chaplain (if Jason and his mother desire)

7. **Jason's mother begins to cry and states that she is afraid her husband "is going to be mad because I brought Jason to the hospital and our insurance doesn't cover emergency room fees." How should you respond to her and the concerns she has voiced?** The nurse must use empathy and therapeutic communication techniques to provide support for Jason's mother. Gather as much information concerning her feelings and clarify her statement about her husband's anticipated response as possible. Collaborate with the social worker and serve as liaison if needed between social worker and Jason's mother.

8. **What client and family teaching should be completed prior to Jason's discharge from the emergency department to home? *NOTE: It is mandatory for health professionals to report suspected child abuse to authorities and environment should be thoroughly evaluated for safety prior to the child's discharge from the Emergency Department!***
   a. Dressing changes and application of antibiotic cream/ointment
   b. Oral antibiotic administration if prescribed, including the importance of completing the entire prescription

- **c.** Taking prescribed pain medication on regular intervals for the first 24-48 hours and then as needed to control discomfort; stress importance of proactively treating pain
- **d.** Signs and symptoms of infection
- **e.** Notifying health care provider of temperature elevation; redness and/or purulent drainage from laceration wounds; numbness, tingling, change in color or temperature of fingers of right hand; discoloration or heat noted on cast; increased pain or pain not controlled
- **f.** Phone numbers of hospital and health care provider
- **g.** Importance of keeping follow-up appointments to monitor lacerations and fracture
- **h.** Information concerning referrals including phone numbers

9. Discuss your own biases about this situation. This will be an individual response by the reader; however, it should include feelings about child abuse, the abusive parent, and feelings regarding caring for a victim of child abuse.

10. What are the benefits and risks of delaying judgment about the father's potential involvement in Jason's condition until all the data and facts are available? Although most of the data lead the reader to the conclusion that Jason is a victim of child abuse, to assume this without a complete social and psychological assessment may falsely accuse the father of abuse. According to the U.S. Department of Social Services Administration for Children & Families, 58% of abusers were female, most commonly the child's mother. Gaining all the facts and data would better ensure an accurate conclusion and appropriate action would be taken. The risks are the greatest because delaying judgment about the father's potential involvement could place Jason in jeopardy of being further abused.

References

ChildhelpUSA: National Child Abuse Statistics. *http://www.childhelpuse.org*

Daniels, R. (2002). *Delmar's manual of laboratory and diagnostic tests.* Clifton Park, NY: Thomson Delmar Learning.

Gahart, B.L. and Nazareno, A.R. (2005). *2005 Intravenous medications* (21st ed.). St. Louis: Mosby.

North American Nursing Diagnosis Association. (2005). *Nursing diagnoses: Definitions & classifications, 2005–2006.* Philadelphia: NANDA.

Potts, N. and Mandleco, B. (2002). *Pediatric nursing: Caring for children and their families.* Clifton Park, NY: Thomson Delmar Learning.

U.S. Department of Health and Human Services Administration for Children & Families. *http://www.acf.hhs.gov*

CASE STUDY 4

Kimberli

GENDER

F

AGE

11

SETTING

- Health care provider's office/hospital

ETHNICITY

- White American

CULTURAL CONSIDERATIONS

PREEXISTING CONDITIONS

COEXISTING CONDITIONS

SIGNIFICANT HISTORY

COMMUNICATION

DISABILITY

SOCIOECONOMIC

- Middle class

SPIRITUAL

PHARMACOLOGIC

- Pain management

PSYCHOSOCIAL

- Client anxiety
- Disturbed body image

LEGAL

ETHICAL

ALTERNATIVE THERAPY

PRIORITIZATION

- Yes

DELEGATION

MODERATE

THE SKELETAL SYSTEM

Level of Difficulty: Moderate

Overview: This case requires knowledge of scoliosis, medical–surgical treatment, growth and development, as well as an understanding of the client's background, personal situation, and family–child attachment relationship.

Client Profile

Kimberli is an 11-year-old school-age child who lives with her parents and 13-year-old brother in a suburban community. She attends school and performs well. During her last physical examination for school, her pediatrician expressed concern about Kimberli's posture, which had a slight right lateral curve. X-ray studies were done at this time. The health care provider instructed Kimberli and Kimberli's parents to encourage proper posture and inform him if they notice any worsening of her condition. The radiological report indicated that Kimberli's curvature was <20%.

Case Study

During a subsequent visit, Kimberli's curvature appears worse and a spinal X-ray film is prescribed. The X-ray film indicates the presence of a >30% lateral curvature of the spinal column at the level of T4–T11. Scoliometric measurements and magnetic resonance imagery (MRI) confirms that Kimberli has scoliosis of unknown etiology. Her diagnosis and treatment plan is explained to Kimberli and her parents.

Questions and Suggested Answers

1. **Describe scoliosis, including the different types.** Scoliosis is a lateral curvature of the spine that forces the rib cage to be misshapened (see Fig. A-15). The body develops a compensatory curve to maintain posture and balance. A <20% curve is considered a slight curve; one that is >40% requires surgery; and a curve >80% results in respiratory compromise. It can occur in any part of the spine, but usually affects the thoracic or lumbar spine and may curve to the right or left. The muscles and ligaments shorten on the concave side of the curvature. As this process continues, the vertebrae become deformed. There are three types of scoliosis: (1) congenital, (2) neuromuscular, and (3) idiopathic. Congenital scoliosis is present at birth and usually is related to a defect in the formation of the vertebrae or fused ribs during fetal development. Neuromuscular scoliosis occurs as a result of muscle weakness and poor muscle control and is associated with conditions such as cerebral palsy, spina bifida, muscular dystrophy, or polio. Idiopathic scoliosis has no identifiable cause.

2. **Discuss the incidence and etiology of idiopathic scoliosis.** Idiopathic scoliosis is the most common type (85%) and affects 2% to 5% of the United States population. This means approximately 6 million people have this disorder. The other two types occur more frequently in underdeveloped countries. Idiopathic scoliosis has no recognized cause and has a peak incidence in the 10- to 15-year-old age group.

3. **How might her diagnosis impact on Kimberli's growth and development?** At the age of 11 years, children are developing a self-esteem based on the response of others to them and their accomplishments. School and interactions with others their age, especially same-sex friends, help provide them with a sense of industry or can lead to feelings of inferiority if they see themselves as different or not belonging. As children approach adolescence, physical appearance becomes increasingly important, especially for girls, and they compare themselves to others their age. Physical coordination reaches its peak during the school-age years. Kimberli's appearance and coordination may be negatively affected by spinal deformity. She will probably feel different from her friends and may not be able to participate in physical activities such as sports.

4. **Describe the medical treatment for idiopathic scoliosis.** For curvatures of <40%, conservative medical management is the standard of care. The child is fitted with a Milwaukee brace, and exercises to be done with the brace on are designed to prevent atrophy of the abdominal and neck muscles and to increase flexibility. The Milwaukee brace is a plastic and metal device that includes a pelvic girdle and a neck ring and is used

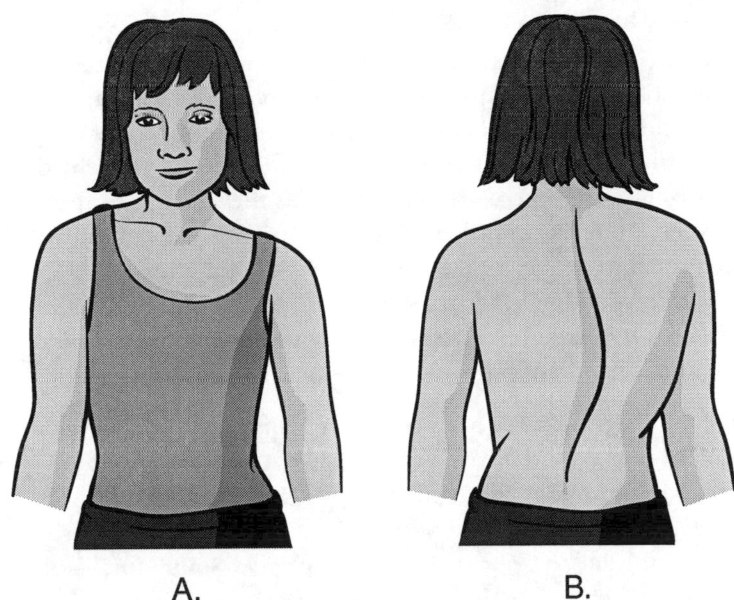

Figure A-15 *Adolescent girl with scoliosis: A. Frontal view; B. Posterior view.*

for high thoracic curvatures. Other devices include the Boston brace and the Wilmington brace (underarm braces used for low thoracic, thoracolumbar, and lumbar curvatures). Although the brace does not reverse the curvature, it does straighten the spine while it is worn to relieve asymmetrical pressure.

5. **Discuss the teaching required for Kimberli and her parents in relation to her medical treatment.** The parents and child are instructed that the brace must be worn for 18–23 hours a day even when sleeping and is to be removed only for the child's hygienic care. The skin must be closely monitored for skin breakdown where the brace makes contact with the skin. Kimberli and her parents should be encouraged to foster her growth and development and provide instructions about normal growth and development for children her age. Turtleneck shirts can be worn to hide the brace.

6. **After Kimberli's scoliosis does not respond to conservative treatment, she is scheduled for a posterior spinal fusion. What are the priorities of care for Kimberli prior to surgery?** Addressing deficient knowledge related to the surgical procedure and postoperative course is the priority for Kimberli. She needs to be taught about respiratory therapy following surgery; pain management; and what she can expect following surgery including the presence of an indwelling urinary catheter until she is able to get out of bed, physical therapy, and monitoring of her vital signs and oxygen saturation.

7. **What is a Harrington rod and how is it used during spinal fusion surgery?** A Harrington rod is a metal rod surgically placed next to the spine to support the fused area. It is left in place indefinitely following surgery unless infection occurs. It is referred to as spinal instrumentation.

8. **Following her surgery, what are the postoperative priorities of care for Kimberli?**
   a. Risk for ineffective breathing pattern related to positioning and pain
   b. Acute pain related to tissue trauma in the surgical site and over the iliac crest where the donor grafts for the fusion are harvested
   c. Risk for impaired gas exchange related to use of fentanyl pain management
   d. Impaired urinary elimination related to placement of an indwelling urinary catheter
   e. Risk for injury, complications related to spinal fusion surgery
   f. Risk for infection related to impaired skin integrity and lack of mobility
   g. Deficient knowledge related to postoperative course and home care

9. **Pulse oximetry reveals that Kimberli's oxygen saturation is 89%. She is receiving 2 L of oxygen per nasal cannula. Discuss the appropriate actions the nurse should take.** The nurse's first action should be to assess Kimberli's breath sounds. The most common cause of a decrease in oxygen saturation postoperatively is stasis of respiratory secretions secondary to general anesthesia, causing a diminished cough reflex and inactivity. In most facilities that perform spinal fusions on children, protocols are present that prescribe oxygen administration to maintain oxygen saturation >94%. This provides the nurse with the autonomy to increase or decrease supplemental oxygen administration to maintain the prescribed saturation. If this is present the nurse should increase the oxygen and titrate it to the prescribed oxygen saturation level. If this protocol is not in place and the surgeon has not addressed this issue in written form, the nurse needs to notify the surgeon for such a prescription. Turning, coughing, and deep breathing exercises should be instituted. If the child is unable to do this, suctioning and chest physiotherapy may be required.

10. **Discuss the importance of pain management for Kimberli and what agent(s) you anticipate will be prescribed to control her surgical pain.** Pain management based on the child's own assessment of the pain is critical to the child's recovery. Pain causes both physiological and psychological stress that inhibits the healing process by utilizing energy reserves needed for healing and negatively impacts on the child's compliance with postoperative therapies necessary to prevent complications of this surgery. Spinal fusion is a very painful procedure and frequently requires nurses to activate multiple interventions to achieve pain control. A reasonable pain level for a postoperative spinal fusion child is 0–2/10. Morphine sulfate administered both on a continuous infusion and patient-controlled analgesia (PCA) dosing is the most common agent and route used for management of moderate to severe postoperative pain. It is both safe and effective, rarely resulting in respiratory distress. However, in recent years, intravenous or epidural fentanyl citrate has demonstrated both its safety and efficacy in the treatment of postspinal fusion pain and is pharmacologically up to 100 times more potent than morphine. However, fentanyl carries an increased risk of respiratory depression. As a result, children receiving fentanyl by the intravenous or epidural rate should be placed on continuous cardiopulmonary monitoring and pulse oximetry and naloxone hydrochloride for injection should be at the child's bedside. Hourly respiratory assessment is also necessary. The use of intravenous dosing of Ketoralac (a nonsteroidal antiinflammatory) as an adjunct to the opioid analgesic regimen offers increased pain management by interfering with prostaglandin at the peripheral level. No medications for pain management should be administered through the intramuscular route, as these medications cause pain when administered and are not as predictable in their analgesic or antiinflammatory action as those administered intravenously.

11. **Discuss the nursing interventions necessary to prevent complications of Kimberli's surgery.** Complications of spinal fusion surgery include risk for damage to the surgical site, impaired skin integrity, hypostatic pneumonia, urinary tract infections, and infection. To prevent damage to the surgical site, Kimberli needs to be log-rolled every 2 hours, ensuring that her spine remains in surgical alignment. Turning also will help prevent skin breakdown over bony prominences although children her age seldom experience skin breakdown because of the elasticity of their skin. Coughing and deep breathing exercises in addition to the use of incentive spirometry help prevent stasis of respiratory secretions, the cause of postoperative hypostatic pneumonia. Meticulous handwashing and indwelling urinary catheter care are the priority nursing interventions to prevent urinary tract infections in addition to ensuring adequate fluid intake. The catheter tubing should be assessed for kinks and stress on the tubing and urinary output should be closely monitored. Catheter care and meeting Kimberli's hygiene needs can be delegated to nonlicensed personnel. Kimberli and her mother may prefer that her mother provide for Kimberli's hygiene needs which should be encouraged but not expected. Monitoring vital signs and assessing Kimberli's surgical incision with each turning will provide information about the potential development of infection as well as providing prescribed incision care to prevent microbial growth at the incision site.

12. **Kimberli has been working with a physical therapist for 3 days and on her 5th postoperative day, you are preparing to get Kimberli out of bed and help her to the chair. What nursing interventions are necessary before getting Kimberli out of bed?** Children with spinal fusions are fitted for a TLS (thoracic, lumbar,

sacral) brace to be worn anytime the child sits, stands, or walks as a standard of care to prevent damage to the surgical site. The brace has a posterior shell and an anterior shell that are fastened together with Velcro straps once the shells are in place. The brace is applied by turning the child on one side and placing the posterior brace against the child's back. The child is then turned to a supine position and the anterior shell is placed on her chest. Then the Velcro straps fasten the brace in place. The nurse needs to move to the foot of the child's bed and assess the brace and the child's body for symmetry and alignment. Once the alignment has been visually confirmed, the child is placed in a sitting position at the side of the bed. At this time the nurse confers with the child to determine that the brace is properly placed. Once the child stands, the same verification process is repeated. Because the child is fitted for the brace during the early postoperative period so it can be adjusted specifically to that child, adjustments frequently need to be made to address such issues as the presence of edema at the time of the fitting and its gradual resolution as the healing process progresses. The child's skin must be closely assessed following her return to a supine position and the brace is removed to detect any areas where the brace may be rubbing and could lead to skin breakdown.

13. **Kimberli has not had a bowel movement since her surgery and Kimberli complains of abdominal fullness. Discuss your impressions of Kimberli's situation including factors that may have precipitated her present condition and the nursing interventions that are appropriate at this time.** Kimberli is probably experiencing constipation. Proper bowel elimination is dependent on activity, adequate fluids, and the presence of food to stimulate peristalsis. In the absence of any of these factors or in the presence of chemical agents that interfere with peristalsis, bowel function is impaired. All three are impacted by the use of opioid analgesics in the management of pain. The most common adverse effect of morphine sulfate is constipation. As with morphine, fentanyl as a central nervus system depressant slows bowel activity. Opioid analgesics lead to a decrease in oral fluid and food intake as a side effect of the decrease in gastrointestinal activity. Kimberli's imposed decreased physical activity following surgery also places her at risk for constipation. Progressing Kimberli to oral analgesics as soon as possible while maintaining pain management acceptable to Kimberli will help bowel function although Schedule II oral analgesics also cause constipation. Encouraging the intake of oral fluids is one of the most beneficial actions to help regain Kimberli's bowel function. Collaborating with the health care provider for a prescription for a stool softener should be done early in the postoperative period to prevent bowel complications. Progressing Kimberli's activity as soon as her condition allows also will be beneficial to restoring bowel function as well as increasing Kimberli's appetite and her food consumption. At the point of this question, the nurse should collaborate with the health care provider for a prescription for a laxative after conferring with Kimberli and her mother regarding their practices at home when constipation occurs. Oral laxatives are preferred; however, if they are not effective, a small volume retention enema may be necessary.

References

Broyles, B.E. (2005). *Medical-surgical nursing clinical companion.* Durham, NC: Carolina Academic Press.

Centers for Disease Control and Prevention. *http://www.cdc.gov*

Gahart, B.L. and Nazareno, A.R. (2005). *2005 Intravenous medications* (21st ed.). St. Louis: Mosby.

The National Institute of Arthritis and Musculoskeletal and Skin Disorders: *http://www.niams.nih.gov*

North American Nursing Diagnosis Association. (2005). *Nursing diagnoses: Definitions & classifications, 2005–2006.* Philadelphia: NANDA.

Potts, N. and Mandleco, B. (2002). *Pediatric nursing: Caring for children and their families.* Clifton Park, NY: Thomson Delmar Learning, pp. 1160–1167.

Reiss, B.S., Evans, M.E., and Broyles, B.E. (2002). *Pharmacological aspects of nursing care* (6th ed.). Clifton Park, NY: Thomson Delmar Learning, pp. 219–223.

Scoliosis Research Society. *http://www.srs.org*

CASE STUDY 5

Ilya

GENDER

M

AGE

14

SETTING

- Hospital

ETHNICITY

- Russian

CULTURAL CONSIDERATIONS

- Recent Russian immigrant

PREEXISTING CONDITIONS

- Osteogenic sarcoma
- Implanted CVAD

COEXISTING CONDITIONS

SIGNIFICANT HISTORY

COMMUNICATION

- Russian-speaking

DISABILITY

SOCIOECONOMIC

- Middle class

SPIRITUAL

PHARMACOLOGIC

- Methotrexate (Trexall)
- Prednisone (Deltasone)
- Doxorubicin (Rubex)

PSYCHOSOCIAL

- Impaired verbal communication
- Anxiety

LEGAL

ETHICAL

ALTERNATIVE THERAPY

PRIORITIZATION

- Yes

DELEGATION

- Graduate nurse and preceptor

THE SKELETAL SYSTEM

Level of Difficulty: Difficult

Overview: This case requires knowledge of osteogenic sarcoma; growth and development; as well as an understanding of the client's background, personal situation, and family relationship; and how to work with non-English-speaking clients.

DIFFICULT

Client Profile

Ilya is a 14-year-old Russian boy who recently came to the United States to receive treatment for osteogenic sarcoma (OS) of his right femur. He was diagnosed 2 months ago in his home country, where he had undergone chemotherapy. His father is a contractor who has worked in the United States for 2 years with plans to have his family join him soon. After his son was diagnosed with OS, he brought Ilya and the boy's mother to the United States for further treatment in a research facility for treatment he is unable to receive in his home country. Ilya is admitted to the hospital for a limb-sparing surgical procedure. He has an implanted central venous access device (CVAD) through which he received chemotherapy during his earlier hospital admission in his home country. The health care provider prescribes continuation of his chemotherapy regimen. Ilya and his mother do not speak English; however, his father, who is fluent in English as well as Russian, is present on admission and provides the nurse with Ilya's medical and social history and translates information for his wife and son. Ilya appears to be a happy and otherwise healthy adolescent whose psychosocial and physical development is appropriate for his age.

Case Study

Ilya is continuing his chemotherapy regime of methotrexate, prednisone, and doxorubicin prior to surgery which is scheduled 3 days from now. His current diagnostic findings are:

- Hematology:
  - Hemoglobin: 10.6 g/dL
  - Hematocrit: 30%
  - White blood cell count: 8,900 cells/mm^3 with a differential of:
    - Neutrophils: 21%
    - Lymphocytes: 65%
    - Eosinophils: 4%
    - Bands: 1%
    - Monocytes: 7%;
  - Platelets: 90,000 cells/mm^3
- Chemistry:
  - Potassium: 3.2 mEq/L
  - Sodium: 130 mEq/L
  - Glucose: 260 mg/dL
  - Calcium: 8.1 mg/dL
  - Uric acid: 6.3 mg/dL

In making assignments for the pediatric unit where Ilya is a client, the charge nurse assigns him to a new graduate nurse, Sally, who is orienting to the unit and Sally's preceptor, John, who has worked on this pediatric oncology unit for 2 years. Sally is excited about working with Ilya and hopes to help him learn some English while she improves her Russian, learned while she was an exchange student in high school.

Questions and Suggested Answers

1. **Discuss your impressions of Ilya's laboratory findings.** Ilya's hemoglobin and hematocrit are below normal for an adolescent boy. This could result in decreased tissue perfusion; however, neither are seriously low. His white blood cell count is within normal range, however, his neutrophil count compromises his ability to fight

infection. His platelets are below normal and could pose a risk of bleeding. Both his potassium and sodium levels are lower than normal, perhaps from the prechemotherapy hydration. Although his potassium level is just below the normal 3.5–5.0 mEq/L, if it continues to drop, he could be at risk for developing cardiac dysrhythmias especially with the use of doxorubicin, which can cause cardiotoxicity. His glucose level is elevated, but this is probably associated with the prednisone in his chemotherapy regimen. His uric acid level is elevated which is an adverse effect associated with methotrexate. His calcium level is below the normal of 8.5–10.5 mg/dL, which could pose both cardiac and coagulation problems.

2. **Identify the nursing concerns related to these findings.**
   a. Risk for infection related to ineffective protection secondary to neutrophil count
   b. Risk for injury, peripheral neuropathy related to elevated uric acid level secondary to methotrexate
   c. Risk for injury, cardiac dysfunction related to potassium and calcium levels
   d. Risk for injury, hyperglycemia related to glucose levels secondary to prednisone
   e. Impaired verbal communication related to client and mother's inability to speak or understand English
   f. Deficient knowledge related to Ilya's condition, surgical treatment and post-operative care, hospital environment secondary to impaired communication

3. **Ilya's father is unable to visit on a regular basis because of his job. Identify nursing concerns related to the language barrier in this situation when his father is not present.** Whenever providing care for a client, the nurse must explain what he or she plans to do to gain the client's consent. Prescribed medications, doses, and uses must be explained prior to administering them so the client and, in pediatrics, the parent or guardian understands what the child is receiving. When receiving chemotherapy, the client is on strict intake and output and the urine must be tested with each void. When drawing blood for laboratory specimens from the client's central venous access device (CVAD), this procedure must be explained to the client. If the client is experiencing discomfort, nausea, and so forth the nurse needs to know that the client is in need of medications so they can be proactively (hopefully) or at least expediently given. When changing the needle and dressing weekly for the implanted CVAD, the nurse wears a mask, which impairs visual and verbal communication. Because the procedures for changing implanted port needles and dressings are standard, Ilya and his mother are probably familiar with these procedures, however. Preoperative teaching would pose a nursing challenge as well.

4. **Why do you think the charge nurse should or should not assign Ilya to the new graduate and her preceptor? Discuss both the benefits and disadvantages.** The preceptor is familiar with the unit and the pediatric population served on the unit, having worked on the unit for 2 years. Sally's knowledge of Russian, however limited because of the time that has passed since her foreign exchange experience, would definitely be of value to Ilya and his mother as well as to other nurses assigned to care for Ilya. In addition, Sally's expressed enthusiasm in wanting to bridge the communication gap is a positive reason for assigning her to Ilya. The main disadvantage in the assignment is Sally's limited exposure to the types of clients on this unit; however, she does have John as her preceptor to help her.

5. **Discuss the incidence and prognosis of osteogenic sarcoma (OS).** OS is the most common bone malignancy, originating in the osteocytes of the long bones. It develops most commonly near the ends of the long bones of the femur (near the knee), the proximal tibia, and the proximal humerus, but can occur in any bone. Ilya's OS is in his femur, which is the most common site. The peak incidence is in 10- to 25-year-olds and is most common in adolescence during the rapid bone growth associated with this growth and development period. Approximately 400 new cases are diagnosed annually in the United States, with this cancer affecting males twice as often as females. As a result of present treatment modalities including limb-sparing the prognosis has improved greatly, with 65% to 75% of clients achieving a long-term survival.

6. **What are the surgical standards of care for a child with this condition?** The surgical procedures used to treat OS of the femur are limb sparing and amputation. In the past three decades, the surgical standard of care has changed from amputation to limb sparing, a procedure in which the bone tumor and a designated

perimeter around the tumor are removed and a replacement prosthesis is placed. This spares the loss of the limb from 7.5 cm (3 in.) above the tumor down, which is the standard for amputations as well as the complexity of prosthetic devices and physical therapy associated with amputations. Amputation of the limb is still performed and in severe cases of OS especially of the shoulder joint, the entire arm, shoulder, scapula, and clavicle (forequarter amputation) are surgically resected. Limb sparing or limb salvage has fewer complications than amputations and much less impact on the child's body image. This procedure is not available in underdeveloped countries and has limited availability in some industrialized countries.

7. **Discuss the appropriate priority nursing interventions for Ilya to prevent the complications associated with his chemotherapy regimen.** In children, intravenous antineoplastics are administered via a CVAD to reduce the risk of extravasation of the chemotherapy. The CVAD must be managed according to facility protocol with dressing changes performed using sterile technique. For Ilya's implanted port, the standard is to change the dressing weekly when the access needle is changed, also using sterile technique. Prior to and following chemotherapy, intravenous hydration is prescribed. This dilutes the antineoplastics as they are collected in the urinary bladder and increases excretion of the agents from the bladder. The nurse monitors the urine every void to ensure that the specific gravity of the urine is maintained at a prescribed level (usually <1.010). Medications including ondansetron and dexamethasone are administered intravenously 30 minutes prior to the administration of antineoplastics to prevent nausea and vomiting associated with chemotherapy with follow-up doses of ondansetron prescribed every 4 hours for 24 hours following chemotherapy. Lorazepam IV is prescribed for breakthrough nausea. Because methotrexate increases uric acid levels, the maintenance fluid administered both as prechemotherapy hydration and following administration of methotrexate is 5% dextrose with sodium bicarbonate. In addition, the nurse must monitor the pH of the urine each void and ensure that it is >7. Also, leucovorin is administered immediately following the infusion of methotrexate as a rescue agent to increase the excretion of the methotrexate in the urine. It acts by competing at the cellular level with methotrexate causing it to leave the cells. Leucovorin is prescribed in follow-up doses every 6 hours until the methotrexate level is <0.05 micromoles. The serum glucose and uric acid levels need to be monitored. The nurse needs to explain all procedures to the client and family and encourage them to ask questions as needed. Ilya's calcium level needs to be monitored and calcium replacements may need to be prescribed. Monitoring of vital signs including auscultating heart sounds should be done every 4 hours and more frequently as needed. Meticulous handwashing is essential to prevent nosocomial infections.

8. **What are Ilya's risk factors for developing an infection?** Ilya has a CVAD that is accessed for the administration of pre- and post-chemotherapy hydration and through which his chemotherapy is administered and his serum laboratory specimens are obtained. Because it is accessed through the skin, it poses a risk of infection. The chemotherapy destroys rapidly multiplying cells and does not differentiate between normal cells and cancer cells. This results in a risk for infection related to decreased leukocytes, especially neutrophils. The hospital environment poses a risk to any compromised client of developing nosocomial infections. This may pose a significant problem from Ilya because he has moved from a country with a possibly different microbial population than the United States and thus may not have developed needed immune defenses.

9. **How will the nurse know if Ilya develops an infection?** The most significant marker for infection is an elevated temperature. Also, Ilya's CVAD needs to be assessed hourly during the routine intravenous assessments for redness, swelling, or drainage. His laboratory values, especially his white blood cell count should be monitored for elevations consistent with the presence of infection. Because Ilya is compromised and at risk for infection, he should be monitored for changes in neurologic status indicative of sepsis.

10. **Five days following his limb-sparing surgery, Ilya's white blood cell count is 6,000 cells/mm^3, his neutrophil count is 49%, and, following transfusion of 2 units of platelets, his platelet count is 120,000. Following the nurse's assessment, Ilya communicates with Sally in broken English that he misses his friends in Russia and would like to make some new friends here. Discuss your impressions of Ilya's request based on his level of growth and development.** For the adolescent who is striving to achieve identity versus role confusion, the

primary sense of belonging comes from peers. Most of the adolescent's waking hours revolve around being with or talking on the phone with friends. Peer input is vital to the adolescent's sense of self-esteem. Ilya's friends are still back in Russia, and he needs contact with other children his age. In many large research facilities, pediatric activity rooms are available for the hospitalized children. Because the interests of adolescents differ greatly from those of younger children, separate activity rooms are designed for children younger than 12 years of age and those older than 12 years of age. Furnishings for these areas should be appropriate for the levels of growth and development of the children served. Child-life specialists or recreational therapists should be available for these children to foster their growth and development during their hospitalizations.

11. John notes that Ilya's mother remains constantly at his bedside and is weepy at times when Ilya is in the adolescent activity room. John has a friend Brett who studied Russian as his second language while he was working on a computer account in Russia. He asks the friend, Brett, to come to the hospital and visit with Ilya's mother. What do you think is John's rationale for this? Nurses should be client and family focused; however in pediatrics this is a must because the way children respond to their condition and hospitalization is based, in part, on their parents' response. John could certainly conclude that although Ilya's mother is happy that her child is receiving the treatment he needs that was not available to him at home, this situation is very difficult for her, especially because of her language barrier. She probably would like to talk to someone in her own language about her home and how she is feeling being away from her familiar environment. She probably feels lost and alone. By providing her with someone she could talk to, John probably hopes he can address Ilya's psychosocial needs. The concern for confidentiality related to Ilya and his condition should be addressed with Brett prior to his visit. John should ask Brett to call him into the room if Ilya's mother has questions about Ilya's care.

References

American Academy of Orthopaedic Surgeons. *http://www.aaos.org*

American Cancer Society. *http://www.cancer.org*

Centers for Disease Control and Prevention. *http://www.cdc.gov*

Daniels, R. (2002). *Delmar's manual of laboratory and diagnostic tests.* Clifton Park, NY: Thomson Delmar Learning.

Gahart, B.L. and Nazareno, A.R. (2005). *2005 Intravenous medications* (21st ed.). St. Louis: Mosby.

Intravenous Therapy. *http://www.nursewise.com*

Josephson, D.L. (2004). *Intravenous infusion therapy for nurses: Principles & practice* (2nd ed.). Clifton Park, NY: Thomson Delmar Learning.

North American Nursing Diagnosis Association. (2005). *Nursing diagnoses: Defintions & classifications, 2005–2006.* Philadelphia: NANDA.

Potts, N. and Mandleco, B. (2002). *Pediatric nursing: Caring for children and their families.* Clifton Park, NY: Thomson Delmar Learning, pp. 942–945.

Wong, D.L., Perry, S.E., and Hockenberry, M.J. (2002). *Maternal child nursing care* (2nd ed.). St. Louis: Mosby, pp. 1573–1574.

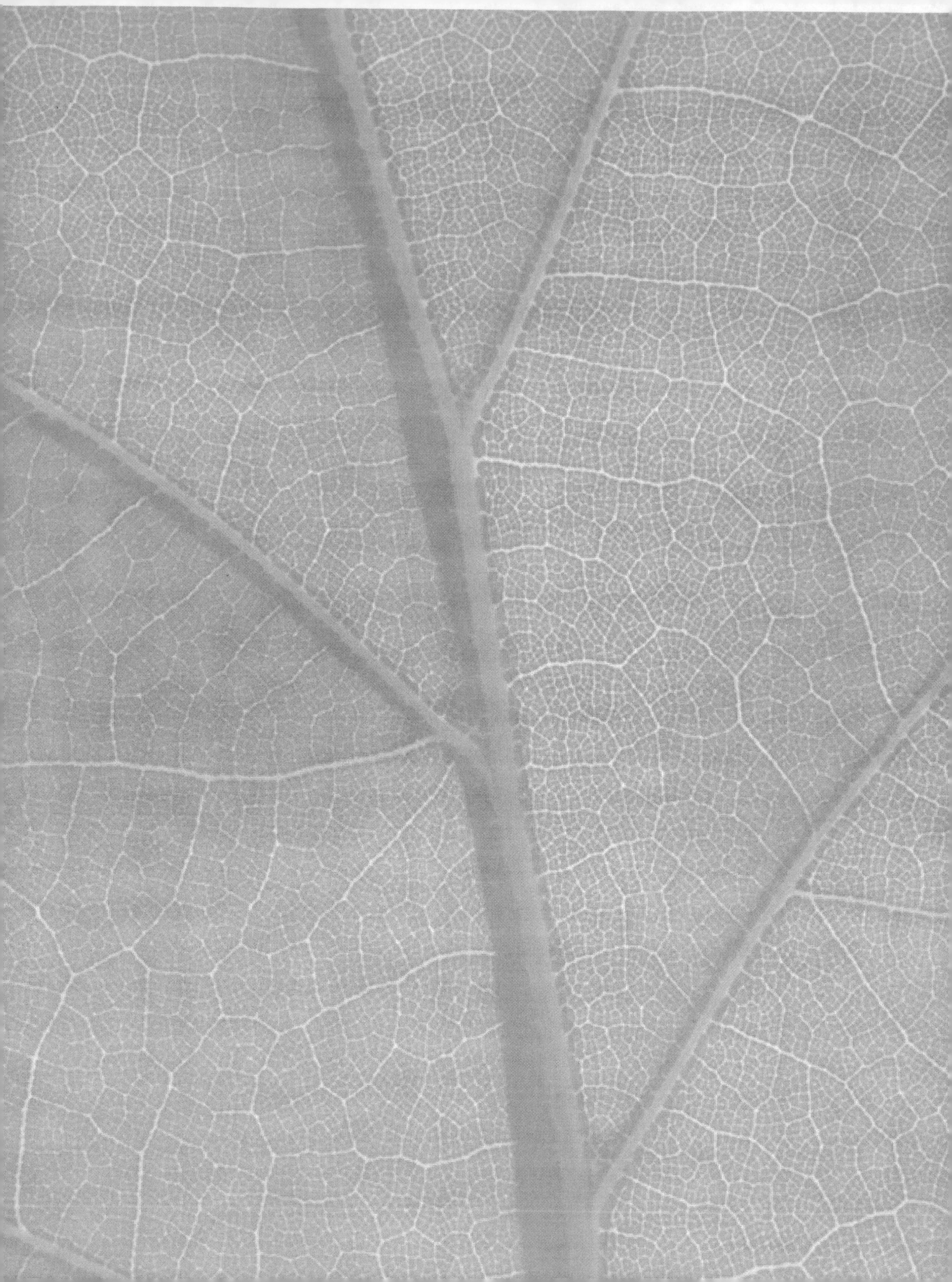

PART FIVE

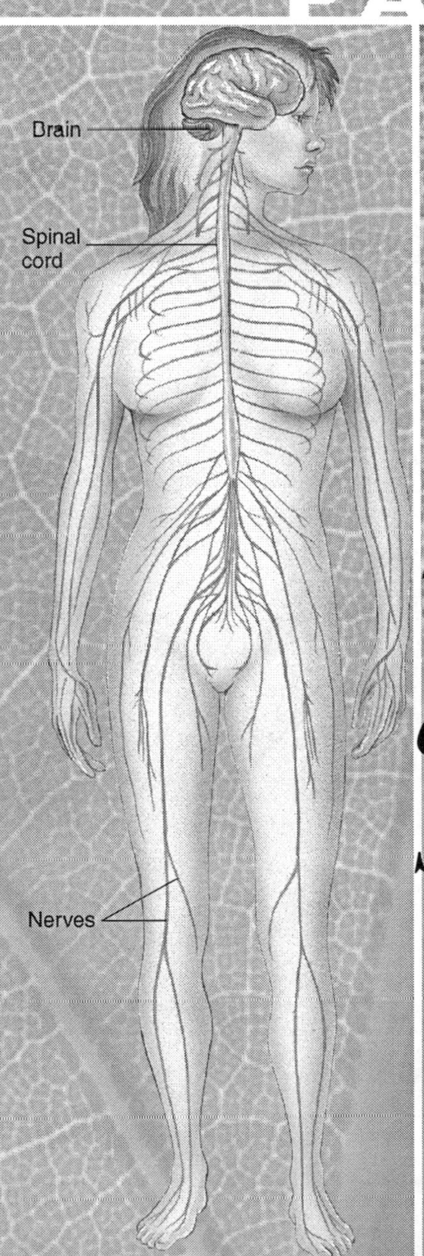

The Nervous and Endocrine Systems

CASE STUDY 1

Andrea

EASY

GENDER

F

AGE

7

SETTING

- Health care provider's office

ETHNICITY

- Spanish American

CULTURAL CONSIDERATIONS

PREEXISTING CONDITIONS

- Congenital hypothyroidism

COEXISTING CONDITIONS

SIGNIFICANT HISTORY

COMMUNICATION

DISABILITY

SOCIOECONOMIC

- Middle class

SPIRITUAL

PHARMACOLOGIC

- Levothyroxine sodium (Synthroid)

PSYCHOSOCIAL

LEGAL

ETHICAL

ALTERNATIVE THERAPY

PRIORITIZATION

- Yes

DELEGATION

- Yes

THE ENDOCRINE SYSTEM

Level of difficulty: Easy

Overview: This case requires knowledge of thyroid dysfunction, growth and development, as well as an understanding of the client's background, personal situation, and mother–child attachment relationship.

Client Profile

Andrea was 3.6 kg (8 lb) and was 50 cm (20 in.) long when she was born. At 2 months of age, she was diagnosed with congenital hypothyroidism. She is now 7 years old and lives with her mother and two siblings. Since her diagnosis she has been treated with levothyroxine. She sees her pediatrician every 6 months for follow-up and at her visit 6 weeks ago her dosage was increased to 125 mcg once every day . She enjoys school and earns a "B" average. For the past month Andrea has experienced difficulty in school and her mother notices that Andrea is irritable and has trouble keeping her attention focused on tasks that normally would not cause any difficulty. She has problems sleeping and for the past week has experienced daily bouts of diarrhea. Her mother makes an appointment with Andrea's pediatrician.

Case Study

Andrea is brought to the pediatrician's office by her mother. The office nurse greets Andrea and her mother and notes that Andrea is fidgety and has difficulty focusing on the nurse's questions. Andrea's vital signs are: temperature, 37.8° C (100° F); pulse, 120 beats/minute; respirations, 28 breaths/minute; and blood pressure, 116/76. She weighs 55 lb and is 112.5 cm (45 in.) tall. Her mother explains that Andrea has had diarrhea for the past week. During the nursing history, Andrea's mother tells the nurse about the other changes that she has noted in her daughter over the past month.

Questions and Suggested Answers

1. **What is congenital hypothyroidism?** Congenital hypothyroidism is the decreased concentration of triiodothyronine (T_3) and thyroxine (T_4) present at birth resulting in reduced metabolic rate. It is believed to result from an embryonic defect in the development of the thyroid gland or an inborn error in thyroid synthesis from an autosomal recessive hereditary trait. It also can result from abnormalities in the pituitary gland, which controls the release of the thyroid-stimulating hormone (TSH).

2. **Discuss the clinical manifestations of congenital hypothyroidism.** The clinical manifestations of congenital hypothyroidism include pallor, difficulty maintaining adequate temperature, hypoactivity, decreased muscle tone and reflexes, enlarged tongue, bradycardia, constipation, feeding difficulties, cool and dry skin, edema of the eyelids, and dull affect. These result from decreased metabolism.

3. **What is the incidence of congenital hypothyroidism and why is it important to diagnose this condition as soon as possible after birth?** Congenital hypothyroidism affects 1 in 4,000 live births. It is important to diagnose and treat this condition as soon as possible after birth to prevent cretinism, which is severe mental retardation. According to Potts (884), "In North America and most of Europe and Japan, mass screening of newborns for CH (congenital hypothyroidism) is routine and identifies the majority of those affected."

4. **Discuss the significance of Andrea's clinical manifestations and their possible causes.** Andrea is manifesting some of the classic symptoms of hyperthyroidism, a complication of thyroid replacement therapy. If an excess of thyroid hormones is present in the body, the metabolic rate increases beyond the normal level. This causes increased sensory stimulation, resulting in irritability, difficulty concentrating, and insomnia. The gastrointestinal system also is stimulated, leading to increased hunger with weight loss and diarrhea. Individually, these manifestations can have other causes; however, the likely reason for the combination of symptoms is that she is experiencing an adverse effect of her thyroid replacement therapy. Irritability and difficulty concentrating can result from attention deficit hyperactivity disorder. Diarrhea can occur secondary to a gastrointestinal parasitic infection or secondary to a respiratory infection or the antibiotics used to treat the infection.

5. **Discuss the significance of Andrea's vital signs.** Compared to the normal ranges of vital signs for a child Andrea's age, Andrea's vital signs indicate her temperature (37.8° C [100° F]) is above normal (36.7°–36.8° C [98°–98.2° F]); she is experiencing tachycardia, tachypnea, and her normal blood pressure is in the 95th percentile for her age. These are all manifestations of hyperthyroidism.

6. **What other assessment data would be helpful for the nurse to have to prepare Andrea's care plan?**
   a. Serum thyroid hormone levels and TSH
   b. Rest of nursing physical assessment data including heart sounds breath sounds, and bowel sounds
   c. Previous thyroid panel results
   d. Presence of other manifestations of hyperthyroidism

7. **What are the priorities of care for Andrea during this office visit?**
   a. Deficient fluid volume related to week of diarrhea
   b. Risk for decreased cardiac output related to tachycardia
   c. Imbalanced nutrition: less than body requirements related to increased metabolic rate
   d. Risk for delayed growth and development related to decreased metabolic function
   e. Disturbed sleep pattern related to increased metabolic rate
   f. Deficient knowledge related to condition, complications, clinical manifestations

8. **The safe dosage range of levothyroxine is 4–5 mcg/kg per day. Is Andrea's currently prescribed dosage safe for her?** Andrea weighs 55 lb that equals 25 kg. Her safe daily dosage range is 100–125 mcg, so her prescribed dosage is safe at the maximum level.

9. **Discuss your impressions of why Andrea's mother did not bring Andrea's other clinical manifestations to the pediatrician's attention earlier.** Perhaps she was not given the appropriate information about adverse effects (hyperthyroidism) of Andrea's drug therapy, or she may have been given this information but did not understand its significance. In addition, Andrea may not have experienced the adverse effects of thyroid replacement therapy before and over the course of 7 years may not have remembered the teaching she received, especially if it was not reinforced at each follow-up visit.

10. **How do you anticipate the pediatrician will treat Andrea's current condition?** After examining the serum thyroid panel, the health care provider will probably lower the dosage of levothyroxine and closely monitor the results. She may decide to discontinue her drug therapy for 1–2 weeks, which is the time frame necessary for the effects of any change of thyroid drug therapy.

11 **Discuss the teaching priorities for Andrea and her mother prior to discharge from the office today.**
   a. Assess Andrea's mother's current level of understanding of Andrea's condition and treatment.
   b. Provide verbal and written information regarding:
      (1) New dosage level of medication
      (2) Signs and symptoms of hypothyroidism (adverse effects of insufficient thyroid replacement)
      (3) Signs and symptoms of hyperthyroidism
      (4) Fluid replacement according to prescribed amount
      (5) When Andrea can return to school
      (6) Importance of 2-week follow-up visit for serum thyroid levels, drug dosage changes
   c. Provide sufficient time for Andrea's mother to ask questions, providing answers or appropriate referrals
   d. Document teaching and Andrea's mother's response

References

Bourgeois, M.J. (2003). Congenital hypothyroidism. *http://www.emedicine.com*

Centers for Disease Control and Prevention. *http://www.cdc.gov*

Daniels, R. (2002). *Delmar's manual of laboratory and diagnostic tests.* Clifton Park, NY: Thomson Delmar Learning.

Neonatal Screening. *http://aap.org*

North American Nursing Diagnosis Association. (2005). *Nursing diagnoses: Defintions & classifications, 2005–2006.* Philadelphia: NANDA.

Potts, N. and Mandleco, B. (2002). *Pediatric nursing: Caring for children and their families.* Clifton Park, NY: Thomson Delmar Learning, pp. 383–387, 884.

Spratto, G.R. and Woods, A.L. (2005). *2005 Edition: PDR nurse's drug handbook.* Clifton Park, NY: Thomson Delmar Learning, pp. 709–710.

CASE STUDY 2

Brent

MODERATE

GENDER

M

AGE

9

SETTING

- School/hospital

ETHNICITY

- White American

CULTURAL CONSIDERATIONS

PREEXISTING CONDITION

- Motor vehicle accident (MVA)/closed head injury (CHI)

COEXISTING CONDITIONS

SIGNIFICANT HISTORY

COMMUNICATION

DISABILITY

- Seizures

SOCIOECONOMIC

- Middle class

SPIRITUAL

PHARMACOLOGIC

- Phenytoin sodium (Dilantin)

PSYCHOSOCIAL

- Client anxiety
- Parental anxiety

LEGAL

ETHICAL

ALTERNATIVE THERAPY

PRIORITIZATION

DELEGATION

THE NERVOUS SYSTEM

Level of difficulty: Moderate

Overview: This case requires knowledge of seizures, growth and development, as well as an understanding of the client's background, personal situation, and parent–child relationship.

Client Profile

Brent is a 9-year-old school-age child who lives with his parents and two siblings. He attends middle school and achieves average performance. Last year Brent and his family were involved in a motor vehicle accident in which Brent experienced a closed head injury. He was hospitalized for 3 months and through therapy has regained his mobility, cognitive functioning, and most of his memory. During his recovery he experienced several seizures and was prescribed phenytoin sodium 50 mg PO t.i.d. When he returned to school, his parents informed the school nurse of Brent's condition. Brent takes one dose of medicine before school, one at lunchtime, and the last dose in the evening at home. This regimen has controlled his seizure activity.

Case Study

This afternoon at school, Brent experiences a seizure involving loss of consciousness, violent spasms, and stiffening with the upper extremities flexed and the lower extremities extended. His classroom teacher moved all the desks away from where Brent was having his seizure, placed a pillow under his head, and sent one of the other students in her class to bring the school nurse to the classroom. By the time the nurse arrived at the classroom about 2 minutes later, Brent's seizure was over and he was lying quietly on the floor. The nurse is able to arouse him and sent the teacher to the office to call 911. His parents were called, and he was transferred to the local acute care facility.

Questions and Suggested Answers

1. **What are seizures?** Seizures are occasional involuntary alterations in consciousness, behavior, movement, and/or sensation caused by excessive disorderly discharge of neuron activity in the brain (Broyles, 2005).
2. **Discuss the different types of seizures that affect children.** According to the Epilepsy Foundation of America (EFA), seizures are classified as partial seizures or generalized seizures with subclassifications under each. Partial seizures are classified as simple or complex. The physical characteristics of a simple partial seizure include jerking or shaking in one part of the body that sometimes progresses as the focus of the seizure tracks through the motor cortex. Loss of consciousness is not seen in the simple partial seizures. However, with the complex partial seizure immediate impairment of consciousness may occur and is frequently exhibited as a blank stare and automatic activities including lip smacking, chewing, picking at clothing, or purposeless walking. Generalized seizures always involve loss of consciousness regardless of whether there is convulsive behavior or not. Absence seizures (formerly called "petit mal" seizures) are most common in children from ages 4–8 years and decrease by the time the child reaches adulthood. These seizures are usually short in duration and are characterized by a blinking and a blank stare and can occur as many as 50–100 times a day. "Myoclonic seizures are characterized by quick, involuntary muscle jerks lasting a few seconds. The movements may be limited to one body part or involve the entire body and are most common in childhood through adolescence. Tonic seizures usually begin in childhood, last less than a minute, and are characterized by a violent spasm or stiffening; most frequently the upper extremities are flexed and lower extremities extended. Clonic seizures are most common in neonates and children and also are characterized by repetitive muscular jerks but at a slower rate. Generalized tonic–clonic seizures (formerly called "grand mal" seizures) are the most dramatic seizure type and the one most commonly identified with a seizure disorder (Broyles, 2005). According to the EFA, "these seizures begin with a sudden-onset tonic phase, typically lasting less than a minute. All skeletal muscles contract at once, and the patient falls stiffly. The diaphragm and chest muscles contract, forcing out air in an "epileptic cry." During the clonic phase, which lasts from one to several minutes, the patient may clench the jaws, biting the inside of the cheek or side of the tongue with the molars. As the clonic phase abates and muscles become flaccid, incontinence can occur. Consciousness may not return for 10–15 minutes; confusion, fatigue, and headache commonly last from hours to days." Finally, the atonic seizure is characterized

by sudden loss of postural tone and is associated with a high risk of injury resulting from falls. Febrile seizures are unique to children and occur when the child's body temperature rises sufficiently to cause increased neuronal activity. They occur secondary to an infection.

3. **How common are seizures in children and what causes them?** According to the EFA, "more than 2.5 million Americans of all ages are living with epilepsy (or seizure disorder). The condition can develop at any time of life, especially in early childhood and old age." Approximately 0.5% to 1% of children will experience at least one seizure during their childhood. Tonic seizures usually begin in childhood. Clonic seizures are most common in neonates and children. The exact cause of generalized seizures may be unknown (idiopathic, 50%) or associated with genetic predisposition or central nervous system conditions (brain tumors, trauma, infection). Febrile seizures typically affect children between the ages of 6 months and 5 years and are caused by a rapid temperature elevation usually associated with an infection.

4. **Discuss the significance of the characteristics of Brent's seizure.** The characteristics displayed by Brent during his seizure are consistent with generalized tonic seizure.

5. **Discuss the possible relationship between Brent's closed head injury and the development of seizures.** Head trauma can lead to seizure disorders as a result of neuron damage secondary to direct assault and/or increased intracranial pressure causing decreased cerebral tissue perfusion and neuron death. For most clients experiencing a severe head injury, anticonvulsant agents are used prophylactically to prevent seizures as well as to treat seizures if they occur.

6. **What assessment data would be helpful for the nurse to have to prepare Brent's care plan on admission?**
   a. Condition of airway, breathing, and circulation (ABCs)
   b. Level of consciousness
   c. Vital signs
   d. Height and weight
   e. Head-to-toe physical examination
   f. Serum glucose and electrolyte levels
   g. Computed tomography of the head
   h. Magnetic resonance imaging
   i. Electroencephalography
   j. Phenytoin sodium serum level

7. **What are the priorities of care for Brent on admission?**
   a. Risk for ineffective airway clearance related to airway obstruction secondary to tongue falling to back of the throat during a tonic seizure
   b. Risk for injury related to tonic activities during seizure
   c. Risk for ineffective cerebral tissue perfusion related to increased intracranial pressure during seizure
   d. Risk for delayed growth and development secondary to chronic condition and altered activities
   e. Deficient knowledge related to condition, treatment, and home care

8. **What is phenytoin sodium and why is Brent prescribed this medication?** Phenytoin sodium is a hydantoin anticonvulsant used to control seizure activity by increasing the seizure threshold in the central nervous system. Brent experienced seizure activity following his closed head injury and was prescribed phenytoin sodium to control these seizures.

9. **Brent's phenytoin sodium level is 4 mcg/mL. Discuss this level and what actions the nurse should take as a result of this information.** The normal therapeutic phenytoin sodium level is 5–20 mcg/mL. Brent's level is below the therapeutic level which could result in seizure activity because the seizure threshold is not high enough. The nurse should notify the health care provider and give her the information about the phenytoin level.

10. **Brent weighs 30 kg (66 lb) on admission. Following diagnostic testing, his health care provider increases Brent's dosage of phenytoin sodium to 75 mg PO t.i.d. Discuss the rationale for this change and whether this dose is**

within the safe dosage range. As noted in the above question, Brent's phenytoin sodium level is below the therapeutic range. The increase in dosage is designed to increase his level to within the therapeutic range. The safe maintenance dosage range for phenytoin sodium is 4–8 mg/kg up to a maximum of 300 mg/day (Spratto and Woods, 2005, p. 975). Brent can receive 120–240 mg/day. His current increase in dosage is 225 mg/day so it is safe. Periodic phenytoin sodium levels must be drawn to determine if the new dose is therapeutic.

11. **What impact might Brent's seizure condition have on his growth and development?** Brent is a school-age child and involved in the task of industry versus inferiority. He achieves his sense of industry through accomplishment of age-related activities. School-age children have a high degree of physical coordination and are involved in competitive activities. They are eager to learn and devote most of their waking time to school and playing with same-sex friends. Brent's seizure disorder will limit some of the activities in which he can participate that would place him in danger of a head injury, especially if he were involved in physical activity when a seizure occurred. Horseback riding usually is discouraged because even with a riding helmet, if Brent were to fall from a horse, the distance of his fall would likely result in a head injury. Other activities including bike riding, contact sports (baseball, basketball, soccer), tag, swimming (except diving), fishing, and so forth would still be permitted. Overprotectiveness on the part of his parents could limit his activities and interfere with his sense of accomplishment and interactions with other children his age. As long as normal safety practices are in place, Brent should be able to achieve his developmental task of industry.

12. **Discuss the teaching priorities for Brent and his parents as he prepares for discharge from the hospital.**
   - **a.** Assess Brent and his parent's current level of knowledge about his condition.
   - **b.** Provide verbal and written information regarding:
     - **(1)** Risk factors for injuries during seizures and instructions as needed to avoid risk factors, for instance, activities that increase his risk of head injury
     - **(2)** Factors that may predispose Brent to seizure activity including noncompliance with his anticonvulsant medication
     - **(3)** How to maintain patent airway and prevent injury during seizure activity
     - **(4)** Instructions for his family on how to monitor length and characteristics of seizure activity
     - **(5)** Medication administration including importance of compliance with the prescribed medication regimen
     - **(6)** Signs and symptoms of adverse effects of medications (drug toxicity)
     - **(7)** Signs and symptoms of worsening of seizure activity
     - **(8)** Contact phone numbers to report signs and symptoms
     - **(9)** The importance of wearing a Medic Alert bracelet or necklace at all times and provide instructions concerning how to obtain one
     - **(10)** Importance of follow-up care with health care provider and periodic drug levels labs
   - **c.** Provide for sufficient time for Brent and his family to ask questions, answering them honestly.
   - **d.** Document teaching and Brent and his family response.

References

Broyles, B.E. (2005). *Medical-surgical clinical nursing companion.* Durham, NC: Carolina Academic Press.

Centers for Disease Control and Prevention. *http://www.cdc.gov*

Epilepsy Foundation of America. *http://www.efa.org*

North American Nursing Diagnosis Association. (2005). *Nursing diagnosis: Definitions & classifications, 2005–2006.* Philadelphia: NANDA.

Potts, N. and Mandleco, B. (2002). *Pediatric nursing: Caring for children and their families.* Clifton Park, NY: Thomson Delmar Learning, pp. 1050–1058.

Seizures in Children: *http://www.webmd.com*

Spratto, G.R. and Woods, A.L. (2005). *2005 Edition PDR nurses's drug handbook.* Clifton Park, NY: Thomson Delmar Learning, p. 975.

Treatment of Epilepsy at Mayo Clinic. *http://www.mayoclinic.org*

CASE STUDY 3

Jessica

MODERATE

GENDER

F

AGE

13

SETTING

- Hospital

ETHNICITY

- White American

CULTURAL CONSIDERATIONS

PREEXISTING CONDITION

- Type 1 diabetes

COEXISTING CONDITIONS

SIGNIFICANT HISTORY

COMMUNICATION

DISABILITY

SOCIOECONOMIC

- Middle class

SPIRITUAL

PHARMACOLOGIC

- NPH Humulin insulin
- 5% Dextrose

PSYCHOSOCIAL

LEGAL

ETHICAL

ALTERNATIVE THERAPY

PRIORITIZATION

- Yes

DELEGATION

- Yes

THE ENDOCRINE SYSTEM

Level of difficulty: Moderate

Overview: This case requires knowledge of diabetes mellitus, nutritional needs of adolescence, as well as an understanding of the client's background, personal situation, and family relationship.

Client Profile

Jessica is a 13-year-old high school student who lives with her parents and younger brother Jonathan (11 years old) in a middle-class neighborhood. Both Mr. and Mrs. Morris work in the community where they live. Jessica has had diabetes mellitus type 1 (insulin-dependent diabetes mellitus [IDDM]) since the age of 7, which has been well controlled with morning and evening injections of NPH Humulin insulin, diet, and exercise. Jessica has been staying up later in the evenings studying for her end-of-year (EOY) exams, and is also the pitcher on her school's softball team, which is playing in the semifinals. Her heavy schedule has contributed to changes in her eating and sleeping habits.

Case Study

Jessica developed a cough, nasal congestion, and a low-grade temperature 3 days ago, but told her parents she felt well enough to go to school and didn't want to miss any of her classes or softball practice. Today Jessica felt worse, so her mother called Jessica's pediatrician, Dr. Sheila Jones, who told Mrs. Morris to bring Jessica into her office. Dr. Jones recommended that Mrs. Morris take Jessica to the emergency department of the hospital, at which point she noted that Jessica's pulse and respirations were elevated, her breath had a fruity odor, and her capillary blood sugar level was elevated. At the emergency department, Jessica's diagnostic test findings are as follows:

Chemistry profile: glucose, 480 mg/dL; sodium, 130 mEq/L; chloride, 79 mEq/L; and potassium, 3.3 mEq/L

Arterial blood gases: pH, 7. 19; $Paco_2$, 25 mm Hg; HCO_3, 10 mEq/L; Pao_2, 92 mm Hg; oxygen saturation, 97%

Questions and Suggested Answers

1. **Discuss your impressions about the above situation.** Jessica's glucose level indicates hyperglycemia; the normal blood glucose level for adolescents is 70–105 mg/dL. Her sodium, chloride, and potassium levels are lower than normal. The normal level of sodium for a child Jessica's age is 135–145 mEq/L. The normal potassium level for children older than 12 years of age is 3.5–5.0 mEq/L., and the normal chloride level is 96–106 mEq/L. The drop in these values probably is caused by the kidney's attempt to excrete the excess glucose in Jessica's blood stream through diuresis. These values also are consistent with hyperglycemia.

2. **How do you explain the abnormal values of Jessica's arterial blood gases?** In diabetes mellitus type 1, elevated blood glucose levels due to insufficient insulin cause the body to utilize fat, which is normally our secondary source of energy to become the body's primary energy source. Metabolic processes increase, as more energy is required to break down fats than carbohydrates. In addition, the action of the kidneys has increased as a result of their attempt to decrease the blood glucose level by excreting it in the urine. Fat metabolism causes an increase in ketone bodies (a by-product of fat metabolism) that results in metabolic acidosis. Jessica's pH of 7.19 indicates acidosis. Normal blood pH is 7.35–7.45. The lungs are the first acid–base buffer; they attempt to return the pH to normal by increasing the output of carbon dioxide from the lungs, which is evident in Jessica's $Paco_2$ of 25 mm Hg, The normal carbon dioxide level is 35–45 mm Hg. The kidneys regulate bicarbonate levels, however they do not effectively buffer the acid–base imbalance until 24 hours after the onset of the imbalance. Jessica's blood oxygen level and oxygen saturation are within normal limits; normal oxygen levels are 80–100 mm Hg and normal oxygen saturation is is 95% to 100%.

3. **What data indicate that Jessica's lungs are attempting to compensate for her present condition?** Her decreased carbon dioxide level indicates that the lungs are attempting to compensate for the acidosis by increasing the amount of carbon dioxide exhaled from the body. The breathing pattern in diabetic ketoacidosis (DKA) is called Kussmaul respirations, which are characterized by rapid, deep respirations that have an acetone smell because of the elevated ketone bodies in the blood stream. Her CO_2 level of 25 mm Hg further indicates the lungs' attempt to compensate to reverse the acidosis.

4. **What factors place Jessica at risk for DKA?** Jessica has a number of risk factors. First, she is an adolescent and involved in the second physical growth spurt of life; this can compromise the regulation of her diabetes. More energy is required during this time of growth and management of insulin requirements becomes more complex. Jessica also has been dealing with her school stressors of preparing for her end-of-year exams and softball. This has caused changes in her eating and sleeping habits. In addition, her body has experienced the stressor of flu-like symptoms including a low-grade temperature that also increases her metabolic needs.

5. **What other data would be helpful to determine whether she has developed other complications of either her DKA or her flu-like symptoms?** A chest x-ray may indicate the progression of the flu to pneumonia, which would further compromise Jessica's health. Listening to breath sounds also would provide data about the status of her respiratory system. Sputum culture and urinalysis could indicate or eliminate sources of infection that would require antibiotic therapy. An electrocardiogram or telemetry would show cardiac electrical conduction that can be compromised by Jessica's serum potassium level.

6. **What medical management should you be prepared to initiate for Jessica?** The standard of care for DKA is the initiation of intravenous access and IV fluids of 0.9% normal saline to provide hydration and replace sodium and chloride electrolytes. This solution is administered at a rate of 250–500 mL/hour. Intravenous insulin infusion is initiated with continuous monitoring of Jessica's blood sugar, not only to monitor the effectiveness of the fluid and insulin therapy, but also to prevent severe hypoglycemia if her blood sugar drops too rapidly. Sodium bicarbonate may be administered to assist in treating the acidosis. Placing a Foley (indwelling) urinary catheter is necessary to provide data about the effectiveness of her IV therapy.

7. **After Jessica has received 2 L of intravenous fluids and her blood glucose level decreases 240 mg/dL, the health care provider prescribes adding 5% dextrose to her intravenous solution. Should you question this prescription? Why or why not?** The nurse should not question this prescription because administration of 1–2 L of sodium chloride intravenous fluids and evidence that Jessica's blood sugar is dropping are indicators that a source of glucose is necessary to prevent a rapid drop in blood sugar with resulting hypoglycemia. As Jessica has no other source of glucose, adding 5% glucose to the intravenous solution provides a standard source of glucose to prevent hypoglycemia. Jessica's blood sugar probably rose to its current level over a period of days or weeks and must not be decreased too rapidly.

8. **What other medical management interventions would you expect to be prescribed to facilitate Jessica's recovery?** According to the 2004 guidelines for management of pediatric hyperglycemic crises in diabetes, "Initial fluid therapy is directed toward expansion of the intravascular and extravascular volume and restoration of renal profusion. The need for vascular volume expansion must be offset by the risk of cerebral edema associated with rapid fluid administration. The 1st hour of fluids should be isotonic saline (0.9% NaCl) at the rate of 10–20 ml $\cdot$ $kg^{-1} \cdot h^{-1}$. In a severely dehydrated patient, this may need to be repeated, but the initial reexpansion should not exceed 50 mL/kg over the first 4 h of therapy. Continued fluid therapy is calculated to replace the fluid deficit evenly over 48 h. In general, 0.45–0.9% NaCl (depending on serum sodium levels) infused at a rate of 1.5 times the 24-h maintenance requirements (5 mL $\cdot$ $kg^{-1} \cdot h^{-1}$) will accomplish a smooth rehydration, with a decrease in osmolality not exceeding 3 mOsm $\cdot$ kg^{-1} $H_2O \cdot h^{-1}$. Once renal function is assured and serum potassium is known, the infusion should include 20–40 mEq/L potassium (2/3 KCl or potassium-acetate and 1/3 KPO_4). Once serum glucose reaches 250 mg/dL, fluid should be changed to 5% dextrose and 0.45–0.75% NaCl, with potassium as described above. Therapy should include monitoring mental status to rapidly identify changes that might indicate iatrogenic fluid overload, which can lead to symptomatic cerebral edema" (*http://www.diabetes.org*). Potassium chloride is added to the intravenous solution to help raise her potassium level to within normal limits. It cannot be added to the rapidly infusing sodium chloride solution during rehydration therapy because it may elevate the potassium level too fast and too high and place Jessica at risk for cardiac dysrhythmias. Continuous cardiac monitoring should be maintained.

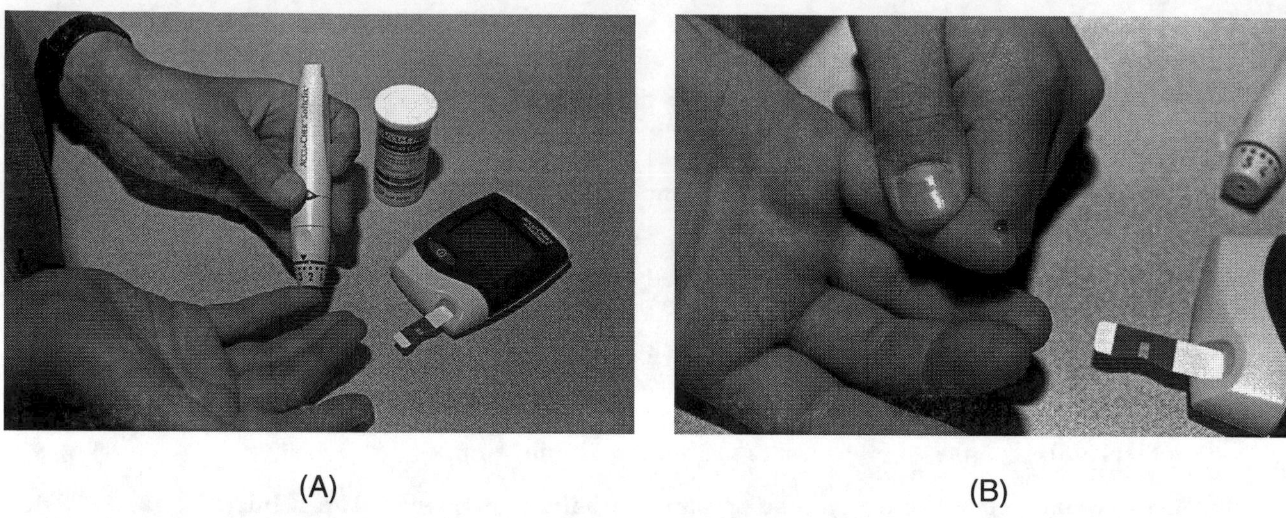

(A) (B)

Figure A-16 *School-aged children are able to perform their own blood glucose monitoring.*

9. **Discuss the potential complications for Jessica if she is not compliant with her medical regimen when she goes home.** Besides DKA, both macro- and microvascular changes occur as a result of consistently elevated blood glucose levels. According to the American Diabetes Association, chronic elevations in blood glucose >140 mg/dL cause vessel sclerosing leading to a narrowing of the vessels. Eventually cells and tissues being supplied by these vessels experience hypoxia and die. The smaller vessels of the eyes are affected, causing diabetic retinopathy and eventual blindness. Diabetes is the leading cause of blindness in persons 20–75 years of age in the United States. People with diabetes are twice as likely to develop heart disease and the disease is the leading cause of renal failure in this country. Because of both vascular changes and neuropathy secondary to the destruction of the myelin sheath that surrounds and protects nerves by elevated glucose levels, people with diabetes are four times as likely to experience amputations. They also are three times as likely to die of complications of influenza and pneumonia. In addition, social and psychological complications related to role performance, self-esteem, employment, and finances can accompany the physiological problems.

10. **In collaboration with the health care provider, what referrals might you obtain prior to Jessica's discharge?** Although nothing in the case study indicates that Jessica has deliberately not managed her diabetes or that her parents are at fault for Jessica's present condition, a child psychologist may be referred to ensure that no problems exist. The guidance counselor, school nurse, and Jessica's teachers at her school should be aware to help Jessica with time management, monitoring her condition, ensuring that she eats before softball practice and/or carries a source of rapidly absorbing glucose (life-savers, soda) with her during practice. This can be done only with Jessica and her parents' consent. A home health nurse referral may be useful to help monitor Jessica's blood sugar and reinforce diabetic teaching. Involvement with a local diabetes support group also might be helpful. Of course, a dietary consult would be appropriate for Jessica.

11. **What are the teaching priorities for Jessica and her parents prior to discharge?**
    a. Assess Jessica and her parents' level of knowledge about diabetes and the importance of compliance with her medical regimen of diet, insulin, and exercise (see Fig. A-16).
    b. Reinforce the basic pathophysiology of diabetes, remembering Jessica's level of growth and development centering on Erikson's "identity versus role confusion." Explain the nutritional need increases with adolescence and incorporate dietician in evaluation and teaching.
    c. Help Jessica with stress and time management by collaborating with her to develop a daily schedule for her to include her studies, softball, time for activities with friends, and compliance with her medical regimen.
    d. Assess Jessica's ability to monitor her capillary blood sugar including how often this should be done daily.

e. Reinforce the following information:
   (1) Insulin storage, preparation, and administration
   (2) Subcutaneous sites for injection including importance of rotating sites
   (3) Signs and symptoms of hyperglycemia and hypoglycemia
   (4) Sources of glucose in the event of hypoglycemia occurrence (orange juice, sugar)
   (5) Preparation and administration of glucagon in the event that Jessica loses consciousness due to presence of too much insulin
   (6) Proper daily foot care
   (7) Importance of an annual eye examination
   (8) Importance of routine medical follow-up/monitoring

f. Evaluate Jessica's ability to perform insulin injections.

g. Provide nutritional guidance regarding exchange list.

h. Provide information concerning referrals and phone numbers to report changes in condition.

i. Provide adequate time for client and family questions.

j. Document teaching and Jessica and her parents' response.

References

American Diabetes Association. *http://www.diabetes.org*

Broyles, B.E. (2005). *Medical-surgical nursing clinical companion.* Durham, NC: Carolina Academic Press.

Centers for Disease Control and Prevention. *http://www.cdc.gov*

Daniels, R. (2002). *Delmar's manual of laboratory and diagnostic tests.* Clifton Park, NY: Thomson Delmar Learning.

Diabetes. *http://www.niddk.nih.gov*

Gahart, B.L. and Nazareno, A.R. (2005). *2005 Intravenous medications* (21st ed.). St. Louis: Mosby.

North American Nursing Diagnosis Association. (2005). Nursing diagnoses: Definitions & classifications, 2005–2006. Philadelphia: NANDA.

Potts, N. and Mandleco, B. (2002). *Pediatric nursing: Caring for children and their families.* Clifton Park, NY: Thomson Delmar Learning.

CASE STUDY 4

Melanie

GENDER

F

AGE

16

SETTING

- Psychiatric unit

ETHNICITY

- White American

CULTURAL CONSIDERATIONS

PREEXISTING CONDITIONS

COEXISTING CONDITIONS

SIGNIFICANT HISTORY

- Interrupted relationships

COMMUNICATION

DISABILITY

SOCIOECONOMIC

- Middle class

SPIRITUAL

PHARMACOLOGIC

PSYCHOSOCIAL

- Recent parent separation
- Recent break-up with boyfriend

LEGAL

- Physical restraints

ETHICAL

ALTERNATIVE THERAPY

PRIORITIZATION

- Yes

DELEGATION

MODERATE

THE NERVOUS SYSTEM

Level of difficulty: Moderate

Overview: This case requires knowledge of anger issues, growth and development, as well as an understanding of the client's background, personal situation, and family–child relationship.

Client Profile

Melanie is a 16-year-old who lived with her parents and two siblings in a suburban neighborhood until her parents separated 6 months ago. At that time her school performance began to decline and she was truant from school, frequently not returning home until after dark. When she arrived home, she was verbally abusive to her mother when asked where she had been. Three days ago, her relationship with her boyfriend of 1 year ended when he told her she had "changed" and he didn't know how to "relate to her anymore." That evening, Melanie became very disruptive at home, breaking lamps and mirrors and turning over furniture. When her mother attempted to talk to Melanie, her daughter threatened her. Melanie was admitted to the children's psychiatric unit of the local inpatient mental health facility.

Case Study

Since her admission, Melanie has refused to attend any group sessions or talk to staff, and spends most of her time in her room. At change of shifts today, the staff heard a loud noise after which the registered nurse and two psychiatric technologists (psych tech) rushed to Melanie's room. There they observed Melanie screaming incoherently and throwing chairs against the wall; clothes were littered across the floor.

Questions and Suggested Answers

1. **Discuss your impression of the situation with Melanie.** With the information given, Melanie seems to be having trouble coping with her parents' separation. The grief process is normal when anyone experiences a loss and part of the grief process is anger. Her truant behavior may be a method of getting her parents to reconcile to help her. Children also commonly feel that they are responsible in some way if their parents' marriage experiences difficulties, especially to the point of separation. Her behavior places stress on her relationship with her boyfriend and culminates in another loss for Melanie. Melanie's coping mechanisms are unable to deal with these losses.

2. **What impact might Melanie's level of growth and development have on her response to life stressors?** Adolescence is a stressful period of growth and development. Melanie is trying to establish her identity, wants to be like her peers, and is experiencing many physiological changes that accompany pubescence. Risk-taking behavior is common and this may be manifesting in her truancy from school. She may be feeling that her parents' separation makes her different from her friends and that jeopardizes her feelings of belonging. The behavior she exhibits toward her mother may indicate that she wants to blame someone for her situation and the human response is to strike out at loved ones who won't abandon her or stop loving her.

3. **What are the priorities of care for Melanie at this time?**
   a. Ineffective coping related to life changing stressors
   b. Risk for other-directed violence related to Melanie's behavior and verbal threats to her mother
   c. Risk for injury related to anger outbursts
   d. Deficient knowledge related to circumstances surrounding her parents' separation and positive coping strategies to assist adjusting to stressors.

4. **What other assessment data would be helpful for the nurse to have to prepare Melanie's care plan?**
   a. Has Melanie experienced previous stressors? If so, how did she respond to those stressors?
   b. Does she have any medical conditions that could contribute to her behavior?
   c. Is there any evidence that would warrant obtaining serum electrolytes and complete blood count?
   d. How did she threaten her mother?
   e. When she is truant, what does she do, where does she go, with whom does she communicate?

f. Does she have support systems available to her?
g. Does she drink alcohol or use drugs?
h. Has Melanie ever been violent to others before?
i. Has Melanie ever been suicidal?
j. Who are her friends and do they support her?
k. How does she feel about her parents' separation (from her own verbalizations)?
l. Does she feel she is responsible for her parents' marital problems?
m. How does she feel about her boyfriend ending their relationship?
n. Has she experienced any additional stressors during this time?
o. Is she receiving any medications at this time?

5. **What factors should the nurse consider prior to approaching Melanie?** The nurse must consider both Melanie's safety and the safety of the nurse and the other staff members. Is Melanie in danger of hurting herself? Has she actually threatened the staff since her admission? What is available to Melanie to use to physically threaten the staff, if anything? Are any of the other clients on the unit in jeopardy? Is there anyone on staff that Melanie trusts? These questions need to be addressed before approaching Melanie. The nurse's response will depend to the individual situation.

6. **When Melanie attempts to throw a chair at staff, the nurse supervisor determines that Melanie needs physical restraint. Discuss the supervisor's decision.** The supervisor has determined that Melanie presents a danger to the staff and needs physical restraint. The supervisor must consider the client's needs, the safety needs of the staff, and maintaining a therapeutic environment for the other clients on the unit.

7. **What precautions must be taken when physically restraining a client?** Laws vary from state to state; however, guidelines for the use of restraints are consistent. Physical restraints require a prescription from a health care provider; however, they can be applied by the nurse without a prescription in a situation in which the client poses a direct threat to self or others (see Fig. A-17). The prescription is then procured from the health care provider as soon as possible. In acute care facilities, this prescription must be reevaluated and renewed every 24 hours. Mental health facilities may have written protocols regarding restraints, leaving more responsibility for the professional nurse. The nurse must be familiar with the statutes that govern the use of restraints in the facility where the nurse works. Neurovascular status must be assessed every 2 hours in clients in physical restraints to prevent compromise. Restraints that are applied around the chest area must be assessed for respiratory compromise.

8. **Do you think that Melanie's behavior at home warranted hospitalization?** This question will be difficult to answer because of lack of sufficient data. Refer to question #4. If Melanie's behavior did pose a direct physical threat to her mother, her mother may have chosen to admit her to the mental health facility rather than involve the police. The student should investigate the laws in his or her state to determine if statutes specific to the admission of children and adolescents to mental health facilities exist. The student also should investigate court cases involving the placement of minors in mental health facilities.

9. **Do you think her present behavior warrants continued hospitalization?** Her present behavior indicates that Melanie may be a threat to others and needs professional evaluation on an in-patient basis until the reason for and extent of her behavior can be assessed. After psychologic and psychiatric evaluation, a plan of care can be developed and decisions made concerning whether she needs continued hospitalization.

10. **Discuss the advantages of waiting until all the data are available before making decisions about Melanie's course of treatment.** Without all the information about Melanie and her physiological and psychological status, the appropriate course of treatment is not possible. Treatment in one situation may be healthful but in a situation with different circumstances may actually make the client's problems worse. For instance, many agents used to treat psychiatric or psychological disorders are not compatible with agents used to treat certain physical conditions. Psychiatric agents used in the absence of actual psychiatric pathology can create psychological dysfunction.

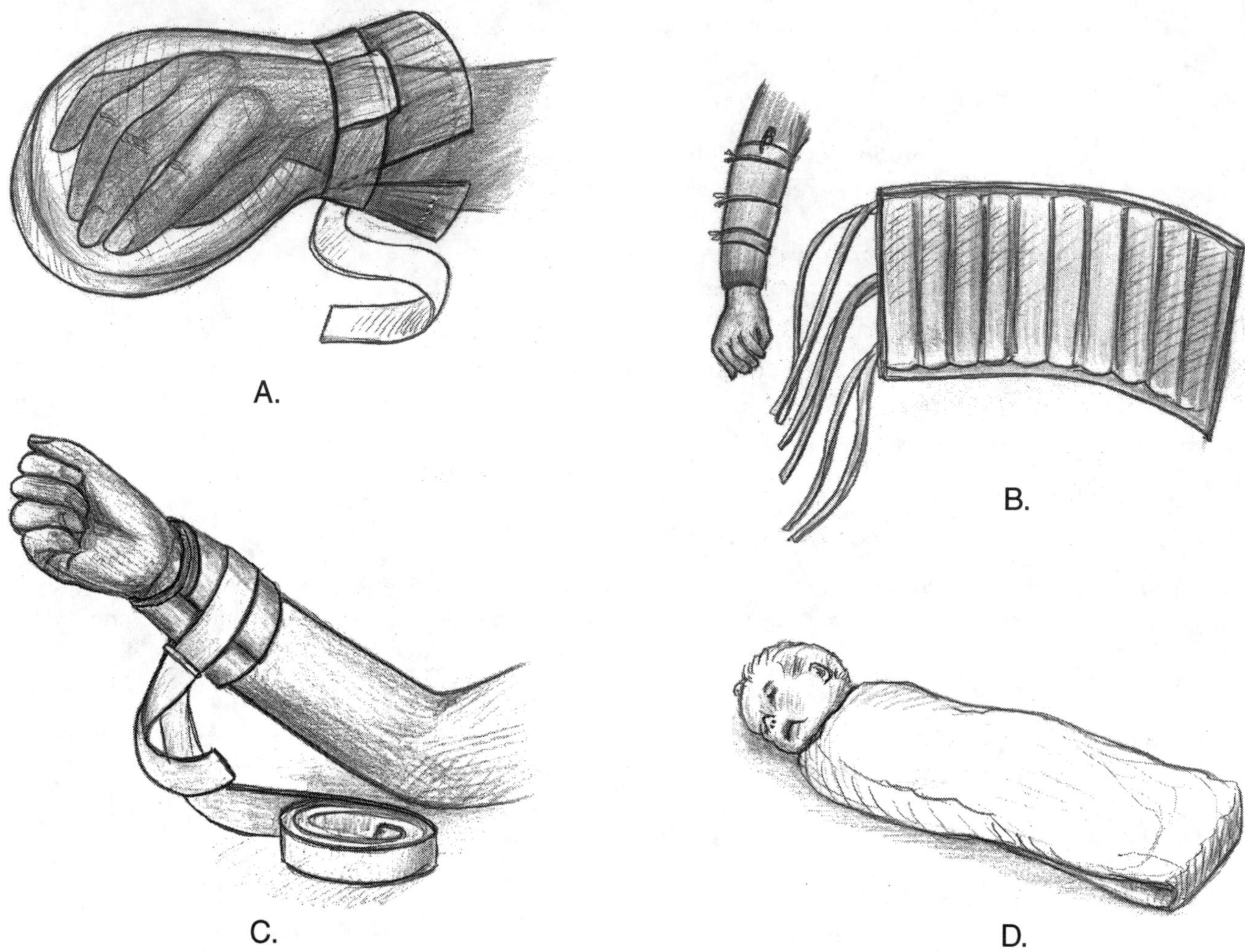

Figure A-17 *Types of physical restraints: A. Mitten or hand; B. Elbow; C. Limb or extremity; D. Mummy*

11. **Melanie's mother calls the unit every day to check on her daughter but is not sure whether she should visit Melanie because, as she says, "I'm afraid I'll upset her. I think she feels that this whole situation is my fault. I love my daughter and I just want her to get well." How would you respond to Melanie's mother?** The nurse should use therapeutic communication techniques such as, restating, validating, and open-ended questions to assess her feelings and the reasons for them. Collaboration with the psychiatric health care provider is necessary and then a multidisciplinary approach with both Melanie and her mother is appropriate.

References

Adolescent Anger Management Program. *http://www.mhcana.org*

American Academy of Child & Adolescent Psychiatry. *http://www.aacap.org*

Centers for Disease Control and Prevention. *http://www.cdc.gov*

North American Nursing Diagnosis Association. (2005). *Nursing diagnoses: Definitions & classifications, 2005–2006.* Philadelphia: NANDA.

Parent Help for Troubled Teens. *http://www.troubledteenhelp.org*

CASE STUDY 5

Andrew

GENDER

M

AGE

10

SETTING

- Hospital

ETHNICITY

- White American

CULTURAL CONSIDERATIONS

PREEXISTING CONDITIONS

- MVA

COEXISTING CONDITIONS

SIGNIFICANT HISTORY

COMMUNICATION

DISABILITY

SOCIOECONOMIC

SPIRITUAL

PHARMACOLOGIC

- Ranitidine (Zantal)
- Metoclopramide (Maxolan)
- Phenytoin (Dilantin)

PSYCHOSOCIAL

- Parental anxiety

LEGAL

ETHICAL

ALTERNATIVE THERAPY

PRIORITIZATION

- Yes

DELEGATION

- Yes

THE NERVOUS SYSTEM

Level of difficulty: Difficult

Overview: This case requires knowledge of head trauma, increased intracranial pressure, growth and development and nutrition, as well as an understanding of the client's background, personal situation, and parent–child relationship.

Client Profile

Andrew is a 10-year-old fifth grader who lives with his parents in the suburb of a large city. He is active in school and enjoys playing with his neighborhood friends. His father (Randy) works in the city and his mother (Joyce) works part-time as a computer programmer from her home office. She takes Andrew to and from school each day and is active in all of his school and extracurricular activities. Andrew is an A–B student who enjoys his school subjects and wants to study to become a doctor one day. The family lives approximately 5 miles from his school. Mr. Burger also is very involved in his son's activities.

Case Study

After picking up Andrew at school 3 weeks ago, Mrs. Burger was involved in a serious motor vehicle accident while driving home. Both she and Andrew had their seat belt restraints fastened. The accident occurred when a van did not stop for a stop-light and struck their car in the side where Andrew was riding. Mrs. Burger sustained lacerations from broken window glass, but Andrew received a closed head injury from the impact. Mrs. Burger was treated in the emergency department of the city hospital and released; however, Andrew was admitted to the pediatric intensive care unit. He was nonresponsive at the scene of the accident, and on admission his Glasgow Coma Scale score was 3 out of 15. He was transferred to the pediatric nursing unit last week. A CD player at his bedside plays music. He focuses and tracks as his parents talk to him, and they perform most of his care, including range-of-motion exercises twice a day. He is receiving oxygen via a tracheostomy collar. He coughs up most of his respiratory secretions, but still requires suctioning every 3–4 hours. He receives enteral nutrition through his gastrostomy tube. This is the first day you have been assigned to Andrew, and during your assessment you find the client awake and able to respond by nodding and shaking his head for "yes" and "no" when questioned. He moves his extremities spontaneously and on command; however; you note bilateral weakness. His Glasgow Coma Scale score currently is 4–1–5; his vital signs are within normal limits for his age; he weighs 77 lb and is 1.5 m (5 ft) tall. His lungs are clear bilaterally and his bowel sounds are present on all four quadrants. He remains incontinent of urine and stool. You overhear Andrew's mother tell him she is "so sorry" about the accident and she begins to cry softly.

Questions and Suggested Answers

1. **Discuss the priorities of care for Andrew on his admission to the pediatric critical care unit.**
   - **a.** Impaired gas exchange related to ineffective airway clearance, ineffective breathing pattern, and impaired spontaneous ventilation related to decreased respiratory drive secondary to increased intracranial pressure (ICP)
   - **b.** Impaired cerebral tissue perfusion related to increased intracranial pressure reducing vessel capacity to supply brain tissue with oxygen and nutrients
   - **c.** Decreased intracranial adaptive capacity related to edema secondary to inflammatory response to tissue trauma (see Fig. A-18)
   - **d.** Risk for injury, seizures related to neuron stimulation secondary to tissue trauma
   - **e.** Risk for imbalanced nutrition related to increased metabolic needs and reduced oral intake secondary to decreased level of consciousness
   - **f.** Total urinary and bowel incontinence related to impaired cognitive function
   - **g.** Ineffective coping, parents, related to extent of Andrew's injuries
   - **h.** Deficient knowledge related to Andrew's condition, treatment, prognosis

2. **What were the priority nursing interventions for Andrew on his admission to the PICU?**
   - **a.** Impaired gas exchange
     - **(1)** Monitor respiratory status continuously.

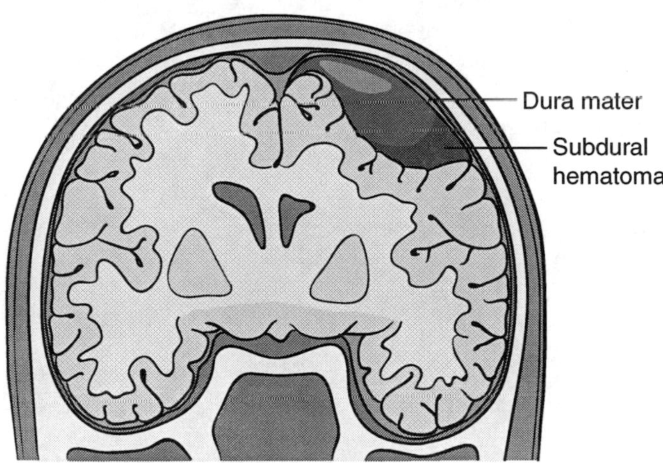

Figure A-18 *Subdural hematoma*

(2) Auscultate lung sounds every 1–2 hours and report adventitious sounds immediately.
(3) Administer oxygen, titrating to maintain oxygen saturation >94% via pulse oximetry.
(4) Assess for manifestations of hypoxia including level of consciousness (LOC).
(5) Maintain airway patency by proper positioning of neck and head and elevating the head as prescribed.
(6) Maintain mechanical ventilator settings as prescribed and according to the client's condition.
(7) Perform endotracheal or tracheostomy suctioning as indicated, being careful to avoid increasing intracranial pressure (ICP) when suctioning.
(8) Perform tracheostomy care at every shift and as needed.
(9) Perform chest physiotherapy as prescribed in collaboration with physical or respiratory therapy.
(10) Monitor arterial blood gases, maintaining patency of arterial access.
(11) Monitor pulmonary artery pressure (PAP) and mean arterial pressure (MAP).

b. Ineffective cerebral tissue perfusion
(1) Monitor cerebral perfusion pressure (CPP).
(2) Assess neurological status every hour and as needed.
(3) Administer medications (osmotic diuretic, antiinflammatory agents) as prescribed.
(4) Position to facilitate reducing intracranial pressure.
(5) Monitor effectiveness of medications by maintaining strict intake and output.
(6) Maintain oxygen saturation >94%.
(7) Assess for potential causes of increased ICP (pain, fear and anxiety, bladder and/or bowel distention, vigorous tracheostomy suctioning).
(8) Adjust nursing care to limit activities that cause CPP to rise >5 mm Hg.
(9) Ensure CPP and ICP return to baseline within 5 minutes after cessation of activity.
(10) Assess for leakage of cerebral spinal fluid (CSF) from eyes, nose, and ears.
(11) Collaborate with health care provider to initiate bowel program to prevent constipation.
(12) DO NOT PLACE IN TRENDELENBURG POSITION.
(13) Maintain patency of intravenous access, monitoring hourly.
(14) Monitor for posturing and report immediately if present.

c. Decreased intracranial adaptive capacity
(1) Monitor neurological status every hour and as needed.
(2) Administer medications as prescribed.
(3) Monitor effectiveness of medications.
(4) Position to decrease intracranial pressure (head of bed elevated 10–15°)
(5) Maintain strict intake and output.

(6) Maintain patency of intravenous access, monitoring hourly.
(7) Assess for potential causes of increased ICP (pain, fear and anxiety, bladder and/or bowel distention, vigorous tracheostomy suctioning).
(8) Adjust nursing care to limit activities that cause CPP to rise >5 mm Hg.
(9) Ensure CPP and ICP return to baseline within 5 minutes after cessation of activity.
(10) Assess for leakage of CSF from eyes, nose, and ears.
(11) Collaborate with health care provider to initiate bowel program to prevent constipation.
(12) DO NOT PLACE IN TRENDELENBURG POSITION.
(13) Monitor for development of posturing and report immediately if present.

d. Risk for injury, seizures
(1) Monitor neurological status every hour and as needed.
(2) Administer anticonvulsants as prescribed, taking appropriate precautions when administering intravenously.
(3) Monitor blood levels of anticonvulsants prescribed.
(4) Institute facility seizure precautions.
(5) Place on EEG monitoring, if available.

3. What is the meaning and significance of Andrew's Glasgow Coma Scale score on admission? The Glasgow Coma Scale is the standard for assessing level of consciousness, the primary indicator of neurological status. The scale measures three categories of cerebral functioning and is broken down into responses with numerical values, as follows:

Category	Response	Score
Eye Opening	Spontaneously	4
	To speech	3
	To pain	2
	No response	1
	Eyes closed due to swelling	C
Verbal Response	Oriented	5
	Confused	4
	Inappropriate words	3
	Incomprehensible sounds	2
	No response	1
	Tracheostomy present	T
Motor Response	Obeys commands	6
	Localizes pain	5
	Flexion withdrawal	4
	Abnormal flexion	3
	Abnormal extension	2
	No response	1

Maximum Total 15; Minimum Total 3

Andrew was nonresponsive according to the scenario, and his Glasgow Coma Scale score demonstrates this. This is common following a traumatic brain injury because of the edema associated with the inflammatory response that occurs with tissue trauma and potential vessel damage leading to intracranial bleeding. His score indicates minimal neurological functioning. Another important indicator of neurological functioning is the presence or absence of posturing, which may be either decorticate or decerebrate. Decorticate posturing is characterized by abnormal flexion of the extremities and indicates bilateral cerebral hemisphere injury. Some nurses refer to the appearance of this posturing as "to the corc" because the extremities assume an inward position toward the body. Decerebrate is rigid extension posturing; it signifies medullary injury and is associated with a poor prognosis. No posturing was noted in Andrew's assessment.

4. **Discuss the differences between the Glasgow Coma Scale used for infants and children and the Glasgow Coma Scale used for adults and which one is the most appropriate one to use when assessing Andrew.** See the previous answer for Glasgow Coma Scale used when assessing adults. The Glasgow Coma Scale developed for assessing infants and children has the same categories and maximum and minimum totals; however, the responses differ. The Glasgow Coma Scale for infants and children is:

Category	Response	Score
Eye Opening	Spontaneous	4
	To command	3
	To pain	2
	No response	1
Verbal Response	Coos and babbles	5
	Irritable cry	4
	Cries to pain	3
	Moans to pain	2
	No response	1
Motor Response	Normal spontaneous movement	6
	Withdraws to touch	5
	Withdraws to pain	4
	Abnormal flexion	3
	Abnormal extension	2
	No response	1

The scale used to assess infants and children focuses primarily on responses of infants and young children and is especially helpful in assessing preverbal children. Given Andrew's age and the evidence of his cognitive ability prior to the accident, the Glasgow Coma Scale used for adults would be most appropriate for his assessment.

5. **Why do you think Andrew has a tracheostomy?** Traumatic brain injury and the increased intracranial pressure that accompanies this type of injury usually results in impairment of spontaneous ventilatory ability that requires mechanical support. This can be achieved by endotracheal intubation or the creation of a tracheostomy. Emergency tracheostomies usually are performed only if needed in the presence of edema that does not allow the passage of an endotracheal tube for mechanical ventilatory support. The scenario does not discuss whether this was the case for Andrew although in the presence of his injury, swelling of the neck area is possible. If not performed as an emergency procedure for airway obstruction, a tracheostomy may be performed when prolonged mechanical ventilation is anticipated.

6. **Discuss your impressions as to why Andrew receives enteral feedings.** In the presence of traumatic brain injury, the normal reflexes including chewing, swallowing, and coughing usually are impaired, especially during the acute period of the injury. Neurogenic shock may occur that dramatically increases metabolic demands as the body attempts to compensate for hypoperfusion. The inability to take oral feedings is present owing to the loss of reflexes; however, as long as gastrointestinal functioning is not impaired, enteral

feedings are preferable to TPN because of the risks associated with parenteral nutrition. Oral feedings are contraindicated in the presence of a tracheostomy, especially as long as the client requires oxygen via the tracheostomy and until the tracheostomy can be safely capped for oral intake.

7. **Why is the radio placed at Andrew's bedside?** Andrew's present Glasgow Coma Scale score indicates he is able to hear. Hearing is the last sense a client loses and the use of music, voice, television, and tape recorders helps to overcome sensory deprivation. The music he is familiar with will help him maintain time reference and usual day and night patterns. The music also can help his orientation and relearn speech, if needed. In addition to his parents' voices, it can be soothing to him as he may be frustrated by his inability to speak.

8. **Discuss Andrew's current Glasgow Coma Scale score.** Andrew's current Glasgow Coma Scale score indicates that his cognitive functioning is returning. The "T" represents that he has a tracheostomy and consequently his verbal response cannot be assessed. He has received 4 points for spontaneous eye opening and 6 points for spontaneous movement. It does not address whether his movements are purposeful or if he moves in response to commands, however, this is a very encouraging score as it indicates much improvement over his admission score.

9. **What are your nursing priorities for Andrew following your assessment?**
   a. Impaired gas exchange related to ineffective airway clearance
   b. Decreased intracranial adaptive capacity related to edema secondary to inflammatory response to tissue trauma
   c. Risk for injury, seizures related to neuron stimulation secondary to tissue trauma
   d. Risk for imbalanced nutrition related to increased metabolic needs and reduced oral intake secondary to decreased level of consciousness
   e. Risk for aspiration related to enteral feedings
   f. Total urinary and bowel incontinence related to impaired cognitive function
   g. Impaired physical mobility related to decreased activity
   h. Ineffective coping of parents, related to extent of Andrew's injuries
   i. Deficient knowledge related to Andrew's condition, treatment, prognosis

10. **Why is it important that Andrew receive range-of-motion exercises?** Clients with impaired physical mobility, especially those who are confined to bed, are at risk for developing joint contractures and muscle atrophy as well as foot drop. The purposes of range-of-motion exercises are to increase and maintain joint flexibility as well as muscle endurance and strength; improve cognitive functioning; increase energy level; and improve cardiorespiratory functioning. For Andrew, the primary purposes are to prevent muscle atrophy and joint contractures. These can lead to permanent physical disabilities that would impede Andrew's overall recovery and are preventable in most circumstances in which actual injury to the muscles and joints was not present at the time physical mobility became impaired.

11. **What risk factors predispose Andrew to infection?**
    a. Immobility places the client at risk for the development of hypostatic pneumonia.
    b. The presence of a tracheostomy and the process of suctioning increase respiratory secretions and increase the risk of respiratory infections.
    c. The presence of a gastrostomy tube and tracheostomy represent breaks in skin integrity and with these, the risk of wound infections. Bowel and bladder incontinence poses a risk of excoriation of skin in the genital area and resultant skin breakdown.
    d. Immobility places the client at risk for skin breakdown and wound infection.
    e. The probability of an indwelling urinary catheter in place increases the risk of urinary tract infection.

12. **Andrew receives all of his medications via his G-tube and is prescribed ranitidine 70 mg b.i.d., metoclopramide 3.5 mg q.i.d., and phenytoin sodium 70 mg b.i.d. Discuss Andrew's medications related to why he is receiving each medication, the safety of the dosages prescribed, and any special precautions needed related to route of administration.** Ranitidine is a histamine-receptor antagonist used to prevent erosion of

the gastric lining from the hydrochloric acid present in gastric secretions. These secretions increase in the presence of impaired mobility. Metoclopramide is a gastric stimulant that increases gastric emptying and works together with the ranitidine to help prevent gastric erosion. Phenytoin sodium is an anticonvulsant that is prescribed to prevent seizures in clients with seizure disorders or, as in Andrew's case, those with head injuries that pose a high risk for seizures. His medication therefore is prescribed prophylactically rather than as a treatment modality. The safe dosage range for ranitidine is 2-4 mg/kg per day in two divided doses (Spratto and Woods, 2005, p. 1055). Andrew can receive 35–70 mg/dose so his dose is safe. The safe dosage of metoclopramide is 0.1 mg/kg per dose administered 30 minutes before meals and at bedtime (Spratto and Woods, 2005, p. 783). Andrew's safe dose is 3.5 mg q.i.d. Phenytoin sodium has a safe dosage range of 3-8 mg/kg per day in two divided doses (Spratto and Woods, 2005, p. 975), so he can receive 52.5–140 mg per dose. Andrew's dose is safe and in the lower dosage range. The precautions related to administering phenytoin sodium to a client receiving enteral feedings is that the feedings must be held for 2 hours before and after phenytoin sodium administration because the enteral feeding formulas decrease the drug's absorption.

13. **What is your priority concern about Andrew's urinary and bowel incontinence?** Risk for impaired skin integrity is the priority concern for the client with incontinence. Prolonged skin exposure to urine and feces can lead to excoriation of the skin in the genital area. Because this area is a perfect environment for bacterial growth, skin breakdown and the development of skin ulcers is a concern. The client should be checked at least every 2 hours for incontinence. This is usually performed during regular turning of the client. Prophylactic skin care products are available for clients at risk for skin breakdown.

14. **How would you explain Mrs. Burger's comments to Andrew and what might your therapeutic interventions consist of?** It is normal for parents to feel guilt if their child is injured. Andrew's mother may think she should have been more careful, should not have been driving so fast, or should not have been talking with Andrew while she was driving, or any number of other probabilities that are not realistic and very likely would not have changed the outcome. The best way to respond to her is to talk with her about your observations and tell her you are available if she wants to talk about her concerns. The best approach is to be an empathetic, nonjudgmental, and an active listener. The nurse needs to be sure to be available if and when Mrs. Burger wants to talk. The nurse should assess whether Mrs. Burger would like to speak to someone else, for instance, a chaplain or her own minister. Your observations should be communicated to other nurses caring for Andrew and his family so continuity of care can be maintained.

15. **How can you intervene to help meet Andrew's growth and development needs?** According to Erikson's psychosocial theory of growth and development, school-age children are focused on a sense of industry to prevent development of a sense of inferiority. They need to be praised for their efforts and to feel a sense of accomplishment. Normally, much of their sense of achievement comes from school, through activities with their friends that are grounded in rules, and through their relationship with their families. Involve Andrew's school teacher or the hospital teacher (present in most large hospitals that provide specialized pediatric care) in Andrew's care by working with him to make up missed work according to his abilities at present. According to the nurse's assessment he is able to move his extremities although weakness is noted. Involve him in computer learning and computer games for recreation, as these can provide both education and a sense of accomplishment and competition. Having him toss wadded up paper towels into the waste basket provides both range-of-motion and a sense of accomplishment with each successful toss. Involving his parents in these activities will provide support for all three of them. Ask Andrew's parents to encourage his friends to call and visit, as this would boost his self-esteem. Even though he can't communicate verbally, he can communicate in writing.

16. **What other health care professionals would be beneficial in Andrew's care?** Social Services should be involved, especially because of Andrew's probable transfer to a rehabilitation facility when he no longer requires acute care. As noted previously, the hospital, school, as well as child-life specialists should be involved in his care. Physical and occupational therapy are needed to assist with mobility and self-care. If available, a speech therapist would be able to assess Andrew's ability to swallow so that he may progress to

oral feedings. The pharmacist is a critical part of Andrew's care team, as is the facility dietician or nutritionist. Consistency of these professionals is very important to his continuity of care, and developing a trusting and therapeutic relationship with them will facilitate Andrew's recovery and his goal of reaching his highest level of growth and development.

References

Bond, C. (2002). Traumatic brain injury: Help for the family. *RN* 65(11). 60–67.

Centers for Disease Control and Prevention. *http://www.cdc.gov*

Chicago Institute of Neurosurgery and Neuroresearch. *http://www.cinn.org*

Daniels, R. (2002). *Delmar's manual of laboratory and diagnostic tests.* Clifton Park, NY: Thomson Delmar Learning.

DeLaune, S.C. and Ladner, P.K. (2002). *Fundamentals of nursing: Standards & practice* (2nd ed.). Clifton Park, NY: Thomson Delmar Learning, pp. 118–122; 956–958.

Gahart, B.L. and Nazareno, A.R. (2005). *2005 Intravenous medications* (21st ed.). St. Louis: Mosby.

MEDLINE. *http://www.nlm.nih.gov*

North American Nursing Diagnosis Association. (2005). *Nursing diagnoses; Definitions & classifications, 2005–2006.* Philadelphia: NANDA.

Potts, N. and Mandleco, B. (2002). *Pediatric nursing: Caring for children and their families.* Clifton Park, NY: Thomson Delmar Learning, p. 1049.

Spratto, G.R. and Woods, A.L. (2005). *2005 Edition PDR Nurse's drug handbook.* Clifton Park, NY: Thomson Delmar Learning.

PART SIX

The Lymphatic System

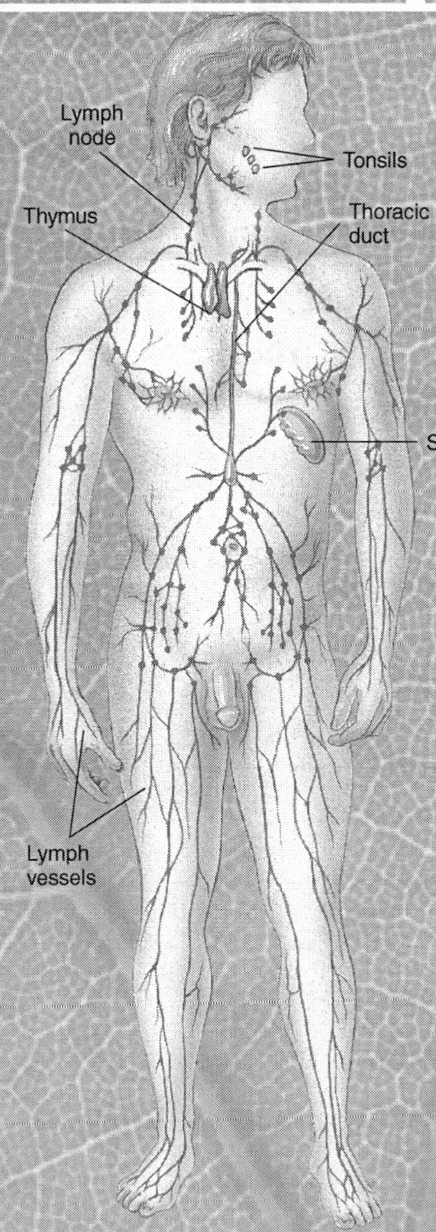

Lymphatic and immune systems
Thymus, bone marrow, spleen, tonsils, lymph nodes, lymph capillaries, lymph vessels, lymphocytes, and lymph.

CASE STUDY 1

David

GENDER

M

AGE

20

SETTING

- Hospital/home

ETHNICITY

- White American

CULTURAL CONSIDERATIONS

PREEXISTING CONDITION

COEXISTING CONDITIONS

- Hodgkin's disease

SIGNIFICANT HISTORY

- Lives with wife

COMMUNICATION

DISABILITY

SOCIOECONOMIC

SPIRITUAL

- Jehovah Witness

PHARMACOLOGIC

- Cyclophosphamide (Cytoxin)

PSYCHOSOCIAL

- Death and dying

LEGAL

- Client's right to die
- Do not resuscitate order

ETHICAL

- Client's right to die
- Possible nurse bias

ALTERNATIVE THERAPY

PRIORITIZATION

- Yes

DELEGATION

- Yes

THE LYMPHATIC SYSTEM

Level of difficulty: Easy

Overview: This case requires knowledge of Hodgkin's disease, chemotherapy, spiritual integrity, growth and development, as well as an understanding of the client's background, personal situation, and marital relationship.

Client Profile

David is a 20-year-old who lives with his wife in a metropolitan area. He received an associate degree in business from a community college and works with his father in the family hardware business. David and his wife are Jehovah Witnesses. Two years ago David was diagnosed with Hodgkin's disease and was treated with chemotherapy (see Fig. A-19). He achieved remission for 18 months, at which time his disease relapsed. For the past 3 months, he has been receiving chemotherapy but has not been able to achieve remission. He has been hospitalized three times for chemotherapy and once for adverse effects of his chemotherapy regimen. Today David is experiencing gross bleeding when he urinates. When he sees his oncologist, the physician admits David to the pediatric oncology unit at the medical center where he has been undergoing treatment for his Hodgkin's disease.

Case Study

David and his wife arrive on the unit for placement of a three-way catheter, continuous bladder irrigation with sterile normal saline, continuous monitoring of oxygen saturation via pulse oximetry, administration of oxygen to maintain saturations >94%, intravenous fluids of lactated Ringer's solution to infuse at 200 mL/hour. His admitting vital signs are: temperature, 36° C (96.8° F); pulse, 110 beats/minute; respirations, 30 breaths/minute; and blood pressure, 90/60. His pulse oximetry reading is 86%. He complains of weakness, dizziness, shortness of breath, and anxiety. His skin is cool and clammy. His admitting laboratory values are:

Complete blood count:

Hemoglobin: 9 g/dL

Hematocrit: 25%

Platelets: 80,000 cells/mm^3

White blood cell count: 4,000 cells/ mm^3

His admitting history reveals that his chemotherapy regimen to treat his Hodgkin's disease is the alkylating agent cyclophosphamide. His urine is bright red with occasional clots present. His wife is visibly anxious and states, "I am so afraid for David even though we have talked about his condition and that he might die as a result of it."

Questions and Suggested Answers

1. **Discuss your impressions of David's clinical manifestations.** Considering the gross bleeding from his urinary bladder, David's clinical manifestations probably reflect hemorrhagic cystitis. His vital signs indicate uncompensated lack of tissue perfusion involving 40% or greater loss of blood volume because the blood pressure does not usually decrease until this amount of volume has been lost. His weakness and dizziness indicates ineffective tissue perfusion to the muscles and brain and represent the presence of hypovolemia and hypoperfusion. His temperature is in the low normal range; his pulse indicates tachycardia; he is tachypneic and hypotensive; and his oxygen saturation is below the normal of 95%-100%. His cool, clammy skin is a sign of shock.

2. **What is the significance of David's laboratory findings?** David's hemoglobin and hematocrit are critically low and indicate severe anemia. This represents a decrease in tissue perfusion. His platelet count also is lower than the normal 150,000–450,000 cells/mm^3. As a result, he is at high risk for bleeding. His white blood cell count is lower than normal.

3. **Discuss the relationship, if any, between David's present condition and his chemotherapy treatment.** An adverse effect of cyclophosphamide therapy is hemorrhagic cystitis. This occurs as a result of contact between this antineoplastic and the sensitive and fragile mucous membrane lining of the urinary bladder. To destroy the lymphoma cells, the agent has the same cellular destructive effect on the bladder lining as it does systemically on the cells of the body. Under the mucous membrane lining of the urinary bladder is the

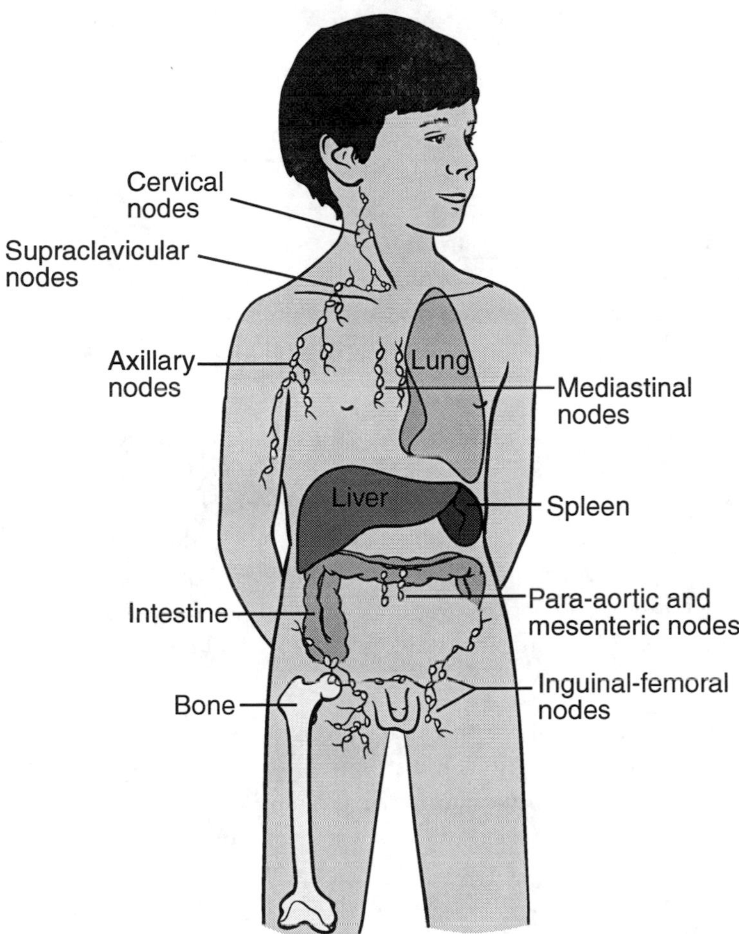

Figure A-19 *Lymph nodes affected by Hodgkin's disease.*

bladder muscle, which is highly vascular and when in prolonged contact with this antineoplastic begins to bleed. Because of the high vascularity of the urinary bladder, bleeding from the urinary bladder wall can be extensive and lead to life-threatening hypovolemia.

4. **What other assessment data would be helpful for the nurse to have to prepare David's care plan?**
   - **a.** When was his last treatment with cyclophosphamide?
   - **b.** Had he been hospitalized for hemorrhagic cystitis previously?
   - **c.** What is his white blood cell count differential?
   - **d.** What are the results of the nurse's physical assessment?
   - **e.** What is his neurologic status?
   - **f.** What are the results of his physical assessment?
   - **g.** When did the bleeding from his bladder begin?
   - **h.** Although his vital signs are abnormal, what is his baseline?

5. **Discuss the rationales for what the oncologist has prescribed for David.** The placement of a three-way indwelling urinary catheter is to provide an access for continuous bladder irrigation (CBI). The CBI is to help stop the bleeding by providing cool sterile normal saline for irrigation to constrict the blood vessels of the bladder. It also helps prevent blood clots from blocking the bladder outlet, which results in the potential for bladder rupture and hemorrhage. Oxygen is administered to provide for adequate oxygenation of body tissues and continuous pulse oximetry monitors the effectiveness of this treatment and also detects life-threatening changes in oxygen saturation. The intravenous infusion is to increase vascular volume to increase tissue perfusion and prevent cardiovascular collapse from hypovolemia. Lactated Ringer's solution

is a volume expander that also acts by converting lactate ions to bicarbonate ions to treat metabolic acidosis that occurs with hypoperfusion.

6. **What are the priorities of care for David on admission?**
   a. Risk for injury, bleeding related to hemorrhagic cystitis and decreased platelets
   b. Ineffective tissue perfusion related to bleeding from the urinary bladder
   c. Risk for injury, falls related to ineffective tissue perfusion
   d. Impaired urinary tissue integrity related to exposure to cyclophosphamide
   e. Anxiety related to the severity of David's condition
   f. Risk for spiritual distress related to severity of David's condition
   g. Deficient knowledge related to David's condition, treatment options, and potential terminal nature of his condition

7. **How would you respond to David's wife and her concern?** An empathetic and nonjudgmental approach is necessary for the nurse, who should ask open-ended questions that encourage David's wife to express her feelings and concerns. The nurse should assume an available affect and actively listen to her. Nurses are not expected to have answers to a client's or family's concerns, but rather listen and therapeutically respond. Phrases such as "Don't worry," "Everything is going to be all right," or "Now don't be upset" should never be used because they offer false hope, block therapeutic communication, and leave the client or family member feeling that the nurse is either uncomfortable with their feelings or simply does not want to address them.

8. **What impact might David and his wife's spiritual beliefs have on his medical treatment plan?** Jehovah Witnesses adhere to a doctrine that prohibits transfusion of someone else's blood into another person. They maintain that it is wrong to sustain life by administering a transfusion of blood or plasma or red cells or other component parts of the blood. This policy originated from a passage in the bible in Leviticus, Chapter 17, verse 14, which states, "You must not eat the blood of any sort of flesh" (*http://www.ajwrb.org*). Recent changes in their doctrine allow for transfusion of hemoglobin but not the cell membrane.

9. **The oncologist informs David and his wife that David needs a transfusion of packed red blood cells and explains why this treatment is necessary. They both refuse this treatment. Discuss your feelings and biases about their decision and why it is important for you to understand your feelings about this situation.** This question asks that students/readers express their own feelings and biases, so the answers will be individualized. They should, however, address the issue of client's right to refuse treatment and recognize religious beliefs as client choices. In addition, under the law, performing care for persons who are cognitively capable of and have refused treatment is considered assault and battery on the client because of lack of client consent and can lead to legal liability. It is important for any health care provider to recognize his or her own biases and deal with them so they do not interfere with therapeutic interactions between the health care professional and the client/family. The nurse may not agree with the decisions that clients and their families make, but must respect their right to make these choices.

10. **Discuss the legality of the decision made by David and his wife.** In some states, 21 years of age is considered the legal age for decision-making and in others, the legal age is 18 years old. Regardless, most states recognize the concept of the emancipated minor who is defined as living apart and independently from the parents. Emancipated minors can make decisions that are legally recognized. Regardless of the state's definition of legal age, David and his wife are living apart and independent of their parents, so their decision in this situation is legal.

11. **David's condition deteriorates as the continuous bladder irrigation is unable to stop the bleeding from his urinary bladder. He and his wife communicate to the oncologist that they don't want him resuscitated if he experiences cardiopulmonary arrest. The oncologist respects their request and initiates "Do Not Resuscitate" and "Discharge to Home" orders. Discuss your feelings about this decision.** Because this question asks for students/readers to express their own feelings, the answer will be individual. The discussion

should include feelings about clients and their families who chose not to pursue "heroic measures" to save clients' lives. It also should address a person's right to make this decision and the fact that it should be respected by health care professionals as long as the client and/or family are cognitively competent to make the decision. Further, the discussion should include the concept of the client's right to die at home if he or she is in a terminal state.

12. **What referrals might be helpful for David and his wife before he is discharged?** Hospice is the most appropriate referral to make since David and his wife have decided not to seek further treatment. Hospice is a national agency that offers psychosocial, emotional, physical, spiritual, and pain management support for the dying client and his or her family in the home (usually) or institution environment. In-patient hospice facilities also are available in some areas.

13. **Later in the day, David is resting with his eyes closed when the nurse enters the room to do her discharge assessment. His wife says angrily, "Can't you people just leave us alone?" Discuss your impression of her comment and how you would respond to her.** Anger is part of the grieving or anticipatory grieving process. Frequently, because of the amount of time nurses spend with clients and their families who are experiencing grief and grieving, they are faced with dealing with this response therapeutically. It is very important that the nurse not become defensive in his or her response to the grieving person, but rather to understand the process they have to work through and be very supportive. The nurse should explain the need for the discharge assessment and then offer to return in 10 minutes or ask David's wife to call the nurse when she is ready for the nurse to return to perform the assessment. Legally the client must be assessed on admission, at least every 24 hours during hospitalization, and prior to discharge, however the nurse can negotiate the timing of the discharge assessment with the client and his wife.

14. **Two weeks after David is discharged, he dies at home with his wife and parents at his bedside. His wife sends a card to the nursing unit to thank them for the "wonderful" care David received and that he had "died peacefully and with dignity." You notice that one of your nursing peers begins to weep. Discuss your feelings about the nurse's response and how you might interact with her.** Nurses have feelings and emotions as human beings. As a nurturing profession that is client focused, the intensity of the emotions can be quite high. This is especially true when the nurse has had repeated contact with the client and family over a period of time. The nurse is expressing his or her own feelings of loss and grief because of David's death. You would respond to the nurse as you would to anyone who is grieving the loss of another human being—with support, therapeutic touch (with permission), active listening, therapeutic silence, or other therapeutic response that is appropriate in the situation. If possible, temporarily assign another staff member to care for the grieving nurse's client to allow the nurse time for the grieving. A misconception among many members of the nursing profession is that manifesting grief by a nurse is inappropriate. On the contrary, it is natural and human.

References

Associated Jehovah's Witness for Reform on Blood. *http://www.afwrb.org*

Centers for Disease Control and Prevention. *http://www.cdc.gov*

Daniels, R. (2002). *Delmar's manual of laboratory and diagnostic tests.* Clifton Park, NY: Thomson Delmar Learning.

Doctrines of Jehovah Witnesses. *http://www.en.wifpedia.org*

Gahart, B.L. and Nazareno, A.R. (2005). *2005 Intravenous medications* (21st ed.). St. Louis: Mosby.

Intravenous Therapy. *http://www.nursewise.com*

North American Nursing Diagnosis Association. (2005). *Nursing diagnoses: Defnitions & classifications, 2005–2006.* Philadelphia: NANDA.

CASE STUDY 2

Jerome

MODERATE

GENDER

M

AGE

11

SETTING

- Hospital

ETHNICITY

- Black American

CULTURAL CONSIDERATIONS

PREEXISTING CONDITION

- Acute myelocytic leukemia

COEXISTING CONDITIONS

SIGNIFICANT HISTORY

COMMUNICATION

DISABILITY

SOCIOECONOMIC

SPIRITUAL

PHARMACOLOGIC

- Chemotherapy

PSYCHOSOCIAL

- Client anxiety
- Parent anxiety

LEGAL

- Informed consent

ETHICAL

- Assent

ALTERNATIVE THERAPY

PRIORITIZATION

- Yes

DELEGATION

- Yes

THE LYMPHATIC SYSTEM

Level of difficulty: Moderate

Overview: This case requires knowledge of leukemia, bone marrow transplantation, growth and development, as well as client's background and personal situation including family relationship.

Client Profile

Jerome is an 11-year-old middle-school child who lives at home with his 13-year-old brother Jason and their parents. Mr. and Mrs. Jones work full time outside the home, and Jerome and Jason stay with a neighbor after school for 2 hours each day until their parents return home from work. Mr. and Mrs. Jones are very devoted to the children and are involved in their activities. Jerome and Jason were healthy children, experiencing only an occasional upper respiratory infection, until 4 years ago when Jerome was diagnosed with acute myelocytic leukemia and was treated with chemotherapy. He achieved remission and remained symptom free for 2 years, at which time he experienced relapse and has been undergoing chemotherapy without achieving remission since.

Case Study

The health care providers discuss Jerome's condition with him and with his family, suggesting that Jerome receive a bone marrow transplantation (BMT). After discussing the procedure and potential risks of BMT, Jerome's parents decide to begin the process of finding a suitable donor. They are very anxious about the procedure but understand that without the BMT, Jerome's prognosis is poor. Once a suitable donor is located, Jerome will be admitted to a research hospital that specializes in transplantation in children. The facility is located a 45- minute driving distance from the Jones' home in a neighboring city.

Questions and Suggested Answers

1. **What types of conditions are treated with BMT?** Bone marrow transplantation (BMT) or peripheral blood stem cell transplant is most commonly used in children whose leukemia has not brought them into permanent remission, and in those with lymphoma, brain tumors, and neuroblastoma who have not responded to first-line treatments including chemotherapy, radiation therapy, and surgery. BMT has proven a successful treatment with 55% to 83% disease-free survival rate for clients with acute myelocytic/myelogenous leukemia (AML). Other conditions include sickle cell disease in children who have experienced a cerebrovascular accident (CVA) or are at high risk for developing one. According to the National Cancer Institute, "The main purpose of BMT and PBSCT (peripheral blood stem cell transplantation) in cancer treatment is to make it possible for patients to receive very high doses of chemotherapy and/or radiation therapy." The Leukemia & Lymphoma Society states that disorders treated with BMT include, "immune deficiency diseases, inherited severe blood cell disease, marrow failure, leukemia, lymphoma, myeloma." The high-dose chemotherapy that is required to destroy disease cells also destroys other rapidly growing normal cells including the client's stem cells. Without these cells, the bone marrow cannot make healthy blood cells.
2. **Discuss the different types of bone marrow transplants.** The three types of BMTs are autologous, syngeneic, and allogeneic. Autologous transplants involve harvesting the client's own stem cells and transplanting them back into the client. In syngeneic transplants, the stem cell donor is an identical twin. Autologous and syngeneic transplants do not pose the risk of rejection that allogeneic BMT do. Allogeneic BMT involves a client receiving stem cells from someone other than the client or an identical twin. The usual donors are others related to the client or can be persons not related to the client. The most common BMT is allogeneic.
3. **Jerome's parents ask the nurse about the difference between bone marrow and stem cells. What is the most appropriate explanation for the nurse to give?** According to the National Cancer Institute, "Bone marrow is the soft, sponge-like material found inside the bones. It contains immature cells called stem cells that produce blood cells." These blood cells include leukocytes (white blood cells), erythrocytes (red blood cells), and platelets. BMT and peripheral blood stem cell transplantation involve different procedures. BMT involves surgery for the donor during which stem cells in the bone marrow are harvested from a bone peripheral site and transplanted into the recipient. Peripheral blood stem cells are harvested using a process called apheresis or leukophoresis.

4. **Discuss the difference between Jerome's assent for the BMT and his parents informed consent.** In 47 of the 50 United States, a child is considered a minor until the age of 18 years. In those three states, the age is 19 years. As a minor, the child cannot legally sign informed consent for surgery or an invasive procedure. The exception to this is most states recognize the status of emancipated minors. These are children under the age of 18 years who live independently and are legally responsible for supporting themselves and for their own decision-making. In Jerome's situation, he would not qualify as an emancipated minor, however, ethically he should have the procedure explained to him with verification that he understands the teaching that has been done. At this point, he verbally or nonverbally gives his assent to the procedure. Informed consent is obtained by the child's legal guardian(s), in Jerome's case his parents, in the form of written consent after the benefits and risks of the procedure have been explained to them (again, with verification that they understand). Their signature on the informed consent means they are giving their legal consent.

5. **Why is it important for Jerome to be involved in the decision about whether he should have a BMT and to give his assent?** Jerome is 11 years old and, according to Piaget's theories, has the cognitive level of concrete operations. His thoughts are increasingly logical, and he is able to understand multiple aspects of a situation simultaneously. Thus, he has the ability to understand the concept of bone marrow transplantation and probably his ability is greater than that of other children his age because of his health history. Children in this age group tend to base their logic on their experiences. By involving Jerome in the decision about receiving a BMT, he will probably be more cooperative in the pre-procedural activities as well as more compliant with the post-procedural regime. If Jerome is restricted in the decision-making, he may be more likely to feel increased fear and anxiety, and believe that this action is being done to him rather than with him.

6. **After testing his family, Jason is determined to be a compatible donor. What process determines a compatible donor?** People usually have different sets of proteins on the surfaces of their cells. These proteins are called human leukocyte-associated (HLA) antigens. The HLA antigens are identified by a blood test called Human Leukocyte Antigen test that is used primarily to determine donor–recipient compatibility. The closer the HLA matches, the better the outcome of the transplant should be.

7. **Discuss the harvesting and processing of donor bone marrow.** With BMT, the donor receives either general or local anesthesia and then several small cuts are made in the skin over the site of the bone from which the stem cells will be harvested. The most common site of harvesting is the iliac crest because of its size and density allowing for the greatest number of stem cells to be harvested from one site. On rare occasions the sternum may be used. A large-bore needle is inserted through the cuts and into the bone marrow. The bone marrow is then removed. This procedure usually involves about an hour for the harvesting of 400–800 mL of bone marrow. Following the harvesting, blood and bones fragments are separated from the bone marrow. The marrow can then be combined with a preservative and placed in a sterile container of liquid nitrogen for freezing. This keeps the stem cells alive until they are needed for transplantation. The stem cells are transplanted into the recipient intravenously. With PBSCT, a central venous access is established using an apheresis catheter. For 4–5 days prior to apheresis or leukophoresis, the donor is given medication to stimulate the production of stem cells. During the apheresis process, blood is removed via the central venous access device (CVAD) and sent through an apheresis machine that removes the stem cells. The blood is then returned to the donor. This procedure does not require anesthesia; however, it usually takes 4–5 hours to complete.

8. **Discuss the adverse effects of high-dose chemotherapy and radiation administered prior to BMT.**
   a. Ineffective protection related to the destruction of leukocytes (including normal ones) and the stem cells that produce them
   b. High risk for bleeding related to the destruction of platelets and the stem cells that produce them secondary to chemotherapy/radiation
   c. High risk for ineffective tissue perfusion (anemia) related to red blood cell destruction and the destruction of stem cells that produce them
   d. Acute pain related to cellular destruction primarily in the mucous membranes
   e. Risk for impaired skin integrity related to full-body radiation burns

Prior to a BMT, the chemotherapy is high dose to destroy all the disease cells. Radiation is especially destructive to the fragile mucous membranes. During the process, normal cells are destroyed, including the normal flora that helps maintain the condition of the mucous membranes. As a result the mucous membranes become inflamed, leading to stomatitis and esophagitis, both very painful conditions requiring intravenous infusion of morphine sulfate to control. As a result of this pre-BMT chemotherapy and radiation, the client is neutropenic, thrombocytopenic, and anemic in addition to the stomatitis and esophagitis. The neutropenic state poses a high risk for life-threatening infection.

9. **Jerome receives his bone marrow transplant. What are the nursing priorities of care for Jerome after his BMT?**
   a. Ineffective protection related to immunosuppression to prevent rejection
   b. Risk for injury, complications related to pre-transplant high-dose chemotherapy/radiation and BMT prior to engraftment
   c. Risk for ineffective tissue perfusion related to destruction of erythrocytes secondary to pre-transplant chemotherapy/radiation and BMT prior to engraftment
   d. Pain related to cellular destruction secondary to chemotherapy/radiation
   e. Risk for injury, graft-versus-host disease (GVHD) related to allogeneic BMT

10. **What is engraftment and how long does it take to occur following BMT?** Engraftment refers to the viability and functional capacity of the bone marrow transplanted into the recipient. Following the BMT it takes approximately 2–4 weeks for the transplanted bone marrow to become functional and begin producing leukocytes, erythrocytes, and platelets. Until engraftment occurs, the recipient is at high risk for infection, bleeding, and anemia, all of which can result in death.

11. **Discuss the short-term and long-term complications of BMT.** The short-term or acute complications of BMT include severe stomatitis, severe esophagitis, nausea, vomiting, diarrhea, hemorrhagic cystitis, and life-threatening infections. The long-term complications include infertility (sterility), pulmonary dysfunction, cardiac dysfunction, liver disease, cataracts, metabolic encephalopathy, secondary malignancies, and hypothyroidism. One of the most serious complications, which can be either acute or chronic, is GVHD.

12. **Discuss the potential impact of the BMT on Jerome's growth and development.** Jerome is a school-age child in late childhood. His task of industry is met primarily in school. He is very involved with schoolmates and most of his activities revolve around school. During his pre-BMT treatment, he will not be able to attend school, nor will he feel like doing any schoolwork because of the effects of the chemotherapy/radiation. Once he has received his chemotherapy/radiation prior to the BMT and for several weeks and months after the BMT, Jerome will be at high risk for developing life-threatening infections. The immunosuppressants given following the BMT (allogeneic) to prevent rejection also produce a high risk of infection by suppressing his immune system which, together with the skin that protects us against microorganisms and infection, is our major system protecting us from infection. Immunosuppressants, including cyclosporine, methotrexate, FK 506, antithymocyte globulin, azathioprine, Sandimmune, and corticosteroids (prednisone, methylprednisolone) frequently produce adverse effects that impact on the client's body image. In Jerome's favor, he has evidently dealt with the alopecia associated with chemotherapy and may not experience difficulty with corticosteroid body changes ("moon face"). Facilities that are specialized enough to perform transplants on children also have hospital schools, school teachers, and child-life specialists. It would be important for Jerome to be referred to these departments so they could help him remain current in his studies. Having his brother help him as well may prove to be very positive for Jerome. Following discharge, Jerome will probably require a tutor until he can return to school unless his school is Internet-connected.

13. **Three months after his BMT, Jerome develops erythema of the palms of his hands, the soles of his feet, and his ears. Discuss your impressions of Jerome's manifestations.** These are symptoms of acute GVHD. It occurs within 100 days of a BMT. GVHD is a potentially life-threatening condition specific to allogenic bone marrow transplants and is the result of the donor bone marrow immune cells developing antibodies against the

recipient's tissue and organs. Occasionally this can occur with autologous BMT as a result of the chemical purging of the client's own stem cells that is done to eradicate malignant cells prior to transplanting them back into the client's body. The immunosuppressant agents used to prevent rejection of the BMT suppress the client's immune cells so they won't destroy the donor stem cells during engraftment. This also makes the client's cells prime targets for the donor T-cells to attack the client's body with antibodies that destroy the client's cells by cell-mediated cytotoxic action of mature "killer cells."

14. Differentiate acute GVHD and chronic GVHD. Acute GVHD occurs within the first 100 days following a BMT and chronic GVHD occurs after 100 days. The pathophysiology of both is the same; however, the complications differ. The complications of acute GVHD include severe stomatitis and esophagitis, hemorrhagic cystitis, infection, and possibly death. Chronic GVHD can result in sterility; damage to the heart, lungs, and liver; hypothyroidism; and death due to severe infection. The clinical manifestations for acute GVHD include erythema of the palms of the hands, soles of the feet, face, and ears. Others include cholestatic hepatitis and enteritis. Chronic GVHD is manifested by blisters on the skin, hair loss, dry eyes and mouth, watery or bloody stools, jaundice, pulmonary compromise, cardiac insufficiency, and hematuria. The goal of treatment is the same for both—prevention of the condition.

15. Discuss the techniques used to prevent GVHD. According to the Sidney Kimmel Comprehensive Cancer Center at Johns Hopkins, two approaches have been recognized to prevent GVHD. These are *elutriation (T-cell depletion)* and immunosuppressant therapy. Elutriation is a technique "where the donor bone marrow is taken to a laboratory and the T-cells which cause GVHD are removed using a sophisticated centrifuge. This centrifuge separates cells on the basis of size and density. Because T-cells are smaller than the stem cells needed to repopulate the bone marrow, most of the lymphocytes can be removed in this manner." This procedure does not remove all T-cells because some are necessary for engraftment. The most frequently used approach is immunosuppressant therapy that decreases the donor cell's ability to develop antibodies that attack the host tissues and organs. Agents used include cyclosporine, methotrexate, FK506, corticosteroids (prednisone), anti-thymocyte globulin, OKT3 (specifically attacks the T3 surface glycoproteins on T-cells), azathioprine, and thalidomide.

The treatment of choice for GVHD is the administration of steroids. Most of the individuals treated with steroidal agents will experience resolution of their GVHD. Anti-thymocyte globulin combined with extremely high dose steroids may be required for those with severe GVHD.

A multidisciplinary approach is used to treat and monitor severe GVHD. These include ophthalmologist, integumentary specialist, cardiopulmonary specialist, bone marrow transplantation team, neurologist, gastroenterologist, nurses, social workers, and physical therapists.

16. Following treatment, Jerome's parents are preparing to take him home. Discuss appropriate client/family teaching needed prior to Jerome's discharge.

a. Assess Jerome and his family's current level of understanding
b. Provide verbal and written information concerning:
   (1) Importance of preventing infection by avoiding large crowds, persons known to have an infection, live flowers and fruits (if neutropenic)
   (2) Medications administration and the importance of compliance with the medical regimen
   (3) Adverse effects of medications and the signs and symptoms of these effects
   (4) Manifestations of worsening of Jerome's condition
   (5) Contact numbers to report manifestations immediately
   (6) Importance of meticulous handwashing and the correct technique, if needed
   (7) Follow-up visits with the health care provider and how important it is to keep these appointments
c. Allow sufficient time for Jerome and his family to ask questions, ensuring they receive appropriate answers.
d. Document teaching and this family's response.

References

Broyles, B.E. (2005). *Medical-surgical nursing clinical companion.* Durham, NC: Carolina Academic Press.
Daniels, R. (2002). *Delmar's manual of laboratory and diagnostic tests.* Clifton Park, NY: Thomson Delmar Learning.
Gahart, B.L. and Nazareno, A.R. (2004). *2004 Intravenous medications* (20th ed.). St. Louis: Mosby.
The Johns Hopkins Oncology Center. *http://www.med.jhu.edu*
The Leukemia & Lymphoma Society. *http://www.leukemia-lymphoma.org*
National Cancer Institute. *http://cis.nic.nih.gov*
National Marrow Donor Program. *http://www.marrow.org*
Spratto, G.R. and Woods, A.L. (2005). *2005 Edition PDR Nurse's drug handbook.* Clifton Park, NY: Thomson Delmar Learning.

CASE STUDY 3

Chad

GENDER

M

AGE

10

SETTING

- Home

ETHNICITY

- White American

CULTURAL CONSIDERATIONS

PREEXISTING CONDITIONS

- HIV

COEXISTING CONDITIONS

SIGNIFICANT HISTORY

COMMUNICATION

DISABILITY

SOCIOECONOMIC

- Middle class

SPIRITUAL

- Strength from spirituality

PHARMACOLOGIC

- Highly active antiretroviral therapy

PSYCHOSOCIAL

- Death of mother 6 years ago
- Client anxiety
- Family anxiety

LEGAL

ETHICAL

ALTERNATIVE THERAPY

PRIORITIZATION

- Yes

DELEGATION

- Yes

THE LYMPHATIC SYSTEM

Level of difficulty: Difficult

Overview: This case requires knowledge of HIV/AIDS, growth and development, grief and grieving, as well as an understanding of the client's background, personal situation, and family relationship.

Client Profile

Chad is a 10-year-old boy who contracted human immunodeficiency virus (HIV) from his mother while she was pregnant with him. She had contracted HIV from a blood transfusion following the birth of Chad's older brother, Steve, when she developed disseminated intravascular coagulation (DIC). His mother died when Chad was 4 years old of complications of acquired immunodeficiency syndrome (AIDS). Chad, his father, and brother were tested for HIV following his mother's diagnosis. His father and brother were HIV negative, but Chad was HIV positive. Chad's father remarried when Chad was 6 years old and Chad's stepmother has been very attentive to Chad during his illness. She recently quit work to stay at home with him as his condition worsened. Chad and his family have a large support network including grandparents, aunts, uncles, cousins, and classmates of both Chad and Steve.

Case Study

During a home health visit the nurse notes that Chad has developed skin lesions, a dry cough, and the presence of crackles on auscultation of his breath sounds. His vital signs are:

Temperature: 38.8° C (101.8° F)

Pulse: 116 beats/minute

Respirations: 28 breaths/minute

Blood pressure: 130/84

She also notes white patches in his mouth. His stepmother says that he has had diarrhea for the past month that he just told her about this morning. She had noticed an increase in his fluid intake, but he told her that he was "just more thirsty" than usual. The nurse notifies the health care provider of her findings, whereupon the physician prescribes a complete blood count and a CDT4 level. Those results are:

CDT4: 186/mm^3, which has decreased from his previous count of 300/mm^3

Hemoglobin: 7.8 g/dL

Hematocrit: 20%

Leukocyte count: 1,200/mm^3 with a neutrophil count of 900/mm^3

Platelet count: 90,000/mm^3

Chad weighs 25 kg (55 lb). He had lost 10 lb in the last month.

Questions and Suggested Answers

1. **Discuss your impressions of the client's assessment data.** It appears that Chad has developed an opportunistic lung infection, probably *Pneumocystis carinii* pneumonia (PCP), which is a common infection that distinguishes the late phase of symptomatic human immunodeficiency virus (HIV) disease. The medication regimen he is prescribed (highly active antiretroviral therapy [HAART]) usually stalls this progression; however, he may have developed a tolerance for his medications, allowing opportunistic infections to attack his body. His temperature elevation, dry cough, and crackles in the lung are manifestations of PCP. The normal temperature for a child Chad's age is 36.6° C (97.9° F). His other vital signs also are elevated from normal values, indicating the stress of the infection. The normal pulse, respiration, and blood pressure for Chad are: pulse, 65–110 beats/minute; respiration, 15–20 per minute; blood pressure, 115–123/75–79. The lesions on his skin may represent an opportunistic skin infection or Kaposi Sarcoma. The oral lesions may be candidiasis, an infection of the mucous membranes that develops in children with moderate symptomatic HIV infection. His hemoglobin and hematocrit indicate anemia; his neutrophil count shows neutropenia, and his platelet count indicates thrombocytopenia. All of these represent moderate symptomatic HIV infection. The CDT4 count indicates the progression from HIV infection to acquired immunodeficiency syndrome (AIDS).

2. What additional information would support your impressions?

a. Chest x-ray
b. Biopsy of skin lesions
c. Serum electrolytes
d. Prothrombin and thromboplastin times
e. Immunological levels
f. Stool for ova and parasite
g. Pulmonary function
h. Oxygen saturation
i. Condition of skin around anorectal area secondary to diarrhea
j. Heart sounds
k. Bowel sounds
l. Intake and output
m. Chad's HAART therapy
n. How long he was able to attend school following his diagnosis of HIV
o. Whether his parents are planning to continue to seek treatment for Chad

3. Discuss the significance of Chad's CDT4 count. HIV uses CDT4 molecules as receptor sites, replicating itself and altering the immunologic function of these cells that normally support the immune system to protect the body from infection. As HIV disease progresses, fewer and fewer of the functional CDT4 cells are present. The Centers for Disease Control and Prevention have established immunologic categories to determine the stages of HIV infection. These categories are:

Immune Category	Age of the Child		
	<12 months	1–5 years	6–12 years
a. Asymptomatic (no suppression)	=1,500	=1,000	=500
b. Moderate suppression	750–1499	500–900	200–499
c. Severe suppression	<750	>500	>200

Chad's CDT4 count indicates that he is experiencing severe suppression meaning he has AIDS.

4. What are the nursing priorities of care for Chad?

a. Ineffective protection related to immunosuppressive state
b. Impaired gas exchange related to presence of opportunistic microorganisms
c. Acute/chronic pain related to myopathy, neuropathics
d. Imbalanced nutrition: less than body requirements related to diarrhea and wasting syndrome
e. Diarrhea related to presence of enteric opportunistic microorganisms
f. Impaired skin integrity related to skin lesions secondary to Kaposi's sarcoma and anorectal excoriation secondary to diarrhea
g. Risk for injury related to central nervous system changes
h. Anticipatory grieving related to terminal stages of AIDS
i. Deficient knowledge related to home care for present condition

5. Discuss the appropriate priority nursing goals for Chad.

a. Client will be effectively treated for opportunistic infections as evidenced by elimination of his present symptoms.
b. Client will regain and maintain adequate oxygenation as evidenced by oxygen saturation >94%.
c. Client will achieve and maintain pain control as determined by client and evidenced by client verbalizations.
d. Client will regain and maintain optimal weight for height and age (approximately 31.1 kg [68.5 lb])
e. Client will experience relief from diarrhea and regain and maintain fluid balance.
f. Client's skin will heal and no further breakdown will occur.

g. Client will not experience injury related to terminal central nervous system changes.
h. Client and family will verbalize feelings and concerns and effectively move through anticipatory grieving process.
i. Client and family will demonstrate understanding of home care for Chad.

6. **Discuss highly active antiretroviral therapy (HAART) and the classifications and examples of agents used in this treatment regimen.** HAART is the standard of care for HIV clients and is the most successful in decreasing the client's viral load. This therapy inhibits viral replication, however, it is not a cure (Jones, 2001). The classifications and examples of these agents are as follows:

Classification	Examples
a. Protease inhibitors	Amprenavir Indinavir Lopinavir Nelfinavir Ritonavir Saquinavir
b. Nucleoside analog reverse transcriptase inhibitors	Abacavir Didanosine Lamivudine Stavudine Zakcutavine Zidovudine
c. Non-nucleoside analog reverse transcriptase inhibitors	Delavirdine Efavirenz Nevirapine
d. Ribonucleotide reductase inhibitors	Hydroxyurea

7. **Discuss the medications used to treat common opportunistic infections.**

Common Opportunistic Infections	Antimicrobials
Pneumocystic carinii pneumonia (PCP)	Trimethoprim-sulfamethoxazole Pentamidine isethionate
Mycobacterium avium complex (MAC)	Ciprofloxacin Clofazimine Ethambutol Rifampin
Candidiasis	Amphotericin B Fluconazole Ketoconazole Metronidazole
Toxoplasmosis	Dapsone Pyrimethamine Sulfadiazine
Cytomegalovirus	Ganciclovir
Herpes simplex, herpes zoster, varicella zoster	Acyclovir (Zovirax)

8. **The home health nurse notes that Chad is withdrawn today during her visit. His parents confirm that he has not interacted with them "much" for the past week and when he does "he bites our heads off." How would you respond to his parents to help them understand Chad's reaction?** Chad's response is probably the result of

a number of factors. He may be going through the grieving response for his loss of normal growth and development (attending school with his friends, being able to participate in competitive sports, having his friends over to his house, and being able to go to their houses to visit). He is supposed to be completing Erikson's industry versus inferiority. The task, which is mastered as a result of feelings of accomplishment and developing positive self-esteem. This is difficult for Chad in his compromised and terminal state. In addition, Chad may be experiencing anticipatory grieving because he has the ability to understand death and its permanence. The first phase is shock and denial followed by anger. Bargaining is experienced followed by depression and finally acceptance. Because of the length of time Chad has been HIV positive and undergoing treatment, but aware that AIDS is a terminal illness, he may have already experienced anticipatory grieving; however, even though acceptance has been reached, clients can vacillate within the last four phases of the grief process.

9. **Discuss Chad's level of growth and development and how his condition may impact this.** Chad is a school-age child with a task of industry versus inferiority. Although his parents are still his primary influence at this stage, most of his waking time during the week should be spent at school learning and playing with his friends. Children Chad's age may be experiencing the beginning of puberty and increased interest in the opposite sex; however, same-sex friends are the ones with whom most of their time is spent. They are involved in active play and are more coordinated than at any other stage of childhood. They enjoy sports and games and are especially aware of rules. Accomplishment is achieved by everyone playing by the same rules. Their activities require balance and strength, and bicycle and skate board riding are common pastimes. They also enjoy fine motor activities including building models, playing musical instruments, and playing computer games. School-age children are increasingly able to accept responsibility for their actions. Clubs (Boy Scouts, 4H, etc.) are very popular. In his compromised state, Chad cannot attend school or participate in activities involving close interactions with other children. His parents can praise him for his accomplishments, but as so many activities of normal school-age children involve other children the same age, Chad will have difficulty because of his limited contact with his friends.

10. **Chad says to the home health nurse that he doesn't want his parents to know that his condition is worse because he doesn't want them to worry and he doesn't want to go back to the hospital. What are your impressions of Chad's remarks?** School-age children are very sensitive to the feelings of their parents, and Chad may want to spare his parents concern. He also may be concerned that if they are aware of his worsening condition, they will want him hospitalized for treatment. His desire not to return to the hospital may be based on his ability to understand the meaning of his condition and that he is going to die, and feeling that if he goes to the hospital, that will verify the seriousness of his condition. He also may have had traumatic experiences in previous hospitalizations. Hospitals are foreign environments and activate the stressors of hospitalization for children. These include separation anxiety, fear of injury and pain, and loss of control. He is with his family at home, home is considered a safe place, and he feels he has more control over what happens to him at home.

11. **On one of the home health nurse's visits, Chad tells the nurse that he misses going to church with his family on Sundays and asks the nurse to pray with him. Discuss Chad's requests and how the nurse might best respond to Chad.** At his age, Chad has an understanding of spirituality and an obvious need to pray. The nurse should assess Chad's religious affiliation and then encourage Chad by staying with him as he prays, asking if he would like his parents involved in the prayer session, assess whether Chad's religious leader (minister, priest [it won't be a rabbi as Jewish services are held on Saturdays]) makes house calls, and encourage parents to have a religious leader come to visit Chad regularly. One might question whether his family is still attending church services or if the entire family is staying home with Chad and perhaps the entire family needs spiritual assistance.

References

Broyles, B.E. (2005). *Medical-surgical nursing clinical companion.* Durham, NC: Carolina Academic Press.
Centers for Disease Control and Prevention. *http://www.cdc.gov*
Centers for Disease Control and Prevention (2000). *HIV/AIDS Surveillance Report.* 12(2). Atlanta: Author.

Daniels, R. (2002). *Delmar's manual of laboratory and diagnostic tests.* Clifton Park, NY: Thomson Delmar Learning.

Daughtry, L.M., Bankston, J.B., and Deshotels, J.M. (2002). HIV meds: Keeping trouble at bay. *RN.* 65(2):31–36.

HIV/AIDS Treatment Information. *http://www.hivatis.org*

Jones, S.G. (2001). Taking HAART: How to support patients with HIV/AIDS. *Nursing 2001.* 31(12): 36–42.

National Institutes of Health. *http://text.nlm.nih.gov/nih/cdc*

Potts, N. and Mandleco, B. (2002). *Pediatric nursing: Caring for children and their families.* Clifton Park, NY: Thomson Delmar Learning, pp. 859 –867.

Wong, D.L., Perry, S.E., and Hockenberry, M.J. (2002). *Maternal child nursing care* (2nd ed.). St. Louis: Mosby, pp. 1384–1391.

CASE STUDY 4

Ashlee

GENDER

F

AGE

4

SETTING

- Hospital

ETHNICITY

- White American

CULTURAL CONSIDERATIONS

PREEXISTING CONDITIONS

COEXISTING CONDITIONS

SIGNIFICANT HISTORY

COMMUNICATION

DISABILITY

SOCIOECONOMIC

SPIRITUAL

- Spiritual Strength

PHARMACOLOGIC

- Acetaminophen (Tylenol)
- Ondansetron (Zofran)
- Dexamethasone (Hexadrol)
- Lorazepam (Ativan)

PSYCHOSOCIAL

- Local extended family
- Client anxiety
- Parent anxiety

LEGAL

ETHICAL

ALTERNATIVE THERAPY

PRIORITIZATION

- Yes

DELEGATION

THE LYMPHATIC SYSTEM

Level of difficulty: Difficult

Overview: This case requires knowledge of leukemia, growth and development, hospitalization of a preschooler and its impact on the family, as well as an understanding of the client's background and family–child relationship.

Client Profile

Ashlee is a 4-year-old preschooler who lives with her parents and two older siblings in a suburban environment. She attends preschool five mornings a week and enjoys playing with her 5-year-old sister and 7-year-old brother. She is very active and enjoys playing outside, riding her tricycle, climbing on the family's jungle gym, and playing on the swing set. Her vocabulary consists of approximately 1,500 words and she speaks using four- or five-word sentences. Her parents are very attentive to their children and spend each weekend doing "family activities." During the week, her parents work, and Ashlee and her siblings stay with their grandmother after school. Their grandmother lives in the same neighborhood. In the evenings, the family eats together and maintains an evening schedule that allows for family play time.

Case Study

During the past 2 months, Ashlee has been less active than usual and has begun taking one or two naps in the afternoon. Her grandmother and parents think she looks pale, reasoning that it is because of her high activity level, until her interest in going outside to play decreases dramatically. When they take her temperature, it is elevated so they administer acetaminophen without effect. At this point they decide to take her to see her pediatrician. Although the health care provider found Ashlee's manifestations consistent with an upper respiratory infection, Dr. Polster is concerned and decides to admit Ashlee to the hospital for tests to rule out leukemia.

Questions and Suggested Answers

1. **What diagnostic tests would you expect to be prescribed for Ashlee?** The diagnostic tests to rule out or confirm a diagnosis are complete blood count, serum electrolytes, bone marrow aspiration, lumbar puncture, and bone scan. The most definitive diagnostic is the bone marrow aspiration. This can not only determine a diagnosis of leukemia but also can microscopically reveal the type of leukemia. The lumbar puncture and bone scan are used to determine central nervous system and bone involvement (see Fig. A-20).

2. **Her admission vital signs are:**

   Temperature: 38° C (100.4° F)
   Pulse: 120 beats/minute
   Respirations: 28 breaths/minute
   Blood pressure: 100/60

   and her admission complete blood count reveals:

   Hemoglobin: 11 g/dL
   Hematocrit: 31%
   Erythrocyte count: 4.6 million/mm^3
   Platelet count: 130,000/mm^3
   White blood cell: 4,000 cells/mm^3
   Neutrophils: 1,600 cells/mm^3
   Lymphocytes: 400 cells/mm^3
   Monocytes: 290 cells/mm^3
   Eosinophils: 120 cells/mm^3
   Basophils: 30 cells/mm^3

   Discuss the significance of Ashlee's vital signs and laboratory findings.

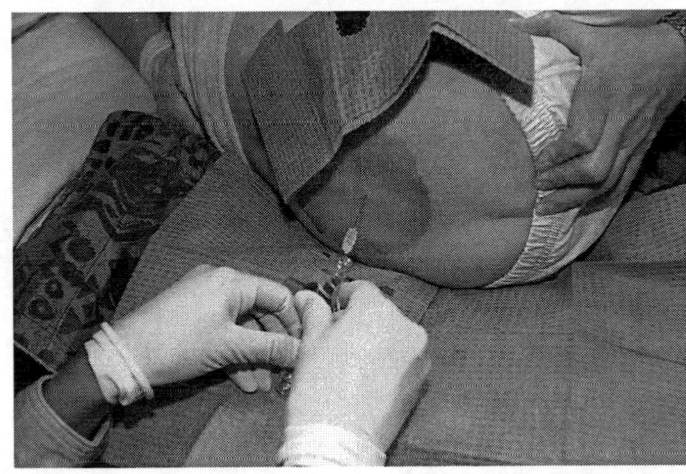

Figure A-20 *A lumbar puncture is performed to detect the presence of leukemic cells in the central nervous system of this child with acute lymphocytic leukemia.*

Ashlee's vital signs are within the normal limit for a 4-year-old except her temperature, which is elevated. The normal temperature for a child Ashlee's age is 37°–37.2° C (98.6°–99° F). The normal complete blood count for a preschooler is:

Hemoglobin: 11–16 g/dL

Hematocrit: 31–41%

Erythrocyte count: 4.5–4.8 million/mm^3

Platelet count: 150,000–450,000/mm^3

White blood cell: 4,100–10,800 cells/mm^3

- Neutrophils: 58–75%
- Lymphocytes: 25–33%
- Monocytes: 3–7%
- Eosinophils: 1–3%
- Basophils: 0–0.75%

Ashlee's leukocyte count is slightly below normal and much lower than one would expect from a child with her temperature, indicating the presence of infection. Normally, one would find an elevated white blood cell count. Her neutrophil count is less than 50% of her total white blood cell count, which should be 58% to 75% and her lymphoblasts account for only 10% instead of 25% to 33%. Her hemoglobin and hematocrit levels are the minimum of the normal range. Her erythrocyte count is below normal, as is her platelet count. These counts pose risks of infection, bleeding, and ineffective tissue perfusion.

3. **The diagnostic tests confirm a diagnosis of acute lymphocytic leukemia. Compare the two most common types of childhood leukemia.** The two common types of leukemia in children are acute lymphocytic or lymphoid leukemia (ALL) and acute myelocytic/myelogenous leukemia (AML) or acute nonlymphocytic leukemia (ANLL). ALL is the most common type (80% of all childhood leukemias) and also is the one with the best prognosis, with 90% of children with ALL reaching a 5-year survival and indefinitely remaining disease free. ALL is characterized by uncontrolled proliferation of immature lymphoblasts (B-cells or T-cells). Under normal circumstances lymphoblasts make lymphocytes in the bone marrow. The lymphocytes then mature and help defend the body against infection. The immature lymphoblasts proliferate to the extent that they almost completely saturate the bone marrow, but are undifferentiated and immature and cannot function as infection-fighting cells. They have a longer life span and do not respond to the body's biofeedback mechanisms. This leaves the client at risk for infection. In addition, the saturation of the bone marrow with these immature lymphoblasts results in the decreased ability of the bone marrow to manufacture

erythrocytes and platelets. This places the client at risk for anemia (decreased tissue perfusion) and thrombocytopenia (risk for bleeding).

AML is acute myelocytic or myelogenous leukemia and it involves the proliferation of immature myeloblasts. The bone marrow produces large numbers of these myeloblasts instead of manufacturing all three types of leukocytes. The myeloblasts then enter the systemic system and are able to cross the blood–brain barrier. They compete with normal cells in the brain, skin, ovaries, testes, and other organs, causing the premature death of the normal cells. Problems similar to those seen in ALL also occur in AML; however, in AML solid tumors may result. The prognosis for AML is poorer, with 20% to 35% achieving a 5-year survival.

4. **Ashlee's mother is at Ashlee's bedside crying. As you approach her, she says, "How could God let my little girl get leukemia? What can I do to make it go away?" How would you respond to Ashlee's mother?** A number of therapeutic communication techniques may be employed here. With an understanding that anger (blame) and bargaining are two phases of the grief process, these are frequently questions the person does not expect an answer to and silence may be the most appropriate response. Ask Ashlee's mother if she would like to speak to the hospital chaplain or have the nurse contact the family's own spiritual leader (minister, priest, rabbi) to come and see them. The nurse also can try to help Ashlee's mother understand that the cause of leukemia in children is unknown and not the result of anything her mother did or didn't do. The mother obviously needs some spiritual support at this point and this need must be addressed.

5. **What are the nursing priorities of care for Ashlee?**
   a. Risk for infection related to decrease in functional white blood cells secondary to ALL
   b. Risk for injury, bleeding, and ineffective tissue perfusion related to decreased platelets and red blood cells secondary to ALL
   c. Risk for imbalanced nutrition: less than body requirements related to nausea secondary to chemotherapy and fatigue secondary to ineffective tissue perfusion
   d. Fear/anxiety related to Ashlee's condition, prognosis, hospitalization, and Ashlee's level of growth and development and magical thinking
   e. Deficient knowledge related to Ashlee's condition, treatment, and home care

6. **Discuss the appropriate priority nursing interventions for Ashlee.**
   a. Risk for infection
      (1) Monitor temperature every 4 hours.
      (2) Place on Compromised Host Precautions.
      (3) Ensure that all persons coming in contact with Ashlee perform meticulous handwashing.
      (4) Maintain and teach Ashlee's parents about the importance of thorough hygiene for Ashlee.
      (5) Avoid invasive procedures including intramuscular injections.
      (6) Monitor white blood cell count.
      (7) Administer antimicrobials as prescribed
      (8) Perform central venous access device (CVAD) dressing changes using sterile technique NOTE: Chemotherapy is the most effective treatment for ALL and should be infused through a CVAD in children.
      (9) If Ashlee becomes neutropenic, place on Neutropenic Precautions following facility protocol.
   b. Risk for injury, bleeding
      (1) Assess all mucous membranes for evidence of bleeding.
      (2) Use soft toothbrush or toothettes for oral hygiene.
      (3) Avoid taking temperatures rectally.
      (4) Avoid foods that may damage oral mucous membranes.
      (5) Monitor vital signs every 4 hours.
      (6) Monitor platelet count.
      (7) Administer platelets as prescribed.

(8) Teach Ashlee to avoid picking her nose (which is a common activity with preschoolers and the leading cause of epistaxis).
(9) Collaborate with the health care provider for a prescription for stool softener.
(10) Encourage quiet preschool activities such as coloring, watching age-appropriate videos, and so forth.
(11) Prevent injury.

c. Ineffective tissue perfusion
(1) Monitor erythrocyte count, hemoglobin, and hematocrit.
(2) Instruct Ashlee's parents to assist Ashlee when she wants to get out of bed or call for assistance.
(3) Administer packed red blood cells as prescribed.
(4) Administer medications to stimulate red blood cell production as prescribed.
(5) Administer oxygen as prescribed, titrating to maintain oxygen saturation of >94%.
(6) Monitor vital signs every 4 hours.
(7) Provide periods of undisturbed rest.

d. Risk for imbalanced nutrition
(1) Collaborate with her parents to determine her favorite foods.
(2) Communicate with the dietician.
(3) Administer antiemetics as prescribed for nausea or collaborate with health care provider to obtain prescription.
(4) Weigh daily.
(5) Offer nutritional supplements as prescribed or collaborate with health care provider to obtain a prescription.
(6) Encourage the family to bring in Ashlee's favorite foods.
(7) Maintain strict intake and output.
(8) Involve Ashlee in food selection.

e. Fear/anxiety
(1) Encourage Ashlee and her parents to express their feelings.
(2) Remember that Ashlee's greatest fear of hospitalization is the fear of mutilation and the nurse must anticipate this.
(3) Encourage parents to bring in Ashlee's favorite toy from home to increase her sense of security.
(4) Encourage the parents to stay with Ashlee, if possible.
(5) Encourage the parents to be active in Ashlee's care.
(6) Communicate the parents' concerns to the appropriate health care professional
(7) Maintain a calm, caring affect.
(8) Use an appropriate growth and development approach when talking and caring for Ashlee.
(9) Collaborate with the health care provider for referral to child life specialist, if available, for Ashlee.

f. Deficient knowledge during hospitalization
(1) Assess parents and Ashlee's current level of knowledge.
(2) Provide verbal and written information concerning:
(a) Medications Ashlee is receiving
(b) Current laboratory values
(c) Procedures for Ashlee
(d) Practices to decrease Ashlee's risks for infection and bleeding
(e) Preschool growth and development including appropriate activities for Ashlee
(f) Hospital visitation policies

7. **Discuss the factors that affect Ashlee's prognosis.** Factors that affect the prognosis of children with leukemia include age at the time of diagnosis, the type of leukemia the child has, gender, white blood cell count at the time of diagnosis, and the child's response to chemotherapy.

Positive factors:

a. Age between 2 and 10 years
b. Female gender
c. White blood cell count normal or slightly below normal
d. ALL

Negative factors:

a. Age <2 years or >10 years
b. Male gender
c. Elevated white blood cell count
d. AML

Ashlee has very positive factors and has a very good prognosis. Ninety percent of children with ALL go into remission following chemotherapy and remain disease free indefinitely with a 5-year survival, which is considered a cure.

8. **Ashlee's mother expresses concern because Ashlee "has been potty-trained for 2 years, but she has wet the bed since she has been in the hospital." How would you respond to Ashee's mother?** One can assume that Ashlee will be receiving chemotherapy and a standard of care prior to and following chemotherapy consisting of hyperhydration with intravenous fluids to ensure that the chemotherapy is dilute as it enters and is then excreted from the urinary bladder. These children do not normally receive 75–100 mL of fluid per hour when at home; however, this is the usual case during hospitalization for chemotherapy. In addition, intravenous fluids do not elicit the same bladder response as taking fluids orally, so the children lack the usual acknowledged stimulation. Given these factors and the fact that preschoolers are very deep sleepers, one would expect an interruption in Ashlee's ability to maintain toilet-training. A suggestion for parents might be to diaper their child at night to avoid both the potential emotional stress to the child (toilet-trained children are very proud of their ability to control their bladders and bowels) and the potential risk to the child's skin by prolonged contact with urine when the child is incontinent. In addition, this allows the child to experience undisturbed rest rather than being awakened hourly either to urinate or to have the bed linen changed. It also is common for hospitalized children to regress in their behavior when experiencing the stressors of hospitalization. Although Ashlee's enuresis in the hospital may, in part, be regression or a response to stress, it is more likely a result of the intravenous hydration associated with chemotherapy.

9. **Ashlee's chemotherapy regimen is started and the oncologist prescribes that she receive ondansetron 2.5 mg IV prior to chemotherapy and the same dose every 4 hours for 24 hours. In addition, she prescribes dexamethasone 16 mg IV prior to chemotherapy and lorazepam 1 mg IV every 4 hours PRN for breakthrough nausea. Discuss these prescriptions including drug classifications, when medications should be administered, special considerations when administering drugs, and safe dosage for Ashlee, who weighs 16.7 kg (36.7 lb).** Ondansetron is the drug of choice to prevent the nausea and vomiting associated with chemotherapy. It should be administered 30 minutes prior to chemotherapy and should be prescribed every 4 hours for 24 hours following chemotherapy. The safe dosage of this drug for Ashlee is 0.15 mg/kg (Gahart and Nazareno, 2005, p. 868), so she is prescribed a safe dose. Dexamethasone is an adenoglucocorticoid that when used as an antiemetic prior to chemotherapy has a safe pediatric dosage range of 4–8 mg/m^2 (Gahart and Nazarone, 2005, p. 365). Ashlee's dose is safe. This agent also is prescribed 30 minutes prior to chemotherapy and can be mixed in the same minibag with ondansetron and administered over 15 minutes. Although ondansetron continues to be administered every 4 hours for 24 hours, this dose of dexamethasone is a once daily dose. The most common agent used for breakthrough nausea and vomiting for clients receiving chemotherapy is lorazepam IV via bolus at a safe dose of 0.04–0.08 mg/kg to a maximum dose of 4 mg per dose every 6 hours (Gahart and Woods, 2005, p. 738). Ashlee's prescribed dose is safe. Lorazepam should be administered over 1 minute.

10. **Discuss Ashlee's level of growth and development and how her treatment may impact this.** A 4-year-old is increasingly competent in gross motor skills and focuses on the development of fine motor skills. The child is very active; constantly on the go; runs well; can catch and throw a ball overhead; jumps, climbs, and swings

well, goes up and down stairs without holding on; walks heel to toe; and hops on one foot. The child can copy a square, tries to print letters, draws a person with two to four parts, can cut on a curved line; and enjoys coloring and drawing pictures. Preschoolers are motivated by socialization and imagination to achieve their task of initiative. If they are not successful, they feel guilt and their imaginations lead them to believe that they are responsible for "bad things" that happen to themselves and their significant others. Their vocabulary is approximately 1,500 words and they enjoy having stories read to them. They know the days of the week and can count to five without assistance. The major complication of chemotherapy is bone marrow suppression with a high risk of infection. This may interfere with Ashlee's socialization outside of the home, negatively affecting her striving for initiative, however playing interactively with dolls, stuffed animals, and puppets with her parents and siblings would be helpful during times that she is compromised by myelosuppression. Her parents and 7-year-old brother can read to her, helping both her vocabulary as well as letter and word recognition. When her blood counts rise, inviting her preschool friends over and/or returning her to preschool would help her regain some of her pre-chemo normalcy. With understanding of growth and development, alternative activities will allow her to master her task of initiative and socialization.

11. **How would you work with Ashlee's parents to help prevent complications associated with her growth and development?** The major focus for the nurse in order to help Ashlee's parents is to assist them in understanding normal growth and development of their preschooler. Close monitoring of Ashlee's laboratory values will help guide them in choosing appropriate activities to foster her fine motor skills while protecting her from infection, bleeding, and ineffective tissue perfusion. The common reaction for parents of these children is overprotection, which frequently interferes with their growth and development. Many facilities that specialize in treating children with cancer who are receiving chemotherapy develop support groups with other parents of similar children. This not only provides for the children's needs, but also serves as a great resource for support for the parents.

References

Daniels, R. (2002). *Delmar's manual of laboratory and diagnostic tests.* Clifton Park, NY: Thomson Delmar Learning.

Gahart, B.L. and Nazareno, A.R. (2005). *2005 Intravenous medications* (21st ed.). St. Louis: Mosby.

Josephson, D.L. (2004). *Intravenous infusion therapy for nurses: Principles & practice* (2nd ed.). Clifton Park, NY: Thomson Delmar Learning.

Leukemia & Lymphoma Society. *http://www.leukemia.org*

Leukemia Research Foundation. *http://www.leukemia-research.org*

North America Nursing Diagnosis Association. (2005). *Nursing diagnoses: Definitions & classifications, 2005–2006.* Philadelphia: NANDA.

Potts, N. and Mandleco, B. (2002). *Pediatric nursing: Caring for children and their families.* Clifton Park, NY: Thomson Delmar Learning, pp. 924–931.

Wong, D.L., Perry, S.E., and Hockenberry, M.J. (2002). *Maternal child nursing care* (2nd ed.). St. Louis: Mosby, pp. 1371–1372.

CASE STUDY 5

Nicole

GENDER

F

AGE

13

SETTING

- Hospital

ETHNICITY

- Middle Eastern

CULTURAL CONSIDERATIONS

PREEXISTING CONDITIONS

- Leukemia
- Alopecia
- CVAD

COEXISTING CONDITIONS

SIGNIFICANT HISTORY

COMMUNICATION

DISABILITY

SOCIOECONOMIC

SPIRITUAL

PHARMACOLOGIC

- Acetaminophen (Tylenol)
- Cyclophosphomide (Cytoxin)
- Gentamicin sulfate (Garamycin)
- Vancomycin hydrochloride (Vancocin)
- Cefoxitin sodium (Mefoxin)

PSYCHOSOCIAL

LEGAL

ETHICAL

ALTERNATIVE THERAPY

PRIORITIZATION

- Yes

DELEGATION

THE LYMPHATIC SYSTEM

Level of difficulty: Difficult

Overview: This case requires knowledge of chemotherapy, growth and development, as well as an understanding of the client's background, personal situation, and parent–child relationship.

Client Profile

Nicole is a 13-year-old with leukemia. She lives at home with her parents and younger siblings and for the past 3 months has been receiving chemotherapy. She has a central venous access device (CVAD) that is cared for by her parents and herself. Nicole has experienced a number of absences from school as a result of her hospitalizations, chemotherapy, and the effects of her chemotherapy regimen, although she has had a tutor at home to keep her current with her studies. Nicole has alopecia and has been hospitalized with a line infection, stomatitis and esophagitis, and bleeding requiring platelet replacement. She refuses to see her friends although she speaks with them frequently on the phone. She tells them her refusal is based on the fact that she is prone to infection and doesn't want to risk exposure and have to be hospitalized again.

Case Study

Nicole is admitted to the pediatric unit of the local hospital with a temperature of 38.8° C (101.8° F) that did not respond to the acetaminophen that she has been taking every 4 hours since yesterday. Her admission assessment indicated the Nicole's lung sounds are clear, heart sounds are strong and regular, she is in no apparent distress, has alopecia, and has evidence of white patches in her mouth. Her laboratory values include:

Hematology:

Hemoglobin: 10.1 g/dL

Hematocrit: 25%

Platelets: 50,000/mm^3

White blood cell count: 2,000/mm^3

Differential: Neutrophils 20%

Questions and Suggested Answers

1. **Discuss the significance of Nicole's laboratory findings.** Nicole's lab values indicate adverse effects of chemotherapy. The most common adverse effect of chemotherapy is myelosuppression. Antineoplastics target fast-growing cells including cells with normal function, erythrocytes, leukocytes, and platelets. This results in anemia, neutropenia, and thrombocytopenia which leads to decrease tissue perfusion, high risk of infections, and high risk for bleeding. Nicole's laboratory findings exemplify all three of the problems. The normal hemoglobin for an adolescent girl is 12–16 g/dL and the normal hematocrit for her age group is 38% to 47%. Nicole's values indicate anemia that occurs when the hematocrit falls below 28%. The normal white blood cell count for Nicole is 4,100–10,800/mm^3 and neutrophils should account for 58% to 67%. Nicole's indicate neutropenia, which is defined as neutrophil count $<$ 500 cells/mm^3. The normal platelet count for 13- to 18- year-old girls is 150,000–450,000/mm^3; Nicole is at risk for bleeding with her platelet count of 50,000, as thrombocytopenia occurs when the platelet count falls below 50,000 cells/mm^3 and creates a high risk for bleeding.
2. **What other assessment data would be helpful for the nurse to have to prepare Nicole's care plan?**
   - a. Urine specific gravity
   - b. Urine for blood
   - c. Hemoccult of stools
   - d. Assessment of central venous access device (CVAD) for redness, swelling, purulent discharge, pain
   - e. Urine culture and sensitivity
   - f. Chest x-ray
   - g. Oxygen saturation via pulse oximetry
   - h. Peripheral blood cultures and cultures from CVAD

3. What are the priorities of care for Nicole on admission?

a. Ineffective protection related to neutrophil count
b. High risk for injury and bleeding related to platelet count
c. Risk for ineffective tissue perfusion related to hemoglobin and hematocrit values
d. Impaired oral mucous membranes related to presence of mouth lesions
e. Acute pain related to presence of mucositis
f. Risk for nausea related to the effects of chemotherapy on gastrointestinal mucosa
g. Disturbed body image related to alopecia
h. Deficient knowledge related to Nicole's current condition, treatment, and home care

4. Discuss the common complications (adverse effects) of chemotherapy. Myelosuppression is the most common complication of chemotherapy and results from the non-differentiating effects of the agents on fast-multiplying cells, both normal and abnormal. As noted in question 1, this results in a risk for neutropenia, thrombocytopenia, and neutropenia. Because antineoplastic are most toxic to rapidly growing cells, hair follicle cells are rapidly destroyed, creating a condition called alopecia. Nausea and vomiting are common because of the toxic action on the epithelium of the gastrointestinal tract and mucositis occurs as a result of the destruction of normal flora in the upper GI tract. In addition, mucositis is a result of the effect of chemotherapy on rapidly dividing cells. These agents are detoxified in the liver and can potentially lead to impaired hepatic function. Also, they are primarily eliminated through the renal/urinary system so may be contraindicated in the presence of renal insufficiency. Because the urinary bladder is the one area in the body in which antineoplastics are not in perpetual movement, they can destroy the urinary bladder lining through constant and concentrated contact. Other complications occur including those that are agent specific, for instance, methotrexate can cause uric acid neuropathy and Adriamycin is associated with cardiotoxicity. Alkylating agents, especially ifosfamide and cyclophosphamide, carry a high risk for hemorrhagic cystitis. Extravasation with the local destruction of tissue can result in amputation or the need for plastic surgery to correct. NOTE: Because peripheral administration of vesicant agents is not appropriate for children, this risk is primarily for adults receiving peripheral chemotherapy, however, it can occur at the site of non-tunnelled CVADs because of the short length of the catheter. Edema and fluid retention are common in the use of corticosteroids as a part of many chemotherapy regimens.

5. What nursing actions address the adverse effects associated with chemotherapy?

a. Myelosuppression
   (1) Place on Compromised Host precautions.
   (2) Monitor temperature every 4 hours during hospitalization.
   (3) Maintain patency of CVAD, monitoring hourly.
   (4) Use sterile technique for CVAD dressing and line changes using approved protocols.
   (5) Monitor laboratory values and report abnormal findings immediately.
   (6) If reddened area on skin appears, notify the health care provider immediately.
   (7) Administer antimicrobials and blood products as prescribed.
   (8) Assess oral mucus membranes, nares for bleeding.
   (9) Monitor platelet count and place on bleeding precautions if platelet counts falls below 50,000.
   (10) Hemoccult stools.
   (11) Collaborate with health care provider for prescription for stool softeners to prevent straining.
   (12) Monitor urine for blood.
   (13) If hematocrit falls below 25%, institute falls precautions.
   (14) Monitor red blood cell count.
   (15) Assess for signs and symptoms of anemia.
   (16) Monitor for bleeding.
   (17) Draw labs from CVAD as prescribed.

b. Nausea
   (1) Premedicate child with antiemetics prior to administering chemotherapy as prescribed.

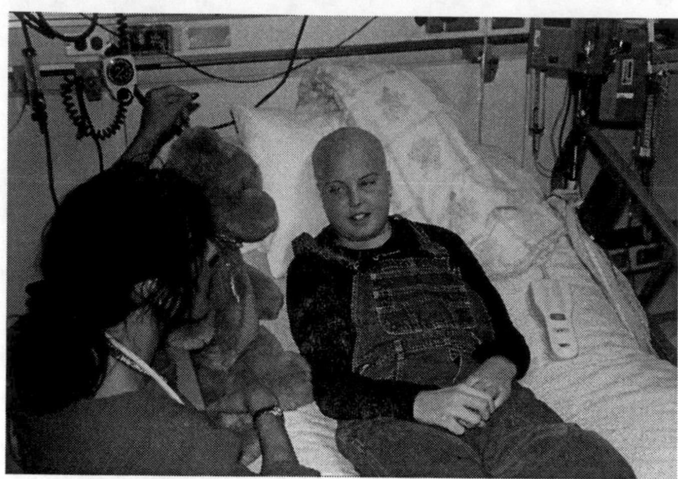

Figure A-21 *Alopecia is a common side effect of chemotherapy and a threat to body image, especially for the older child.*

(2) Administer prescribed proton pump inhibitors every 4 hours for 24 hours following chemotherapy.
(3) Administer lorazepam as prescribed for breakthrough nausea.
(4) Eliminate offensive odors in environment.

c. Alopecia (see Fig. A-21)
(1) Assess child and parent's knowledge of alopecia.
(2) Stress to child that alopecia is temporary and following chemotherapy, hair will grow back.
(3) Encourage child and family to express feelings and concerns.
(4) Actively listen, providing empathetic therapeutic responses to questions.
(5) Provide information concerning local wig retailers if appropriate, depending on child's desire.
(6) Discuss use of scarves or turbans as alternatives to wearing a wig.

d. Acute pain associated with mucositis (stomatitis, esophagitis)
(1) Assess oral mucous membranes.
(2) Administer nystatin swish and swallow or swish and spit as prescribed.
(3) Assess pain level baseline using appropriate pain assessment tool.
(4) Administer morphine sulfate (drug of choice) PCA (patient-controlled analgesia), using both continuous intravenous infusion and PCA dosing as prescribed until acute pain controlled, which usually takes 48–72 hours.
(5) Assess pain level hourly to evaluate effectiveness of prescribed analgesic.
(6) Encourage intake of cool liquids during the acute phase, if possible.
(7) If the child has esophagitis, enteral feedings may be required.

e. Vesicant extravasation risk with peripheral intravenous administration of chemotherapy
(1) Assess intravenous site for patency and placement prior to administering chemotherapy.
(2) Monitor intravenous site every 15–30 minutes during chemotherapy infusion.
(3) Caution the client to inform the nurse immediately if intravenous site causes any discomfort or swelling.
(4) If vesicant extravasation occurs, **stop infusion immediately, remove access, flush site with sterile fluid (as determined by facility protocol), notify the health care provider.**

6. **Nicole is receiving cyclophosphamide intravenously. Discuss this agent including any nursing interventions necessary specifically related to its use?** Cyclophosphamide is an alkylating neoplastic agent that acts by inhibiting DNA synthesis that works in all phases of the cell cycle; however, it is most effective in the S cycle and changes the internal acid–base balance in the cell. It is used as a component of numerous chemotherapy regimens to treat acute and chronic leukemia in children. Alkylating agents cause myelosuppression, with their greatest impact on the production of white blood cells (leukocytes), especially neutrophils, resulting in neutropenia. Because these agents are most toxic to rapidly growing cells, hair follicle cells are rapidly

destroyed, creating a condition called alopecia. Nausea and vomiting are common because of the toxic action on the epithelium of the GI tract and mucositis occurs as a result of the destruction of normal flora in the upper GI tract. These agents are detoxified in the liver and can potentially lead to impaired hepatic function. Because of the toxic effects on epithelial tissue that line the mucous membranes, two alkylating agents, ifosfamide and cyclophosphamide, can result in hemorrhagic cystitis, a potentially life-threatening bleeding complication, especially in the presence of thrombocytopenia. Because of its potential for extravasation, cyclophosphamide should be administered via a central venous access (CVAD). As a result of the risk of hemorrhagic cystitis, the rescue agent mesna should be prescribed and the first dose administered immediately following the completion of each cyclophosphamide administration. Mesna rescues the urinary bladder from the effects of cyclophosphamide. Mesna dosing is continued for 24 hours following the first dose. The urine should be tested each void for blood as well as specific gravity. In addition, the hyperhydration prior to and following administration of the agent is critical. Antiemetics, ondansetron (or other serotonin blocking setrons) should be prescribed prior to cyclophosphamide administration in addition to dexamethasone. Ondansetron dosing should continue every 4 hours for 24 hours following cyclophosphamide administration. Lorazepam is the drug of choice for breakthrough nausea and vomiting. Laboratory values must be monitored closely (at least every 24 hours) to detect myelosuppression and the child should be placed on compromised host precautions. Alopecia can have a potentially harmful effect on the child's body image, especially for adolescent girls. Teenage boys have fared better with alopecia because of the impact of professional sports where the participants often shave their heads and it is a part of their image (Broyles, 2005).

7. **Nicole is diagnosed with a CVAD line infection. Discuss how these infections occur and why.** Although tunneled CVAD catheters have an antibacterial filter to protect the line from microorganisms traveling down the catheter from the insertion site, line infections are a risk with any CVAD. The primary source of line infection is pathogenic organism growth at the proximal tip of the catheter and is fostered by fibrin formation that can occur at this site. Fibrin provides an excellent media for bacterial growth. These can be prevented by proper flushing of CVAD and maintaining positive pressure at the proximal tip of the catheter. Infection is the greatest risk with CVADs and in the presence of myelosuppression, the risk increases.

8. **Nicole's mother is staying with Nicole during her hospitalization and expresses concern about Nicole refusing to see her friends and that Nicole seems "down" since her last chemotherapy. Discuss your impressions about Nicole's mother's statements, considering Nicole's level of growth and development.** Although Nicole's reason for not wanting to see her friends (risk of exposure to infection) is plausible, her level of growth and development would support that Nicole is having difficulty adjusting to her alopecia. For adolescents, peers are the primary source of a sense of belonging and it is vital to them to be like their peers to foster this belonging. Girls at this age are particularly sensitive about their appearance, and hair styles are a major focus. Baldness is not an acceptable trait for them. Although teenagers can make cruel and hurtful comments about other teenagers, they also can express sensitivity. The greatest fear of teenagers is being ostracized by others their age. School represents a time of continuous contact with peers and Nicole probably feels that by staying at home, she can protect herself from being shunned by her friends. Talking with Nicole about her concerns should be suggested to her mother so that she can realize that true friends accept people as they are. If Nicole remains convinced that her friends would not accept her with her alopecia, encouraging her to purchase a wig or wearing a hat may result in improved self-esteem. The scenario does not address how Nicole's family reacts to her appearance. If they are not accepting, the nurse should focus on their perceptions first.

9. **Nicole tells the nurse that her mouth and throat are so sore she cannot drink or eat anything. Discuss your impressions about Nicole's complaints and the appropriate nursing actions to help Nicole.** The lesions in Nicole's mouth probably represent mucositis, a very painful condition resulting from the destruction of oral normal flora by chemotherapy. Collaborating with the health care provider for prescriptions including nystatin swish and spit (for stomatitis) or swish and swallow (for esophagitis) and intravenous morphine sulfate, both continuous infusion and PCA dosing, have proven effective in treating mucositis. Her hydration can be maintained with intravenous fluids until her pain is controlled, at which time cool liquids should be offered.

These should include supplements of high-protein and high-carbohydrate drinks; citrus fruits should be avoided because their acid content is irritating to the sensitive and injured mucous membranes of the mouth and esophagus.

10. **Nicole is prescribed intravenous antibiotic therapy to treat her line infection. The health care provider prescribes gentamicin sulfate 100 mg IV q8h, vancomycin hydrochloride 500 mg IV every 6 hours, and cefoxitin sodium 1 g IV every 6 hours. Nicole weighs 44 kg (96.8 lb). Discuss these agents and if the doses prescribed are safe for Nicole.** Gentamicin sulfate is an aminoglycoside that acts as an antimicrobial by inhibiting protein synthesis in the bacterial cell wall. This causes the cell to die. The adverse effect specific to this classification is ototoxicity. Vancomycin hydrochloride is classified as a miscellaneous antimicrobial or tricyclic glycopeptide that is a highly potent antimicrobial used to treat many gram positive infections that are not responsive to other less toxic agents. The most serious complication specific to this agent is renal failure. Cefoxitin sodium is a second-generation cephalosporin that acts on gram-positive and some gram-negative bacteria by interfering with the cell wall synthesis. The most serious adverse effect of cephalosporins is allergic or sensitivity reaction that can lead to anaphylaxis. All of Nicole's dosages are safe. The safe dosage range for gentamicin is 6.0–7.5 mg/kg every 24 hours (Gahart and Woods, 2005, pp. 592–593), so Nicole's safe dose every 8 hours would be 80–100 mg IV. The safe dosage range for vancomycin for children is 60 mg/kg every 24 hours (Gahart and Woods, 2005, p. 1145). Nicole's safe dose should not exceed 600 mg every 6 hours. The safe dosage range for cefoxitin is 13.3–26.6 mg/kg per dose (Gahart and Woods, 2005, p. 254). Nicole's safe dose is 532–1,064 mg.

11. **The pharmacy schedules Nicole's antibiotic therapy as follows:**

Gentamicin	**2400h**	**0600h**	**1200h**	**1800h**
Vancomycin	**0200h**	**0800h**	**1400h**	**2200h**
Cefoxitin	**2400h**	**0600h**	**1200h**	**1800h**

Discuss this schedule and what alterations the nurse should make, if any. This schedule is possible; however, changing the cefoxitin schedule to 0100–0700–1300–1900 would eliminate the overlap of drug administration. Nurses must realize that the time of administration for medications is part of the seven rights of medication administration—Right Time. Some nurses do not want to use this schedule because of the 0700 dose being at the time of morning change of shifts, and on units where nurses work 12-hour shifts, it affects both shift times; however, nurses should first consider what is best for the client. In most health facilities, a 30-minute window for administration is policy (drugs can be administered 30 minutes prior to or after the scheduled time) so if the aforementioned schedule above cannot be changed, the nurse should administer the cefoxitin sodium before the gentamicin because it infuses in 15 minutes versus the 30-minute administration time for gentamicin, thus both could be administered within the 30-minute window.

12. **Calculate the rates of administration via a volumetric intravenous infusion pump for the following:**
Gentamicin sulfate 100 mg in 100 mL of 5% dextrose in water to infuse over 30 minutes
Vancomycin hydrochloride 500 mg in 250 mL of 0.9% normal saline
Cefoxitin sodium 1 g in 50 mL of 5% dextrose in water to infuse over 15 minutes
Using the formula of

$$\frac{\text{Time}}{\text{Volume}} = \frac{\text{Time}}{\text{Volume}}$$

The hourly rate for gentamicin is 200 mg/hour:

$$\frac{30 \text{ minutes}}{100 \text{ mL}} = \frac{60 \text{ minutes}}{X}$$

The hourly rate for vancomycin is not stated in the prescription because the nurse should note that to prevent renal adverse effects, it must be administered over a minimum of 60 minutes (250 mL/hour). Common practice in pediatrics is infusing it over 2 hours so the rate should be 125 mL/hour. The hourly rate for cefoxitin is 200 mL/hour.

References

Broyles, B.E. (2005). *Medical-surgical clinical companion.* Durham, NC: Carolina Academic Press, pp. 183–186.

Centers for Disease Control and Prevention. *http://www.cdc.gov*

Daniels, R. (2002). *Delmar's manual of laboratory and diagnostic tests.* Clifton Park, NY: Thomson Delmar Learning.

Gahart, B.L. and Nazareno, A.R. (2005). *2005 Intravenous medications* (21st ed.). St. Louis: Mosby.

Intravenous Therapy. *http://www.nursewise.com*

Josephson, D.L. (2004). *Intravenous infusion therapy for nurses: Principles & practice* (2nd ed.). Clifton Park, NY: Thomson Delmar Learning.

North American Nursing Diagnosis Association. (2005). *Nursing diagnoses: Definitions & classifications, 2005–2006.* Philadelphia: NANDA.

Potts, N. and Mandleco, B. (2002). *Pediatric nursing: Caring for children and their families.* Clifton Park, NY: Thomson Delmar Learning.

Reiss, B.S., Evans, M.E. and Broyles, B.E. (2002). *Pharmacological aspects of nursing care.* (6th ed.). Clifton Park, NY: Thomson Delmar Learning, pp. 760–797.

Wong, D.L., Perry, S.E., and Hockenberry, M.J. (2002). *Maternal child nursing care* (2nd ed.). St. Louis: Mosby, p. 1376.

CASE STUDY 6

Katie

GENDER

F

AGE

11

SETTING

- Health care provider's office

ETHNICITY

- Black American

CULTURAL CONSIDERATIONS

PREEXISTING CONDITIONS

COEXISTING CONDITIONS

SIGNIFICANT HISTORY

COMMUNICATION

DISABILITY

SOCIOECONOMIC

SPIRITUAL

PHARMACOLOGIC

- Acetaminophen (Tylenol)
- Nystatin (Mycostatin)
- Prednisone (Deltasone)
- Ibuprofen (Motrin)

PSYCHOSOCIAL

- Client anxiety

LEGAL

ETHICAL

ALTERNATIVE THERAPY

PRIORITIZATION

- Yes

DELEGATION

- Client teaching

THE LYMPHATIC SYSTEM

Level of difficulty: Difficult

Overview: This case requires knowledge of systemic lupus erythematosus (SLE), growth and development, as well as an understanding of the client's background, personal situation, and parent–child relationship, and of interaction with antagonistic parents.

Client Profile

Katie is an 11-year-old school-age child who lives with her parents and 13-year-old sister in a suburban neighborhood. She has a 2-year history of frequent upper respiratory infections (URI) accompanied by joint pain, headaches, and mouth ulcers. Her parents are frustrated because even though Katie's pediatrician has treated her recurrent URIs, no definitive diagnosis has been made to explain her other clinical manifestations. They treat her headaches and joint pain with acetaminophen and the mouth ulcers with nystatin, but they continue to recur. Her symptoms have caused Katie's school performance to decline, and now over the past 2 days, Katie has developed a malar rash in the shape of a butterfly. Determined to find out what is wrong with Katie, her parents make another appointment to see her pediatrician

Case Study

Katie is brought to her pediatrician's office by her parents. As the nurse approaches them, Katie's mother says, "We haven't seen you here before but either you people find out what is wrong with Katie and effectively treat her or we are going to find another pediatrician who knows what he is doing." During her assessment, the nurse notes that Katie is pale and holding her head in her hand. When questioned, Katie says, "Oh, it's just another one of my headaches. I probably have a brain tumor like my friend Alisha." Katie's vital signs are: temperature, 37.7° C (99.8° F); pulse, 115 beats/minute; respirations, 24 breaths/minute; and blood pressure, 112/70.

Questions and Suggested Answers

1. **Discuss your impression of Katie's history and clinical manifestations.** Katie is exhibiting manifestations of systemic lupus erythematosus (SLE). The clinical signs of SLE include the malar "butterfly" rash or discoid rash (see Fig. A-22), photosensitivity, oral and nasal ulcers, arthritis, serositis, pleuritis, pericarditis, renal dysfunction, neurological disorders (seizures, psychosis, headaches, personality changes), hematological disorders (leukopenia, lymphoma, thrombocytopenia, anemia), and immunological disorders. The diagnosis of SLE is usually made in the presence of four or more of the clinical manifestations.
2. **What other assessment data would be helpful for the nurse to have to prepare Katie's care plan?**
   - a. The results of her previous diagnostic testing
   - b. Her history of upper respiratory infections (URIs) prior to 2 years ago
   - c. Height and weight
   - d. Physical assessment data (especially breath sounds, heart sounds)
   - e. Serum chemistry values
   - f. Complete blood count
   - g. Autoantibody (ANA) results
   - h. Electrocardiogram
   - i. Gamma-globulin and sedimentation rate
   - j. Tissue biopsies
3. **Discuss her parents comment to the nurse and how the nurse can best respond to them.** Her parents obviously are frustrated because of the lack of a definitive diagnosis after watching their daughter experience her clinical manifestations, especially the ones that caused her pain. Having their child in pain is a very difficult thing for parents, and very frustrating when the cause of the pain cannot be identified and effectively treated. Anger results. The nurse must not be defensive and consider this as a personal attack. He or she must be nonjudgmental and understanding of their frustration, encouraging them to continue to verbalize their feelings and frustrations with open-ended questions or therapeutic silence. It is important to be empathetic perhaps saying, "I think I can understand how frustrating this is for you and Katie." (Never say, "I understand how you

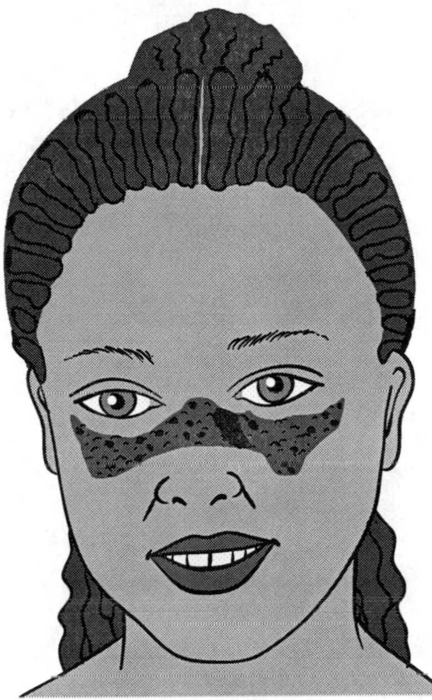

Figure A-22 *Butterfly rash often seen in SLE.*

feel" because you are not one of these parents so you can't completely understand their level of frustration. This comment would be a block to therapeutic communication.) The nurse must collaborate with the pediatrician, explaining the interchange between the nurse and the parents prior to his or her talking to them so that he or she is prepared.

4. **Discuss Katie's comment and how the nurse can best respond to her.** Katie obviously is frustrated as well and fearful that she may have cancer "like my friend." In the absence of a definitive diagnosis, and even if the diagnostic testing done previously ruled out a brain tumor, Katie's feelings and frustrations are fueled by her friend's diagnosis. Her feelings also are associated with her level of growth and development and the effects her clinical manifestations have on her ability to achieve her task of industry versus inferiority.

5. **Katie is diagnosed with SLE. What is SLE and why is it so difficult to diagnose?** SLE is an autoimmune disorder that is associated with many abnormalities in the immune system. T-suppressor cells are insufficient in numbers to protect the system and this results in the formation of ANAs against the proteins in the cell nucleus of the body's connective tissues. This initiates a dysfunctional immune complex response, producing inflammation and damage to the connective tissues of the skin, joints, heart, lungs, kidneys, brain, and circulatory vessels. The difficulty in diagnosing SLE exists because each of the manifestations can result from other causes. They must be investigated collectively after ruling out more common etiologies of each symptom. The "red flag" for most health care providers to pursue the diagnosis of SLE is the presence of four or more of the manifestations occurring simultaneously causing them to draw a serum ANA.

6. **How common is SLE in children?** "The Lupus Foundation of America estimates that approximately 1,500,000 Americans have a form of lupus. Although lupus can strike men and women of all ages, 90% of individuals diagnosed with the disease are women, and 80% of those afflicted with systemic lupus develop it between the ages of 15 and 45. Approximately 70% of lupus cases are systemic. In about 50% of these cases, a major organ will be affected. About 5% of the children born to individuals with lupus will develop the illness." The foundation further states, "Lupus is two to three times more prevalent among people of color, including African Americans, Hispanics, Asians, and Native American" (*http://www.lupus.org*). Onset in childhood usually occurs after the age of 5 years, with a peak incidence between 11 and 15 years. Girls are affected

8–10 times more frequently than boys. The average pediatric incidence is 5.56/100,000 (Potts and Mandleco, 2002, 857).

7. **Discuss the potential complications associated with SLE.** Complications of SLE may involve one body system or be multisystem. Arthritis, pericarditis, chronic renal failure, seizures, psychosis, personality disorders, headaches, infection, bleeding, and cancer (lymphoma). Although the complications can be devastating, the Lupus Foundation states, "...the idea that lupus is generally a fatal disease is one of the gravest misconceptions about the illness... With current methods of therapy 80-90% of people with non-organ threatening lupus can look forward to a normal lifespan."

8. **What are the priorities of care for Katie during this visit?**
   a. Altered protection related to immune dysfunction
   b. Disturbed body image related to clinical manifestations and treating SLE
   c. Activity intolerance related to fatigue and disease process
   d. Acute/chronic pain related to inflammation of connective tissue
   e. Risk for ineffective therapeutic regimen management related to noncompliance secondary to complications associated with therapy and growth and development
   f. Deficient knowledge related to Katie's condition, treatment, and home care

9. **Discuss the impact of Katie's clinical manifestations and diagnosis on her growth and development.** At the age of 11, Katie is pursuing a sense of industry and entering pubescence. In the presence of frequent illnesses, her primary source of a sense of accomplishment (school) is interrupted by the manifestations of SLE including pain, frequent visits to the pediatrician, and diagnostic studies. School-age children are at their childhood peak of physical coordination and involved in physical activities including running, jumping, and even competitive sports. Success with these activities enhances the child's sense of industry and belonging. The joint pain and headaches will interfere with Katie's ability to participate in these activities. Best friends are important to the school-aged child's sense of belonging, and participating in activities with these friends is important to maintain these friendships. The butterfly rash and the complications associated with treatment for lupus can cause the child to experience a disturbed body image, making her feel different and as though she doesn't belong.

10. **Katie is prescribed prednisone 5 mg by mouth each day, ibuprofen 200 mg by mouth every 6 hours as needed for pain, and acetaminophen 320 mg by mouth every 4–6 hours (alternating with ibuprofen as needed for pain). Katie weighs 35.5 kg (78.1 lb). Discuss these prescriptions including drug classifications, use in treating SLE, and whether the prescribed doses are safe for Katie.** Prednisone is a corticosteroid used to treat moderate to severe inflammation. Ibuprofen is a nonsteroidal anti-inflammatory (NSAID) prescribed to treat inflammation by blocking the synthesis of COX 1 and COX 2 prostaglandins. Acetaminophen is a non-opioid analgesic and potent antipyretic. This combination of agents is the first-line management for SLE. If prednisone is not effective, an immunosuppressant, such as cyclophosphamide, is prescribed. The safe dosage range for prednisone is 0.1–0.15 mg/kg per day. At 35.5 kg, Katie can receive 3.5–5.3 mg each day. Ibuprofen is usually prescribed at 30 mg/kg per day in four divided doses. Katie can receive up to 266 mg/dose. Although her prescribed dose is lower than the usual range, this may be because of the potential gastric upset associated with both prednisone and ibuprofen. The usual dose of acetaminophen for a child Katie's age is 325 mg every 4 hours as needed for pain or fever. All of her doses are safe (Reiss and Evans, 2002, pp. 272–276).

11. **Discuss the pre-discharge teaching priorities for Katie and her parents.**
    a. Assess Katie and her parents understanding of SLE.
    b. Provide verbal and written information regarding the following (NOTE: Keep in mind their current state of frustration and anxiety and the potential effects these emotions may have on their perception and retention of teaching):
       (1) Importance of following a well-planned individualized exercise program for Katie
       (2) Need for Katie to rest at least 8 hours at night and take naps during the day as needed
       (3) Minimizing Katie's stress as much as possible including use of stress management strategies

(4) Dietary management including a well balanced diet high in antioxidants, fruits, vegetables
(5) Need to avoid direct sunlight if Katie develops photosensitivity
(6) Taking appropriate precautions to prevent infection including handwashing
(7) Importance of compliance with prescribed medication regimen
(8) Importance of notifying health care provider if pain management is inadequate
(9) Signs and symptoms of adverse effects of medications
(10) Signs and symptoms of worsening condition
(11) Contact phone numbers to report signs and symptoms or for questions
(12) Support group—The Lupus Foundation of America (800) 558-0121
(13) Importance of follow-up with Katie's team of health care providers (pediatrician, rheumatologist, specialists in the presence of organ-specific SLE manifestations)

c. Provide for sufficient time for Katie and her parents to ask questions, answering them honestly and referring them to appropriate sources if the nurse is unable to answer the question(s)

d. Document teaching and Katie and her parents' response.

References

Broyles, B.E. (2005). *Medical-surgical nursing clinical companion.* Durham, NC: Carolina Academic Press.

Centers for Disease Control and Prevention. *http://www.cdc.gov*

Daniels, R. (2002). *Delmar's manual of laboratory and diagnostic tests.* Clifton Park, NY: Thomson Delmar Learning.

The Lupus Foundation of America. *http://www.lupus.org*

North American Nursing Diagnosis Association. (2005). *Nursing diagnoses: Definitions & classifications, 2005–2006.* Philadelphia: NANDA.

Potts, N. and Mandleco, B. (2002). *Pediatric nursing: Caring for children and their families.* Clifton Park, NY: Thomson Delmar Learning, pp. 857 –859.

Reiss, B.S. and Evans, M.E. (2002). *Pharmacological aspects of nursing care* (6th ed.). Edited by Broyles, B. Clifton Park, NY: Thomson Delmar Learning, pp. 272–276.

Spratto, G.R. and Woods, A.L. (2005). *2005 Edition: PDR nurse's drug handbook.* Clifton Park, NY: Thomson Delmar Learning.

Wong, D.L., Perry, S.E., and Hockenberry, M.J. (2002). *Maternal child nursing care.* (2nd ed.). St. Louis: Mosby, pp. 1578–1579.

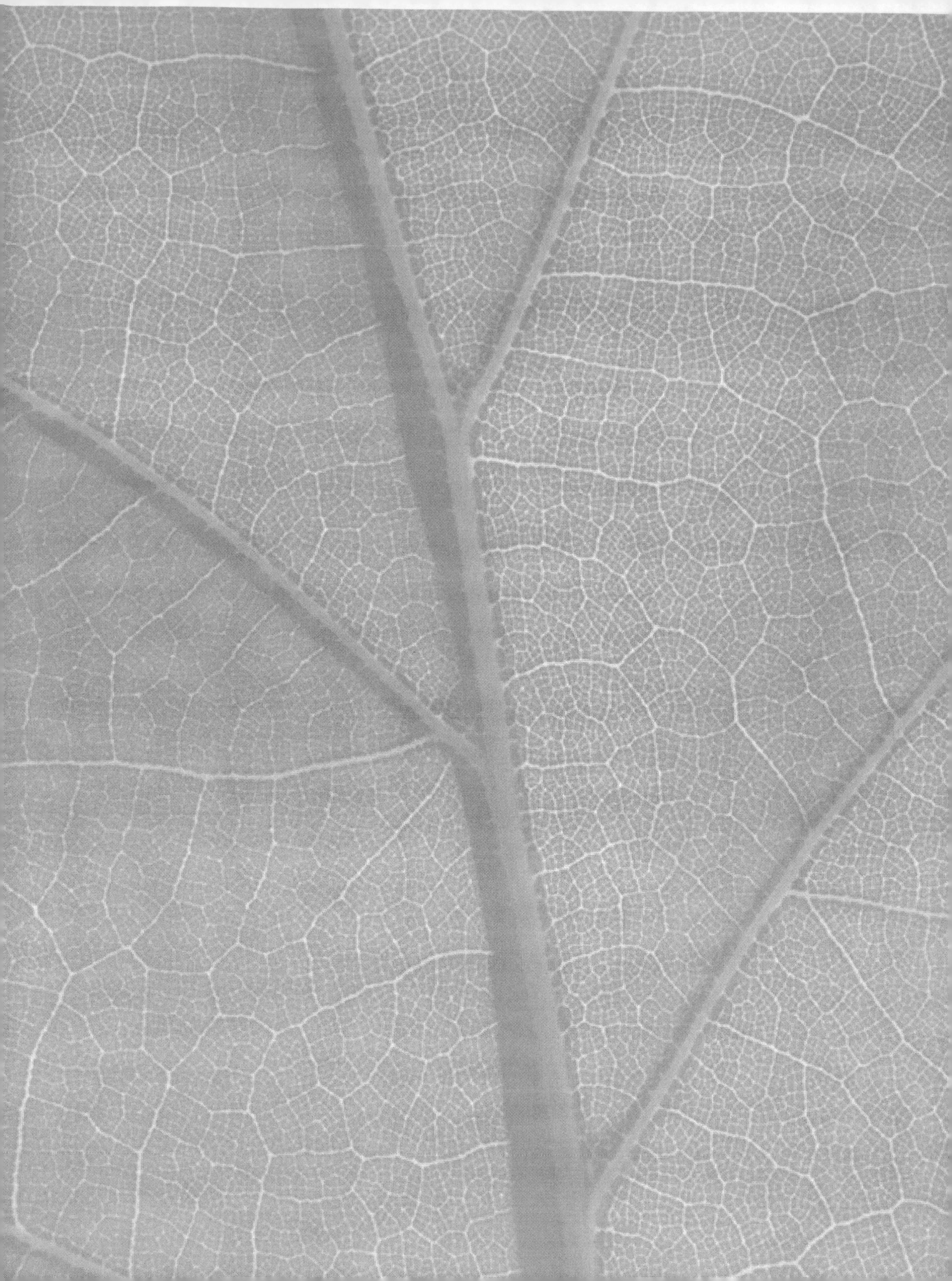

PART SEVEN

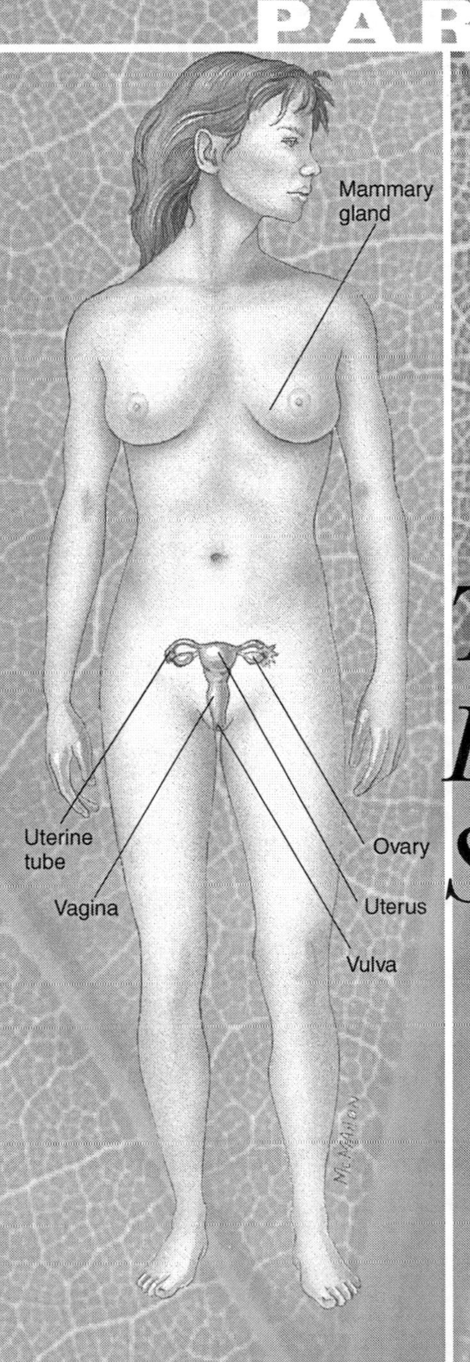

The Reproductive System

EASY

CASE STUDY 1

Sriah

GENDER

F

AGE

3 weeks old

SETTING

- Home

ETHNICITY

CULTURAL CONSIDERATIONS

- Iraqi

PREEXISTING CONDITIONS

COEXISTING CONDITIONS

SIGNIFICANT HISTORY

COMMUNICATION

DISABILITY

SOCIOECONOMIC

- Middle class

SPIRITUAL

- Muslim

PHARMACOLOGIC

PSYCHOSOCIAL

- Breastfeeding support

LEGAL

ETHICAL

ALTERNATIVE THERAPY

PRIORITIZATION

DELEGATION

THE REPRODUCTIVE SYSTEM

Level of difficulty: Easy

Overview: This case requires knowledge of breastfeeding and alternative options as well as an understanding of the client's culture, background, personal situation, and mother–child attachment relationship.

Client Profile

Sriah is a 3-week-old infant who was born at 37 weeks' gestation following premature labor. She weighed 2.3 kg (5 lb, 1 oz) at birth. Her mother immigrated to the United States from Iraq 8 months ago shortly after becoming pregnant. She had studied English in her home country before immigrating. In the United States she attended prenatal classes with her husband, followed her prescribed nutritional program, and during her prenatal classes decided to breastfeed her baby. Sriah is nursing every 2–3 hours for 20 minutes each feeding and has eight wet diapers a day. Because of her low birth weight, she is seen at her pediatrician's office, at which time she weighs 2.6 kg (5 lb, 11 oz). She receives weekly visits from the home health nurse to monitor Sriah's growth progress.

Case Study

Sriah's mother tells the home health nurse that her mother-in-law came to visit during her seventh month of pregnancy and remains with them to "help with the baby." She states that her mother-in-law is very concerned that Sriah is not getting enough nutrition with the breastfeeding and repeatedly tells her son and daughter that Sriah should be on formula. Sriah is frequently fussy after eating, and her grandmother states that the breastfeeding is responsible for Sriah's discomfort and Sriah's father is not supportive about the breastfeeding, agreeing with his mother. As a result, Sriah's mother is considering stopping the breastfeeding and starting formula feeding because "it would probably be better for Sriah."

Questions and Suggested Answers

1. **Discuss your impressions about the above situation.** The student (reader) should consider what impact the family's culture has on this situation including the strong relationship between the husband and his mother, the maternal domination of the home in this culture with the paternal figure usually spending long working hours away from the home each day, how being in a foreign country may impact on Sriah's mother and father's response to her grandmother's attitude about breastfeeding, and the normal psychosocial adjustment of new parenthood.

2. **Discuss the normal weight gain for an infant Sriah's age and compare it to Sriah's current weight.** Neonates usually lose 8% to 10% of their birth weight within the first 3–5 days following birth as a result of loss of meconium and amniotic fluid. Following this loss, they usually gain 20–30 g (0.7–1 oz) per day or 120–210 g (4.3–7.5 oz) per week. This means the neonate should regain his or her birth weight by 2 weeks of age. Sriah has regained her birth weight and gained an additional 0.35 g (10 oz) during her first 3 weeks of life. This is normal.

3. **Discuss the advantages of breastfeeding including those specific to Sriah's situation.** The changes that occur during the birthing process that stimulate breast milk production (drop in estrogen and progesterone that stimulates the release of prolactin from the anterior pituitary, stimulation by oxytocin for milk let-down, and the resulting ejection of milk from the nipples on stimulation by the suckling neonate [see Fig. A-23])and also occur in preterm births, however, the composition is specific to the needs of the neonate. Breast milk contains antibodies that provide the neonate with protection against a variety of viruses, bacteria, and protozoa. Colostrum is rich in immunoglobulins that facilitate the binding of bilirubin. Its laxative effect encourages the passage of meconium. Breast milk has a high concentration of proteins, fats, vitamins, minerals, and fluid that changes during each feeding with higher concentrations occurring in the first 5–10 minutes of the feeding during which time the nursing infant receives approximately 90% of his/her nutritional intake for that feeding. The high fluid content facilitates fluid balance, which in turn assists both gastrointestinal and renal function. Although closer bonding with the infant who is breastfed has been cited as an advantage, this bonding can be achieved with equal intensity when formula feeding an infant.

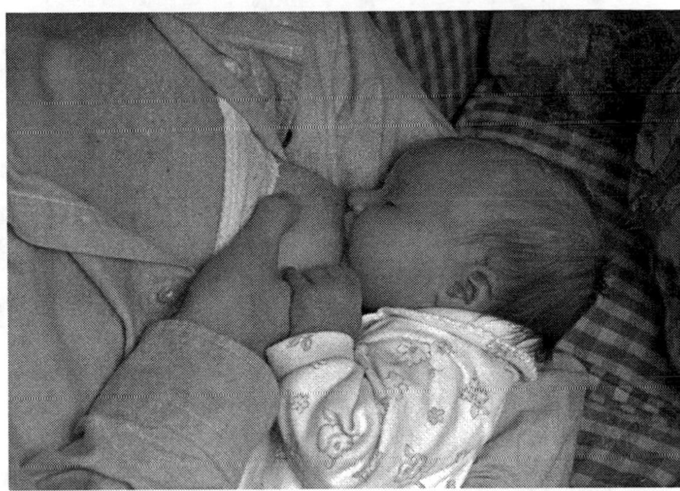

Figure A-23 *Full-term and pre-term neonates are capable of breastfeeding; the composition of the breast milk is specific to the needs of the individual neonate.*

In Sriah's situation, breast milk is the ideal food for premature and low-birth-weight neonates. In addition to the advantages noted previously, breast milk enhances the maturation of the neonates retinas and facilitates neurological maturation.

4. **What factors indicate that Sriah is receiving adequate nutrition from her mother breastfeeding?** Sriah has regained her birth weight plus an additional 0.35 g (10 oz) above her birth weight. The standard for measuring the adequacy of intake for an infant is six to eight wet diapers per day as the norm. According to Sriah's mother, Sriah has eight wet diapers a day. In addition, breastfeeding infants should have 8–12 feedings per day to receive adequate nutrition. Sriah is feeding every 2–3 hours which is normal.

5. **Discuss the possible relationship between Sriah's discomfort following feedings and breastfeeding in this family situation.** Maternal anxiety can have a negative effect on breastfeeding. It can slow the let-down of the milk, causing the infant to become frustrated and to start crying and swallowing excessive amounts of air which can lead to increased gastrointestinal gas and pain. It can cause maternal excretion of epinephrine, resulting in overstimulation of the infant, causing crying and increased gastrointestinal air intake that leads to gas discomfort. Environmental stress caused by family disagreements translates to the infant in terms of sensory overload with similar effects on crying and gas production.

6. **Given the dietary intake consistent with Sriah's family's culture, what, if any, relationship might this have on Sriah's discomfort following feedings?** Most individuals from the Middle East practice the Muslim faith. The dietary laws are based on religious prohibitions of certain foods or methods of preparing these foods and the promotion of other foods. These laws are based on the Islamic teachings of the Koran. Milk products are permitted at all times and Muslim diets contain all fruits and vegetables as long as they are not fermented or poisonous. Certain foods in their diet that may aggravate infants if consumed by a breastfeeding mother include broccoli, cauliflower, spiced beans, onions, and cabbage. Seafood is a staple food as well as beef, chicken, and turkey; however, pork is prohibited. Although no evidence is apparent in the case study that Sriah's mother eats chocolate or consumes beverages with caffeine, these also may cause gastrointestinal distress in the infant. According to Middle Eastern customs, coffee is a favorite beverage and is usually consumed at all meals.

7. **Discuss the significance of family support when a mother wants to breastfeed her infant.** Because of the demands of breastfeeding including frequent interruptions in the mother's sleep pattern as well as the energy demands on the mother related to breastfeeding, fatigue is common. When combined with the normal hormonal changes associated with the postpartum period and the energy expenditure related to the physiological return of the body to its prepregnant state as well as the psychosocial adjustments of parenthood

as described by Reva Rubin, the mother may be very sensitive and vulnerable to criticism during this time. Breastfeeding is the right way to feed an infant, only if it is the right way for all of the individuals intimate to the situation—infant, mother, and father. Otherwise the mother's attempt to breastfeed is prone to sabotage by family, friends, and health care professionals.

8. **Identify the priority nursing diagnoses pertinent to this situation.**
   a. Risk for ineffective breastfeeding related to lack of support from the father and mother-in-law, lack of maternal self-confidence, presence of anxiety
   b. Deficient knowledge related to the current factors indicating effective breastfeeding

9. **Discuss how the nurse could intervene in this situation to support the mother's desire to breastfeed Sriah.** First, the nurse should discuss with Sriah's mother regarding whether she wants her husband and mother-in-law involved in the discussion. The nurse should then assess the reasons Sriah's mother wants to breastfeed her. The benefits of this include not only the nurse gaining important assessment data but also Sriah's mother reinforcing why she chose to breastfeed. The nurse should interview Sriah's father and grandmother to determine their reasons for not supporting her mother's desire to breastfeed Sriah. The nurse could then determine if Sriah's mother and her husband and mother-in-law have any inaccurate information about the benefits of breastfeeding and provide appropriate accurate information. The nurse should discuss the benefits of breastfeeding and the impact that family support or lack of support has on the success of breastfeeding for both Sriah and her mother. Finally, the nurse must support whatever Sriah's mother decides about whether she continues to breastfeed or changes to formula feeding.

10. **During the visit, Sriah's mother decides to continue breastfeeding with her husband and mother-in- law's support. What, if any, professionals should the nurse collaborate with regarding this situation to ensure adequate and consistent follow-up for Sriah and her family?** Following this home visit, the home health nurse should collaborate with the pediatrician and the nurse practitioner about what transpired during the visit, including the client and family teaching, to get their input into the most effective way to support Sriah's mother's decision.

References

Eat Ethnic. *http://www.eatethnic.com*

The Learning Space. *http://www.learningspace.org*

North American Nursing Diagnosis Association. (2005). *Nursing diagnoses: Definitions & classifications, 2005–2006.* Philadelphia: NANDA.

Potts, N. and Mandleco, B. (2002). *Pediatric nursing: Caring for children and their families.* Clifton Park, NY: Thomson Delmar Learning.

Williams, S.R. and Schlenker, E. (2003). *Essentials for nutrition and diet therapy* (8th ed.). St. Louis: Mosby.

Wong, D.L., Perry, S.E., and Hockenberry, M.J. (2002). *Maternal child nursing care* (2nd ed.). St. Louis: Mosby, p. 857.

CASE STUDY 2

Alexis

MODERATE

GENDER

F

AGE

16

SETTING

- Prenatal clinic

ETHNICITY

- White American

CULTURAL CONSIDERATIONS

PREEXISTING CONDITIONS

COEXISTING CONDITIONS

SIGNIFICANT HISTORY

COMMUNICATION

DISABILITY

SOCIOECONOMIC

SPIRITUAL

PHARMACOLOGIC

PSYCHOSOCIAL

- Single pregnant teenager

LEGAL

ETHICAL

- Possible nurse bias

ALTERNATIVE THERAPY

PRIORITIZATION

DELEGATION

- Yes

THE REPRODUCTIVE SYSTEM

Level of difficulty: Moderate

Overview: This case requires knowledge of growth and development, pregnancy, parenting, prenatal mental health, as well as an understanding of the client's personal situation and family relationships.

Client Profile

Alexis is a 16-year-old high school sophomore who is single and living at home with her parents. Her boyfriend, Matt, who is the father of the child she is carrying, is an 18-year-old senior at the same high school Alexis attends. Alexis and Matt, who also lives at home with his parents a few houses away from Alexis and her parents, have been going together since he was a sophomore and she was in eighth grade. They both have excelled in school and were very popular with their classmates until the last semester, at which time their grades began to falter and their popularity diminished. They appear to care a great deal for each other, but both had plans to attend college after high school graduation, and in the past month they have argued frequently. Both Matt and Alexis' parents have been very supportive, although initially they were devastated by the news of the pregnancy.

Case Study

During her prenatal visit during her 32nd week of her first pregnancy, Alexis states she has been experiencing low back pain and "tightening in my tummy" for the past week. When a vaginal examination is performed, it reveals that her cervix is 0 cm dilated, thick, and high with no evidence of effacement. Alexis appears irritable, stating, "I just want this to be over. I'm tired of being big and fat while my friends are pretty and doing all the things I want to be doing. Can't you just take the baby now? A friend of mine had her baby early and she and the baby are just fine." Alexis is accompanied by her parents and Matt, who have attended all of her prenatal visits with her.

Questions and Suggested Answers

1. **Discuss your impressions about the above situation.** The lower back pain and "tightening" of the uterus are normal in the third trimester of pregnancy. Especially in light of the vaginal examination results, the tightening probably represents Braxton Hicks contractions. Alexis' statements about wanting the baby to be delivered early may represent a very present and self-oriented level of growth and development as well as immaturity in believing that delivering the baby early won't hurt anything and will take care of her present discomforts. Both sets of parents appear to be very supportive of their children after their initial devastation.
2. **What additional data would be helpful in developing a plan of care for Alexis?**
   - **a.** An abdominal ultrasound would provide information about the fetus's maturity.
   - **b.** Do Alexis and Matt plan to parent their baby or place it for adoption?
   - **c.** Fetal heart rate
   - **d.** Are Alexis and Matt attending prenatal classes, Lamaze, etc?
3. **How do Alexis' growth and development needs differ from those of a 28-year-old woman?** As an adolescent, Alexis is focused on establishing her own identity as a person. Her primary support system should be her peers as she needs this sense of belonging for her self-esteem. This tends to be a very egocentric time of development because in order to develop a personal identity separate from her parents, her focus is on herself. She tests the established rules, may participate in risk-taking behavior (her pregnancy may be evidence of this), and at times has an adversarial relationship with the same-sex parent. She needs to be with her friends, participating in teen activities. She wants and needs to be like her friends, but the pregnancy makes her different in her own perception. At a time when she is so self-focused, it is very difficult to focus on the needs of another (the fetus). A 28-year-old woman is well established in developing intimacy, making a permanent personal romantic relationship, marrying, and establishing a home and family. The developmental focus has shifted from self to others (husband and children), a career, and activities with other couples of the same age and interests. For a 28-year-old, having children is a "normal" part of this developmental stage.

4. **Given their psychosocial level of growth and development, discuss how you think Alexis and Matt are feeling about their situation.** Although this is a normal time for developing relationships with opposite-sex peers, these relationships are not generally permanent relationships. Each still needs same sex friends for the development of autonomy and identity. The scenario shows evidence of the changes in their sense of belonging as their "popularity" has declined (at least in their perception) as the evidence of her pregnancy becomes more obvious. This places both of them "out of circulation" with their peers. Alexis' physical condition makes participation in some teen activities difficult or inappropriate (cheerleading, gymnastics). The continuation of this struggle for identity usually continues as adolescents enter college and are "on their own" for the first time. Matt and Alexis may feel that the pregnancy has ruined all of their plans and dreams, which also may be the basis for their frequent disagreements. With the progression of her pregnancy, the hormone changes, the discomforts (including back pain), and the changes in body image are causes of mood swings and irritability during the last trimester of pregnancy.

5. **How would you respond to Alexis' statement about premature births?** First, the nurse needs to consider that her statement may reflect her needs rather than the needs of the fetus. Alexis is uncomfortable; she can no longer ignore or deny the pregnancy to herself or others; and she is no doubt frustrated given her circumstances. Again, it is very difficult for Alexis to be focused on the health and welfare of her unborn child when her developmental task is to be focused on herself and her own needs. The nurse needs to provide Alexis with information concerning the development of a 32-week fetus and the risks of premature delivery including respiratory conditions related to insufficient surfactant, sensory development, growth needs, prolonged hospitalization, financial impact, and so forth. Because Alexis' statement also may be in response to her back discomfort, information concerning elevating her feet when she is sitting, avoiding standing in one place for more than 10–20 minutes, placing a pillow at her back when she is sitting, having a significant other rub her back when she is lying down, applying a heat source to help relax the back muscles, and so forth.

6. **How effective do you think your teaching about premature births would be to Alexis at this time?** Because we don't know exactly how Alexis and Matt perceive their present situation, it is difficult to say how effective the teaching will be. However, the teaching approach may need to focus on the impact of premature labor or a surgical extraction of the fetus on Alexis rather than focusing on the fetus. Also, during psychosocial stress, the comprehension and retention of information is decreased, so involving Alexis' parents and Matt and his parents in the teaching will dramatically increase the understanding and reinforcement of the information. If teaching Alexis alone, she may retain 50% of the information; by involving Matt and her parents, the retention dramatically increases.

7. **Discuss your impressions of Alexis and Matt's parents' response to the pregnancy.** Both Alexis and Matt's parents appear to be very supportive of their children. The case study does not project any "hidden agendas" on the part of either set of parents. They seem to genuinely care for their children and want whatever is best for them.

8. **Discuss your biases, if any, toward Alexis' situation.** This nurse should consider any biases about adolescent pregnancy, Alexis and Matt not being married; and concepts of adoption versus the impact on Alexis, Matt, their parents, and the child if they decide to raise the child themselves. How will this impact on Alexis and Matt's relationship? What about plans for college and the need for higher education to get better jobs in today's economy?

9. **What impact would your biases, if any, have on your approach to Alexis and Matt?** Biases can negatively impact teaching. Understanding one's biases is the first step in preventing them from interfering with the focus on the client's needs. The approach needs to be supportive and nonjudgmental. The nurse must be empathetic to Alexis's discomfort and provide information regarding methods of reducing her back pain. Explaining to Alexis the normal process of pregnancy and the rationale behind why her back is uncomfortable as well as information concerning what to expect as the pregnancy progresses would be helpful.

10. Discuss your teaching plan for Alexis and her significant others at this visit.

a. Assess their level of understanding about Alexis' present condition (32-week gestation).
b. Explain diagnostic findings, providing information concerning the progression of cervical dilation and effacement.
c. Suggest techniques to ease third-trimester discomforts.
d. Discuss activities that Alexis and Matt could still pursue with their friends.
e. Emphasize the importance of communication and support to Alexis, Matt, and their parents.
f. Allow sufficient time for them to ask questions, providing information as appropriate.
g. Document teaching and Alexis' and her significant other's response.
h. Explore how connected Alexis (and Matt) feel to the baby.
i. Explore how prepared Alexis is for taking on the role of mother; does she have a realistic view of being a mother?

References

Daniels, R. (2002). *Delmar's manual of laboratory and diagnostic tests.* Clifton Park, NY: Thomson Delmar Learning.

North American Nursing Diagnosis Association. (2005). *Nursing diagnoses: Definitions & classifications, 2005–2006.* Philadelphia: NANDA.

Potts, N. and Mandleco, B. (2002). *Pediatric nursing: Caring for children and their families.* Clifton Park, NY: Thomson Delmar Learning.

Solchany, J. (2001). *Promoting maternal mental health during pregnancy.* Seattle: HCAST Publications.